More praise for *Mutual Accompaniment and the Creation of the Commons*

"In this wide-ranging, thoughtful, insightful, and infinitely generative book, Watkins crystallizes, distills, analyzes, and augments the long history of the practice that has become known as accompaniment. She illuminates diverse and varied places of origin and implementation of different forms of accompaniment connected to struggles for dignity, decency, and democracy. . . . It is a book for our time that is right on time."—From the Foreword by George Lipsitz, author of *How Racism Takes Place*

"A groundbreaking book that reveals the heart of an activist. Mary Watkins' wonderful and accessible stories of accompaniment have the potential to transform the very structures of human service provision."—Lynne Layton, Harvard Medical School

"In this book, 'accompaniment' is presented as a preferred approach to psychotherapy; as recognition of the web of life; and as an alternative to capitalism. An absorbing read."—Staughton Lynd, author of *Accompanying: Pathways to Social Change* and co-editor with Alice Lynd of *Nonviolence in America: A Documentary History*

"An original and significant intervention that will have far-ranging appeal to students of psychology, anthropology, and cultural studies. This book holds the potential of becoming a classic."—Deanne Bell, University of East London

"Watkins speaks about the need for providers to go beyond their privileged comfort levels and address the real needs of the people we aim to serve and support."—Chakira M. Haddock Lazala, Ph.D.

"Quite creative and amazingly integrative."—Darcia Narvaez, University of Notre Dame, author of *Neurobiology and the Development of Human Morality: Evolution, Culture, and Wisdom*

Mutual Accompaniment and the Creation of the Commons

Mutual Accompaniment and the Creation of the Commons

Mary Watkins

With a Foreword by George Lipsitz and
a Contribution by G. A. Bradshaw

Yale

UNIVERSITY PRESS

New Haven & London

Published with assistance from the foundation established in memory of James Wesley Cooper of the Class of 1865, Yale College.

Yale University Press books may be purchased in quantity for educational, business, or promotional use. For information, please e-mail sales.press@yale.edu (U.S. office) or sales@yaleup.co.uk (U.K. office).

Set in Bulmer type by IDS Infotech Ltd., Chandigarh, India.
Printed in the United States of America.

Library of Congress Control Number: 2018960645
ISBN 978-0-300-23614-9 (hardcover : alk. paper)

A catalogue record for this book is available from the British Library.

This paper meets the requirements of ANSI/NISO Z39.48-1992 (Permanence of Paper).

10 9 8 7 6 5 4 3 2 1

*To all those who have deepened into lives graced by mutual accompaniment,
who have rejected disregarding their neighbors, human and other-than-human,
who have nurtured their courage and perseverance, shared the risks of resistance,
and created in the face of difficulty: thank you.
Your loving solidarity prefigures the commons-to-come,
providing us bread for our journeys.*

If you have come here to help me, you are wasting your time.
But if you have come because your liberation is bound up with mine,
then let us work together.

—Aboriginal Activist Group, Queensland, Australia, 1970s

Contents

Accompaniment as a Way of Life

George Lipsitz

IN ONE OF HER TYPICALLY scintillating, self-reflexive essays, author, activist, and filmmaker Toni Cade Bambara argued that in her attempts to change society, she discovered the need to transform herself. It was not enough for Bambara simply to envision more decent and democratic social relations. It was necessary instead to learn how to become a person capable of experiencing those relations in the present by seceding from the dominant norms and values of the self-centered, materialistic, and aggressively competitive society in which she had been raised. Bambara described her quest for self-transformation as a collective effort based on augmented connections with others, as a persistent struggle that necessitated "rising above my training, thinking better than I've been taught, developing a listening habit, making the self available to intelligence, engaging in demystification, and seeking out teachers at every turn."[1] Bambara emphasized that the teachers she needed were not necessarily credentialed experts offering instruction in classrooms. While expressing due respect and appreciation for people with advanced knowledge, she delineated the many different kinds of lessons that she had learned from many different kinds of people, especially those who had developed an augmented capacity for love in a world that so often makes people unloving and even seemingly unlovable.

Bambara did not use the term "accompaniment" to describe her practice, but her art and activism revolved resolutely around the ideas and ideals that Mary Watkins associates with accompaniment in this book. Bambara's employment history before she became known as a writer placed her in the consciously chosen company of the poor, the shunned, and the segregated, and with those diagnosed as dangerous, dysfunctional, and damaged. She labored inside some of the very institutions that Watkins identifies as historically generative crucibles of accompaniment, such as settlement houses and psychiatric wards. Through Bambara's employment as a youth case worker for the New York City Department of Welfare, director of recreation in the psychiatric division at the Metropolitan Hospital Center in Harlem, and program director for the Colony Settlement House in Brooklyn, she learned to discern value in undervalued people, to experience the joys of accompanying people who created beauty and found joy in the midst of misery and suffering. The people she encountered—and learned from and with—inside these grim institutional settings resonated with the capacities for resistance and resilience that Bambara had recognized early in life in the Harlem of her childhood among what one of her biographers describes as her neighborhood's "longshoremen, union activists, communists, the beauty-parlor women and the barbershop men, the ladies of the night, tap dancers, be-bop musicians, chitlin' circuit women, the numbers runners, the Rastafarians, the Abyssinians, the church women, the m'dears, the Father Divine workers, the barmaids, and the rappers on speaker's corner."[2] Bambara consistently presented her quests for personal and societal transformation as an innately collective and social process that required creating horizontal relations based on mutual respect and recognition. Born Miltona Cade, she adopted the name Bambara because she admired the ritual Chiwara masks of the Bambara people of Mali, but also to augment the identity she inherited from familial bloodlines by fusing it with the identity she shared with entire groups like the Bambara people due to their linked fate of dispossession, displacement, and enslavement, but also of African retention and New World invention in slavery and in freedom.

In *Mutual Accompaniment and the Creation of the Commons*, Mary Watkins reveals the pressing urgency in the present for creating the forms of personal and social transformation that Bambara championed four decades ago. In this wide-ranging, thoughtful, insightful, and infinitely generative book, Watkins crystallizes, distills, analyzes, and augments the long history of the practice that has become known as accompaniment. She illuminates diverse and varied places of origin and implementation of different forms of accompaniment connected to struggles for dignity, decency, and democracy. She explains how at the most intimate and personal levels of existence, experience, and understanding, accompaniment emerges from "looking at" rather than "looking away," from listening rather than speaking prematurely, and from promoting cooperation rather than competition.

The pressing need for accompaniment today is all too evident. In a society that elevates the love of gain over the well-being of both the social and the natural commons, people come to feel alone and disconnected. In Doris Sommer's deft formulation, they become "inured to suffering and afraid of love."[3] This seemingly solely personal state of alienation has public and political consequences. As Hannah Arendt astutely observed, "What prepares men for totalitarian domination in the non-totalitarian world is the fact that loneliness, once a borderline experience usually suffered in certain marginal social conditions like old age, has become an everyday experience of the ever-growing masses of our century."[4] Yet this new marginality and vulnerability among people who previously presumed themselves to be secure in the center means that they now have a great deal to learn from people they may despise, from subjugated communities whose insurgent knowledges emanate from and depend on accompaniment. In this book, Watkins introduces us to teachers at every turn, people in places where new forms of horizontal relations across difference are being envisioned and enacted.

The accompaniment that Watkins champions rests on the cultivation of collective capacities for noticing others and connecting with them. It entails concentrated efforts to cross over the often invisible barriers that divide differently situated people. It involves learning from the experiences of others, listening for the kinds of assistance they might need, and inhabiting an ethos of openness and inclusion. It defines responsibility as a collective commitment to respond-ability, to hear the cries of the excluded and to respond to them honorably and decently, to see *their* problems as *our* problems.

Watkins envisions accompaniment as a tool for realizing and expanding recognition of our mutual dependence on the commons. Drawing deftly on the historical scholarship of Peter Linebaugh, she notes how the enclosures of common lands in eighteenth-century England set in motion a pattern of pairing privatization of public resources with criminalization of the survival strategies of the dispossessed. This pattern continues to shape the exploitive, extractive, cruel, competitive, rapacious, and racist capitalism that dominates the world today. Watkins shows how the struggle to preserve a sustainable commons has a long history, how it infused the settlement house movement of the Progressive era, the hospitality houses and alternative communities of the mid-twentieth century, the base communities that coalesced around liberation theology in the 1960s and 1970s, and the movements to live in harmony with the nonhuman world emanating from Indigenous communities, environmentalists, and animal rights activists in the late twentieth and early twenty-first centuries. In its survey of practices of accompaniment in support of a sustainable commons, Watkins's book is a declaration of independence from outmoded ways of living, and a passionately and persuasively argued provocation to think and act freely, boldly, and differently.

Yet it is not easy to envision, much less enact, a new and better world under current conditions. The book appears at a time in history when callousness, contempt, and cruelty pervade political and commercial culture. Times like these provide ample reasons for despair. What is the work we are now called upon to do? Do we sit back and watch in sorrow as the world unravels? Do we seek to scramble to a site of private refuge? Will we be content to author ever more indignant or ever more eloquent descriptions of the suffering that surrounds us while the suffering continues unabated? In a world that perpetually encourages us to *have* more, how do we learn to *be* more? In an age of the calculated abandonment of entire populations, how can the people of the world find each other and help each other?

It is precisely the dire nature of our present problems, however, that makes Watkins's excavation of the tools of accompaniment so important. At a moment in history when neoliberal economic, political, and cultural policies increasingly divide the world into a small group to be treated as exceptional and large numbers of people to be dismissed as disposable, identifying and preserving the commons has never been more important. In an age where even modest ameliorative reforms seem unlikely to be adopted, it is time to explore, learn from, and participate in advancing the survival strategies and social imaginations of the most aggrieved, despised, and shunned social groups. The people who hold power in this world cannot fix the things they have broken. They cannot repair the damage they have done to the planet and its people. They have created a crisis that requires a collective response. The crisis has discredited the authority of experts and the legitimacy of leaders. It has exposed the mean-spirited mendacity of those in power. In this context, the practices of accompaniment that Watkins documents and analyzes are, as she argues, a potential pathway to another world.

Mutual Accompaniment and the Creation of the Commons ranges widely across situations, centuries, countries, and continents for its objects of analysis. It is a book for our time that is right on time. Its delineation of the many different forms of accompaniment in the defense of the commons that have shaped the past can infuse the present and the future with an augmented potential to discover and deploy usable truths. Watkins's evidence, ideas, and arguments equip us with valuable tools for the tasks Toni Cade Bambara advised us to carry out, the tools of rising above our training, thinking better than we have been taught, developing a listening habit, making ourselves available to intelligence, and seeking out teachers—from all backgrounds and all walks of life—at every turn.

Mutual Accompaniment and the Creation of the Commons

Introduction

TRAGICALLY, WE LIVE IN A time when divisions are being grievously deepened, neighbors turned against one another, strangers denied at the door. It is a time when the accumulation of immense excess wealth by a few and the absolute destitution of the many tragically coexist. It is an unprecedented time of capitalism-induced ecocide, when our earthly home can no longer absorb the effects of our waste and plunder. It is a time when acts of helping have been increasingly professionalized following the dictates of capitalist engagement, serving ever more privileged sectors of society and largely failing to understand sufferings within their historical and sociopolitical contexts.

It is this time that has called me to focus on our accompaniment of each other, both of those within the communities we call our own and of those on the other side of the many lines we draw that divide us, including divisions of race, class, ethnicity, sexuality, disability, and nationality. With the help of Gay Bradshaw, I have also turned to our accompaniment of and by other-than-human animals and the Earth.

My focus on accompaniment rather than on the provision of psychotherapy or social services signals an intentional move away from models based on individualism and unidirectional helping to those that acknowledge our inherent interdependence and potential mutuality. I turn away from expertism and toward mutual, dialogical, participatory, and horizontal relations. I am eager to differentiate accompaniment from normative practices of psychotherapy, which too often proceed from an individualistic orientation, stripping human beings of the wider social, economic, environmental, and political contexts in which their lives develop and which give meaning to their distress and symptoms. Through the assumption of professionalized roles based in "expert" knowledge, these practices too often usurp the understandings and agency of those they intend to help.

"Accompaniment" is a term used in arenas as diverse as social medicine, peace activism, human rights, pastoral support, social psychology,
animal rights, and liberation psychology. The concept is used when speaking of accompanying the ill who are also poor,[1] those caught in prison and
detention systems,[2] political dissidents,[3] refugees,[4] those suffering under
occupation,[5] victims of torture and other forms of violence,[6] those forcibly
displaced,[7] those suffering violations of human rights,[8] and those attempting to live peacefully in the face of paramilitary and military violence. In
countless other situations of human and environmental duress, accompaniment is engaged in without recourse to the term. In this book I seek to bring
accompaniment into sharp relief by tracing its history and that of some of
the movements that rely on its principles. I hope to lift up the practice of
accompaniment so it can become a North Star orienting us in our creation
of relationships that help us build intercultural commons where justice,
peace, and ecological well-being can flourish.

It is crucial that we claim and strengthen our human capacities to
stand with one another, animals, and the Earth in the existential difficulties
of life and in the particular local and global sociocultural and environmental
challenges of this historical period of capitalist-induced coloniality. Developing the sensitivity to hear others' legitimate calls for assistance and nourishing our desire and commitment to respond to them are essential to the
pursuit of loving and caring relationships, as well as to our own integrity.

If our professional work includes responding to human needs, we
have often sequestered ourselves in offices and work schedules, attempting
to keep the shape of our private lives intact. Too often we have narrowed our
understanding of distress to the most local context, failing to open our vision to the psychological, community, and ecological sequelae of the last
five hundred years of colonialism, capitalism, racism, and ongoing neoliberalism. For those within the human services professions, this book advocates
for a move toward the activity and ethics of ecopsychosocial accompaniment that takes into account this long arc of history. At times I focus on
psychology, the discipline that has preoccupied me for four decades of my
life, but I understand this shift as relevant to many other kinds of human
services providers and nonprofessionalized accompanists.

Chapter 1 defines and describes psychosocial accompaniment and helps to situate the reader. It addresses my own position with regard to accompaniment and underscores the importance of the practice of reflexivity for accompaniers. Because accompaniment is both a human necessity and an existential reality, one could construct multiple genealogies from different cultural standpoints and positions. I am choosing from those that have inspired me and that I have found useful, aware that while my own orientation enables me to open some windows to see into accompaniment, it leaves others closed. This yields ample room for you to offer your own examples, critiques, and possible genealogies. The initial chapters draw together exemplars of psychosocial accompaniment that can help us see what is distinctive about it as an approach and an ethical commitment. I have engaged storytelling to invite you into understanding how accompaniment begins and evolves in a person's life and within a community. Chapters 2 to 6 unfold roughly historically, while drawing examples of how accompaniment looks when addressing the concerns of immigrants and refugees, the homeless, those with intellectual challenges, the ill who are also poor, those who have suffered genocide, those who have been displaced by violence, and those who live with a diagnosis of serious mental illness.

The first strand of genealogy I trace in chapter 2 is the practice of accompaniment in settlement houses in the United States during the Progressive era, focusing on Jane Addams and Hull-House, Victoria Earle Matthews and the White Rose Society, and Georgia Washington and the People's Village School. Settlement house work strove to create strong bridges between struggling communities and communities with resources, hoping to build a common "we." There is a lot we can learn today from the history of settlement houses as we try to bridge between communities that have their needs met and the internal colonies and sacrifice zones spawned by neoliberal practices.[9]

Houses of radical hospitality exemplify a second strand of accompaniment, considered in chapter 3. We explore both those for the homeless poor, founded by Dorothy Day, Peter Maurin, and the Catholic Worker Movement, and those for people with intellectual disabilities, the L'Arche communities begun by Jean Vanier. Both settlement houses and houses of hospitality illustrate the importance of creating places where people who are usually socially separated can discover common ground and purpose. Both early settlement houses and houses of hospitality engender and exemplify the mutuality of accompaniment, replacing the vertical hierarchy that is an ingredient in normatively understood "helping." They are also exemplars of how to create networks of small commons that are inclusive, generate a sense of belonging, and meet needs while enjoying the sharing and conviviality of communal life.

The third strand of genealogy for psychosocial accompaniment, discussed in chapter 4, arises from the migration of values and practices from liberation theology in Latin America to social medicine and liberation psychology. It is within this strand that the concept of psychosocial accompaniment is explicitly developed, and where we can witness its capacity to radically transform the provision of human services into mutual efforts of liberation.

The fourth strand addresses how accompaniment, rather than psychotherapeutic and psychiatric treatment, radically transforms how we interact with those among us who suffer diagnoses of severe psychiatric illness. This is accomplished by reflecting on multiple approaches that highlight accompaniment as essential—that is, the centuries-long tradition in Geel, Belgium, and the recent Family Care model in Sweden, where those with mental illness have been welcomed into families; the community living models pioneered by R. D. Laing and Loren Mosher at Kingsley Hall and Soteria House; and the more recent effects in Italy of the deinstitutionalizing reforms of Franco Basaglia and others, all examined in chapter 5. The following chapter turns to the shift to peer accompaniment, enclave models, and finally the experience of being accompanied by the natural world.

Drawing inspiration from such examples of accompaniment, we then turn in chapter 7 to look at the path of accompaniment for accompanists who work with individuals and groups from communities other than their own. Liberation psychologist Hussein Bulhan analyzes coloniality as consisting of multiple, ongoing colonizations: the colonization of space, time, values, knowledge, compassion, language, identity, religion, medicine, and madness.[10] It is crucial to attend to how accompaniers, living within the ongoing coloniality of our time, can mindfully strive to position themselves in ways that do not replicate colonial relationships but that prefigure a decolonial future. In addition, we explore the kinds of education, apprenticeship, and principles that are useful to many on the path of accompaniment.

Accompaniment is desperately needed not only by human individuals, groups, and communities but also by animals, species, and ecosystems. The human plundering and desecration of animals, earth, air, and waters have overwhelmed the capacity of many animal communities and ecosystems to restore themselves. Western scientists have now openly admitted what many Indigenous communities have long known, that sentience is not a distinctly human possession but a gift we share with other creatures. How are we to live in the light of this knowledge? The fifth lineage traced in chapters 8 and 9 is the extension of the idea of accompaniment to our relationships with other species and to the Earth itself—mountains, trees, rivers, and oceans. G. A. Bradshaw, founder of the Kerulos Center for Nonviolence and key theorist of trans-species psychology and human-induced animal trauma, has contributed chapter 8. She lends her deep personal experiences of accompaniment of nonhuman animals and their communities, as well as her wide grasp of trans-species sanctuary work worldwide.[11]

Finally, in chapter 10, "Mutual Accompaniment and the Commons-to-Come," I turn to how the historical forces of capitalism and colonialism have given rise to the present coloniality that deepens the tears in the psychic, social, and ecological fabric of our lives. I seek to illuminate the relationship between mutual accompaniment and the creating and sustaining of commons, those places—small and large—where we build relationships with one another and with nature that are caring and mutual. Here we see liberating transformation come about through dialogue, consensus building, shared imagination and action, and commitment to the sustainability of the natural world. Through accompaniment that creates commons, human material desires are tempered in the light of the shared needs of others: humans, other-than-human animals, and the Earth. Here, communality—a spirit of cooperation, neighborliness, sharing, mutual aid, and belonging—can thrive.[12]

Different societies have different names and definitions for what the British called "commons," that is, right relations, beloved communities, the common pot. By the use of the term "commons" I do not sidestep the most important issue to Indigenous societies: the return of land. One group's "commons" should not be built on the eradication of other groups' commons. First Nations scholar and Yellowknives Dene Glen Coulthard reminds us that there is a forgetting that commons belonged to someone: "The commons not only belong to somebody—*the First Peoples of this land*—they also deeply inform and sustain Indigenous modes of thought and behavior that harbor profound insights into the maintenance of relationships within and between human beings and the natural world built on principles of reciprocity, nonexploitation and respectful existence."[13] English colonists brought to their "new" world experiences of both the commons and of the enclosure of commons. Their idea of commons clashed with that of Natives, undermining Natives' traditional ways of tending "the common pot."[14] This clash underscores the need for mutual accompaniment and understanding as we work to restore Native commons and to create intercultural commons. The building of right relationships must include the appropriate just reparations from settler to Native societies.

Commons historian Peter Linebaugh urges us to think of the commons as an activity, as "commoning." When we do so, says Max Haiven, "[commoning] is something we do rather than something we have. If this is the case then the 'right to the commons' is, in actuality, the rights we take to struggle for the commons. I think here we are speaking of a 'right' in the beautiful double sense that this word gives us in English: both a legal entitlement and something virtuous or correct. In that sense, the right to the commons is the obligation 'to common': to make and make anew the commons, to reclaim and reinvent the commons."[15]

I place mutual accompaniment at the heart of commoning. When we do so, relationships of accompaniment and solidarity become the needed scaffold to help us build commons each day. Mutual accompaniment is a way of living that mends the gaps and tears in our interdependency from which we suffer so dearly and tragically. In doing so, it creates some of the psychological, social, and ecological integrity we deeply desire and desperately need.

ONE

Accompaniment

Existential, Psychosocial, Ecological

IT IS A GRAY DECEMBER DAY. I emerge out into the cold with a heavy heart and stare back at the stark grounds of the Elizabeth Detention Center in Elizabeth, New Jersey. I have been visiting with Karun, a young man who is a prodemocracy advocate in his homeland, a place worlds away from where he is now being held.[1] We met as part of a detainee accompaniment program in which I have been volunteering. During this first meeting, he haltingly tells me bits and pieces of his life: how he was kidnapped, tortured, and imprisoned by his country's ruling dictatorial regime as a result of his activism. During his last frightening interrogation, Karun was told that if he remained in his country, he would be killed. His wife and young children were also threatened with murder. He fled to the United States with reluctance. He is sick with missing his loved ones but knows that the only chance to get his family to safety is if he can be granted asylum himself.

I am his first external visitor. Karun has been imprisoned in this building for three months with three hundred other detainees who have come seeking asylum from around the world. He was detained upon his arrival at JFK Airport. The Elizabeth Detention Center is one of hundreds of detention prisons that constitute an American gulag archipelago. Every detainee has traveled an unimaginable, tortuous path, full of twists and turns, danger and death, for the shared purpose of finding asylum and safety for themselves and often for their families. Their stories are staggering testaments to the inhumanity of man to man in our common world. Some have even undertaken the long voyage from Africa to Brazil and then made their way to the United States on foot. When they arrive at the border "gate," they are imprisoned for months, even years, until they gain asylum or are returned to their countries of origin. Under U.S. law, asylum seekers have no right to legal representation. As most have no or insufficient funds to pay for representation, the majority will lose their cases and be forcibly returned to their countries of origin and faced again with the consequences from which they had fled. They will often be punished more harshly, even put to death, for their fleeing. Karun will be one of these if asylum is denied.

The door shuts behind me, and I am released outside into the empty cold. Karun's soft voice is still with me. I pause and look back at the building before walking on. It used to be a warehouse where boxes and crates were stored. "And it still is," I say under my breath, "but now its contents are human beings." There are no windows, no way to see the sky, no outside space for the men to walk and feel fresh air on their faces or to glimpse a star in a cosmos larger than this place where their lives are arrested. Other warehouses in this rundown and partially deserted part of the city surround the detention center. All of a sudden, I am flooded by the visceral sense of what "detaining a life" means: to separate loved ones, impose deprivation, withhold meaningful action, and deny exercise of even the smallest liberty. The deep contrast with my own freedom—my ability to leave while others are condemned to stay—is not lost on me.

I turn toward the van that brought us, the "accompaniers," to the center. The van will return us to our lives and families, leaving Karun and the other detainees locked behind these walls and into states marked by desperate uncertainty and fear about their life fates.

Over the next months, I visit him when I can. We write letters to each other. I send him novels to read and paper and stamps so he can write his loved ones. He sends me different versions of his asylum application. I research how to help find him a pro bono lawyer and how to obtain a letter from Amnesty International that supports his plea. He asks me to read his country's local paper and keep watch for any news that may help his case. At the beginning, when I first visited Karun, I knew next to nothing about the political situation in his country. These days, I scan the papers daily and pray for political change so that if he is returned, he will not be killed.

When we meet, he smiles warmly and asks after my children and grandchildren. He requests a photo of them. I send it, feeling some pain in my heart. My children are safe and close, his are in danger and far away. I listen to his sorrow. He misses his wife and children. He wonders and worries about their safety. It remains unsaid, but we can both hear the unanswerable question, "Will I ever see them again?" Sorrowful days turn into sorrowful weeks and months. Letters sent home infused with love and hope only thinly veil the desperation he surely feels. His life, their lives, have become a part of mine. A special place has grown in my heart for Karun and his family.

I have spent the past fifteen years along a winding path of accompaniment with immigrants like Karun and their communities. Each time, I find myself at a familiar gateway, a potential opening where two people and, at times, two communities can meet. Too often the door is never seen. It remains closed as those in marginalized communities are separated from those who live in more privileged conditions, such as me. It has been normalized to look away and to walk on by. They are marginalized not only by the oppressions and lack of opportunity suffered, not only by being pushed out into the far rims of cities, into prisons and detention centers, but marginalized in the consciousness of more privileged neighbors, eliminating the possibility of mutual accompaniment.

Accompaniment begins with stopping and noticing, crossing over the invisible lines that separate us, making time to connect, to understand, and to respond. It depends on learning about the experiences of people and listening for the kinds of assistance that are welcomed, if any. It also crucially depends on understanding that as far apart as our individual fates seem from one another, they are ultimately intimately connected. To walk right by, to pretend that others do not exist, to develop blind spots for large portions of our communities and our neighbors—human and other-than-human animals—compromises our personal integrity. Walking right by negates the potential solidarity we could achieve and strands us as nonresponsive bystanders to those around us. Those of us who hold various privileges have too often become accustomed to two options: keeping ourselves apart from situations where others are in need, as though our engagement would compromise our own happiness, or entering into situations naively unaware of the historical context that has created the suffering and the structural changes that are necessary to address it.

In a formal sense, my professional work did not start off with accompaniment. I was trained as a developmental and clinical psychologist and practiced psychotherapy in hospitals, clinics, and private practice for two decades. Once I learned to see human suffering and psychological theory in their sociocultural contexts, however, I set out on a different path, closing the door of private practice behind me and leaning into what the public practice of psychology might look like.

But in an informal sense, the relationships I had with those with whom I worked were rooted in a nascent sense of accompaniment. In 1970, when I was nineteen, without much more instruction than being told to conduct "occupational therapy," I was given the keys to the wards of autistic boys at Creedmoor State Hospital. At the time, Creedmoor was a massive state mental hospital in Queens, New York, with seven thousand patients. Many of the boys who were diagnosed as autistic were the victims of abandonment, institutional life, and multiple electroshock treatments before they had even reached the age of twelve. They were lost and helpless in an overcrowded and misconceived system that was unable to provide for their needs. Their families despaired of taking care of them; accordingly, most boys were abandoned to institutional situations where they became prey to older, stronger, and equally disturbed children and subject to staff neglect and abuse. Before deinstitutionalization, they too often simply passed from the child wards to the adult ones, where they lived out lives with few, if any, words, visitors, or hope.

I despaired about where their futures might take them. Lacking any knowledge of or stature within the system, I decided that the best I could do was to follow each child's lead, play with him, listen to and respond to his communications, and create a space in which we could enjoy each other's company. I faithfully conveyed what I learned in notes and comments at the change of staff each afternoon. I had no illusions about the long-term benefit of what I was to later understand was a kind of accompaniment. I intuited that while it had limited lasting value, it held intrinsic worth. Reflecting on my experience years later, I gradually saw that appropriate and effective support needed to be linked to an understanding of an entire array of subjects and to actions that corresponded to them. To better understand the boys at Creedmoor, I needed not only a better grasp of the rise of autism and its historical construction as a diagnosis but of the intersection of poverty and mental illness, the often-destructive sequelae of mental health diagnoses, the history of asylums, the practice of experimenting on vulnerable human subjects, and the oncoming crashing wave of deinstitutionalization and its unintended effects. The latter would open the hospital doors, in hopes that those inside could construct lives in ordinary neighborhoods. Too few found welcome and accompaniment. Now too many reside on the street and in prisons, a situation sadly parallel to what their fate might have been three hundred years ago in Europe.

My next position was living in a halfway house with young people diagnosed as schizophrenic. We were living together in a community-minded model, and I was the dinner cook. I was also working at a city psychiatric hospital during the night, where I talked in quiet tones with those who could not sleep. I was not yet professionalized. I was simply available to listen, to be present.

As my clinical training got under way, I was more frequently pulled away from these kinds of informal encounters and into therapy offices to conduct psychological assessments and treatment of "individual" psychological difficulties and pathologies. But in addition to what I learned in the confines of consulting rooms, I often learned even more when I went beyond them. Whether visiting a child in his home, school, or playground; meeting his teachers; taking walks with him in the woods; pretending to fish together in the nearby pond, I appreciated the importance of sharing in his world for both our evolving understanding and his feeling of being accompanied. I saw how the professional world of tightly bound and orderly clinical hours had little relationship to the complexity of my clients' homes, communities, and neighborhoods, where their struggles and their resilience were rooted. This view, of course, is contrary to the conventional, evidenced-based practice that informs much of psychotherapy. Human services providers are expected to act within their professions' delineated roles, with strict explicit and implicit boundaries. We are cautioned never to depart from these norms for fear of ethical complications with, at times, legal ramifications. If we stray from sanctioned practices and roles, we learn not to speak about it. But we need to speak about such departures, particularly departures that point toward needed practices of psychosocial accompaniment.

Beyond a gathering flexibility with regard to place and time, I was learning the necessity of moving between levels of organization in order to affect the roots of the suffering I was witnessing. For instance, while working in a women's clinic with mothers who were abusing their children, I was struck by the normative cultural ideologies about motherhood they had unquestioningly incorporated as mothers and under which they suffered. I began to study the history and anthropology of motherhood across cultures, and the economic and political functions of twentieth-century Western European and U.S. constructions of motherhood. This enabled me to see how cultural parenting norms were knit into developmental theories that influenced these mothers and their children, often placing the mothers in extremely lonely, highly responsible, and overly stressful positions.

I began to meet with small groups of mothers to open a space where they could inquire into their own knowledge about the conditions under which they mothered in ways they most wanted and which they deemed best for their children. We wondered together: How might they alter their daily lives and support each other to enhance their access to these conditions? What would need to change in the community around them to help support them and their motherhood? Looking at how differently mothers in divergent cultures parented helped to open our imagination about how the role of mother could be enacted in ways that were more conducive to the thriving of both mothers and children. I began to understand how the psychopathologies of a given culture need to be understood so that distress is not pathologized as wholly individual. Often this could be seen more clearly when working with people in small groups, where they could witness others struggling with the same dilemmas.

Most chillingly, I began to inquire not only into what was deemed pathological but into what was taken for granted as normal. This helped me to see the variety of psychic mutilations that are wrought by living in a highly individualistic and materialistic culture, where violence and greed are normalized. It was clear that conventional Western psychotherapy was ill suited to address these deep-seated dysfunctions, and I turned my eyes south to learn from practices of liberation psychology. I entered into a study of the work of Brazilian pedagogist Paulo Freire, who worked with community groups to create together sites of self- and societal-critical knowledge, as well as places to formulate action in concert with others for the purpose of transforming the social structures that give rise to great suffering.

I realized that I needed to set out on a different path, one that included the individual in the context of his family but that also saw the individual and the family in the context of the neighborhood, the school, the city or town, the nation. This path sought to clarify the interrelated cultural and ecological systems in which our lives unfold and by which they are marked. Walking through the door to public practice, to places of dialogue and collaboration with others, set me on the path that wound its way to the Elizabeth Detention Center.

My heart was heavy as the warehouse door shut behind me. The brutal and isolating imprisonment of human beings seeking asylum is morally wrong. It is a living contradiction to the oft-stated historical value of welcoming immigrants in need to this country, the United States. To disable these institutions, it is necessary to act at the community and federal levels, and I try to do so. But I also believe that, while such oppression exists, citizen neighbors need to stand by the detainees: to visit them, welcome them, assist them with their cases, forge needed contacts that they are unable to make themselves from within detention, and lighten their sorrow through everyday sharing with a fellow human being. We must open the door and extend past the tidy boundaries set by our professions and daily living. When we stand by someone who is experiencing great difficulty, we necessarily bring in who we are as a person and what we know about the issues and conditions that have contributed to their suffering. But we need to learn more than what we already know, even at times stretching beyond places of comfort within ourselves, to adequately understand and then to address the needs of those who seek support. It is this offering of human connection, sociocultural understanding, and action on political and cultural levels against oppression and for liberation that I am calling psychosocial accompaniment. When we succeed in thinking and feeling our interdependence with one another, psychological well-being no longer appears as an individual matter. The psychological becomes visible as social, and the social as psychological. "Psychosocial" as a term conveys this interpenetration that refuses a separation between the social and the psychological or a prioritization of one over the other. To think psychosocially and to act in the light of psychosocial understandings, many human services providers need to transform their therapeutic and research practices.

Accompaniment: Another "Tradition That Has No Name"

Mary Field Belenky, Lynne Bond, and Jacqueline Weinstock studied a variety of women's community centers in Europe and the United States.[2] Each center was distinctive, but all shared a common approach. Their female founders were good listeners, not preachers. They practiced inclusivity, welcoming all members of a community and taking special efforts to make sure each person had a medium through which they could offer their voice. The founders encouraged people to raise their voices and to engage the arts as forms of expression and intergenerational communication. These women worked to hear common dreams expressed in poetry, song, theater, and conversation. They thought alongside others to co-create strategies to pursue and embody these visions. They practiced shared and horizontal leadership that was empowering to those around them and displaced focus from themselves. Belenky and her colleagues argued that there was a long tradition of such places in the United States, particularly in African American communities, but that "the tradition had no name."

Borrowing from cultural critic bell hooks's use of the term "homeplace," they proposed naming these various community centers "public homeplaces," emphasizing how the valued virtues of well-functioning and loving homes—care, inclusivity, stability, safety, love, and regard—were essential ingredients in these more public community settings.[3] They hoped that by describing and then naming these places and this tradition, a sharper light could be shone on the importance of their work and the strategies by which they accomplished it—work based on remarkable community-building, support, solidarity, and the transformation of social conditions in the light of shared vision.

Once I heard the term "public homeplace" twenty years ago, the constellation of such places throughout the world became more visible to me. For instance, in Santa Barbara, California, where I live, I was moved by an organization called City @ Peace, founded by Nancy Davis. Bringing together youth from different economic, ethnic, and racial experiences, the adolescents share their lives and create theater together to educate the community about their challenges, experiences, and dreams. This community of youth and adults is a public homeplace. I began to work with Alternatives to Violence, a group approach often used in prisons and community groups to help individuals learn the tools of nonviolent communication and living. During the course of a workshop at a prison, I could witness a public homeplace being built within a punitive and austere prison environment. It was woven together by intimate sharing, laughter from brief periods of playing together, and the common desire to create a kinder and more humane world in prison, in our families, and in our communities. I was and am inspired by the literal presence and multiplicity of such homeplaces. I understand in my body and heart the important goal of creating and sustaining them. This constellation of public homeplaces began to guide me in my community work, including that in classrooms and other kinds of learning communities.

Such is the potential power of creating and claiming generative words. Brazilian pedagogist Paulo Freire, who focused on how to link literacy training with the decoding of everyday reality, was clear that we must give special attention to those words and ideas that can help us see more clearly into the important themes of our daily living. These two generative ideas—public homeplaces and psychosocial accompaniment—are kindred. Although Belenky and her colleagues did not thematize accompaniment per se, all of the public homeplaces they chronicled began and proceeded with the deep listening to community members that is at the heart of accompaniment. Their work, however, did not stop with listening but continued by partnering with their fellow community members, and ultimately with kindred souls and groups far away, to transform the deleterious conditions afflicting their communities.

Toward Decolonial Mutual Psychosocial Accompaniment

While this book is a praise song for accompaniment, it is also an attempt to see into the potential shadows of accompaniment as a practice when power differentials mark our relationships and remain unexamined and unchanged. While psychosocial accompaniment strives for horizontal relationships, when the accompanist holds more social power and privilege than those accompanied, such horizontality and equality are aspirational but also elusive.

Accompaniment practices can themselves be expressions of and imbedded within structures of coloniality that perpetuate unjust patterns of inequality persisting in the aftermath of historical colonialism. A psychosocial accompanist needs to pay attention not only to the psychosocial context of the one being accompanied but to that of oneself. Liberation psychologist Hussein Bulhan searingly describes the colonization of compassion: citizens of First World countries that have wreaked havoc on others then show up and display compassion as though it is their individual preserve.[4] Such displays of compassion can obscure the degree to which they serve identity functions for the accompanists, positioning the accompanists in a positive light, as though their own privileges are unrelated to the structures that are causing misery. White colonists in the United States represented themselves as rescuers and saviors to Native Americans, whom they saw as primitives in need of white people's interventions. Roxanne Dunbar-Ortiz understands this savior mentality as key to U.S. militarism and critiques that it "seeps in and even guides much of our oppositional projects."[5] What should be offered as reparations for unjust and violent historical (and present) harms is packaged as charity, enhancing the image of the one who "gives" at the expense of the one who "receives." Freire cautions us to differentiate false from true generosity, describing false generosity as flowing from and dependent on maintaining injustice, while true generosity "consists precisely in fighting to destroy the causes" of it. It strives to turn hands that have been forced into supplication into "human hands which work and, working, transform the world."[6]

As this book seeks to clarify, psychosocial accompaniment across national, racial, class, and gender lines is a complex ethical practice. In transnational situations, white, First World accompaniers may use their racial, class, and citizenship privilege to assist the publicizing of violent struggles and to give pause to attackers of activists because those attackers do not want to draw First World attention and intervention. The irony, of course, is that one uses power and privilege in an attempt to undermine the effects of power and privilege. While hoping to join in solidarity, it is one's privilege and power that is deployed, the very things that otherwise undermine human solidarity. Even more problematic, as Gada Mahrouse ably points out, is the way that the use of white, First World bodies in situations of protective accompaniment of communities under attack casts Third World bodies of color in need of assistance as victims.[7] Mahrouse underscores the elision of racial privilege from the discourse of many efforts of transnational solidarity. The accompaniers, while identified with antiracism, may in fact be deploying their First World white bodies to assist or protect embattled activists. While organizations that seek white, First World accompaniers rarely make explicit the role of racial and citizenship privilege, the effectiveness of some aspects of their work relies on it. Mahrouse is careful to point out the difference between the accompanier's narrative of the effects of his or her presence and the understandings offered by those within a community that has requested accompaniment.

Clearly, accompaniment with a decolonial agenda must rest on a persistent foundation of critical reflexivity, taking pains to understand one's own positionality with a focus on intersectionality and the effects of this on those with whom one works. A commitment to reflexivity is a crucial partial antidote to naive relationships that are insufficiently conscious of power differentials and unwittingly reinforce the structures causing suffering. Attention to reflexivity encourages us to problematize our encounters with others and interrogate how we might be benefiting from our privilege at others' expense. It commits us to seeking out and challenging our assumptions and questioning our representations of self and other, a focus of chapter 7.

I am a white, cisgender, heterosexual woman with economic and professional privilege. If I accompany other white professional women in a white affinity group attempting to disrupt racial privilege, the power dynamics are quite different from my accompaniment at Elizabeth Detention Center. In the detention center, racial, social, citizenship, sexual preference, and economic privilege differentials create an appreciable degree of variance in life experiences, understandings, power, and needs. As mentioned earlier, the fact that my privileges allow me to choose to come and go, to return or not to return, creates an essential difference between myself and those I meet. While some accompanists may want to focus on the importance of the human relationship in such a situation of duress, for the detainee there are also important questions about how accompanists might be able to deploy their privilege to increase the likelihood of the awarding of asylum. I can phone Amnesty International, assemble supportive newspaper articles from the internet, explore pro bono legal assistance with an e-mail—all symptomatic of my freedoms of mobility and access in contrast to the detainee's state of forced incarceration.

This book examines both accompaniment from within a community and accompaniment from outsiders. Some "inside" accompaniers, those from the same community, may enjoy some power and privilege differential, that is, economic, educational, or social standing that positions them to have the time and resources to devote to accompaniment. Many do not but live lives of accompaniment nonetheless.

The embodied practice of psychosocial accompaniment requires a reorientation of human subjectivity, of interpersonal practices, and of the critical understanding of the accompanier so that she or he can stand alongside others who desire listening, witnessing, advocacy, and space to develop critical inquiry and joint action to address desired and needed structural and other changes. To accompany, rather than to "treat" or "advise," requires psychic decolonization, becoming mindful of entrenched proclivities to reenact vertical hierarchies based on colonial categories and experiences, including those from experiences of formal education and professionalization. Indeed, efforts to decolonize our work with others requires careful attention to our own psychic decolonization and to the cultivation of decolonizing interpersonal practices that provide a relational and ethical foundation for joint inquiry, restorative healing, and reparative and transformative action. Such practices endeavor through dialogue to build mutual respect and understanding, to create effective solidarity, and to contribute to the empowerment of those who have been marginalized. This empowerment includes the accompanist discerning when to step out of the spotlight, refusing to be the mouthpiece and declining to be the leader when those from the community are quite able to do so themselves. This decolonization of "helping" professions should enable practitioners of accompaniment to be more effective in working for increased social, economic, and environmental justice, peacebuilding and reconciliation, and local and global ecological sustainability.[8]

Existential Accompaniment: A "Bread" for Life

To accompany someone is to go somewhere with him or her, to break bread together, to be present on a journey with a beginning and an end. There's an element of mystery, of openness, of trust, in accompaniment. The companion, the *accompagnateur*, says: "I'll go with you and support you on your journey wherever it leads. I'll share your fate for a while—and by 'a while,' I don't mean a little while." Accompaniment is about sticking with a task until it's deemed completed—not by the *accompagnateur*, but by the person being accompanied.

—Paul Farmer[9]

The root of *acompañamiento* is *compañero,* or friend. It draws from the Latin *ad cum panis,* to break bread with one another. In the daily course of our lives, we enjoy the friendship of family, friends, and colleagues, and share the labors and joys of living life with one another. There is often an easy back-and-forth relationship with these others. We "break bread" with them. Inevitably, however, daily life is interrupted by crises—both acute and chronic—that call on us for extraordinary efforts. At times, we are the subject of such crises and need to call on others for help and assistance. At other times, we are aware of the need of others who are facing challenges. In these situations, they request accompaniment, our coming alongside them in an intentional way to be of whatever assistance they might request and that we are capable of offering.

Accompaniment, one by another, is central to human life, for instance, the parent's accompaniment of the baby and the child, the partner's or close friend's accompaniment of his or her partner or friend in a time of illness or duress, the adult child's accompaniment of an aging or dying parent. Each of these requires a sacrifice of other desires and intentions, and an ongoing commitment of care, attention, resources, and time. Without such accompaniment, we as human beings could not thrive and in many cases could not even survive. With such existential accompaniment, we are able to deepen into and count on necessary interdependencies and intimacies that grow from experiences of accompaniment. From this strengthening web of attuned connections, we gather a strong sense that life is possible, meaningful, and worthwhile, and that we are not alone in facing its challenges and enjoying its nectar. Indeed, it is through these connections with others that love, care, humor, and joy become possible and can be enjoyed. We experience the beauty of being met in our need as we are and of being supported in care, all the while finding our own attunement to others and a capacity to respond to their needs in challenging situations.

The fabric of our lives is woven with that of living others, humans and other-than-humans, giving rise to a complex weave of relationships that sustain and support us, and at times defeat and imperil us. Most of us are involved in accompaniment in one way or another, and to one extent or another. For many of us, this accompaniment spills over the borders of our private lives into our neighborhoods, schools, and town halls, taking up some of the critical issues of our day. Accompaniment is part of the way humans are in the world. It is intrinsic to us as deeply relational beings. And when it is greatly diminished or fails, the fabric of life—rent and unmended— fails to support us.

In the midst of such accompaniment, one becomes aware of the convergence of two or more lifelines, one's own and others'. A common path is created for a time during which lives intermingle, often in radically interpenetrative modes. Our kinship and friendship relationships draw on us and sustain us through our engagement in a flexible flow of mutual accompaniment.

In some cultures, this draw is experienced in a wider circle of neighbors and cultural "kin" than is the case in most Westernized cultures. In individualistically oriented cultures, many of our neighbors fall outside the narrow circle of care that is extended only to our closest friends and relations. This leaves many outside constricted circles of social support that are necessary to human thriving and survival: prisoners, detainees, the homeless, those with disabilities and mental illnesses, the abandoned sick and elderly, those caught in abject poverty, refugees displaced by violence and environmental catastrophes (acute and chronic), and immigrants displaced by global economic inequities, to name but a few.

Paradoxically, it is when this false separation between us and our "brothers" and "sisters" collapses that joy is often released. Staughton Lynd, activist-accompanier and self-proclaimed "guerilla historian," shares that his own "source of quiet joy" is imagining and experiencing the transition to "an unending creation of self-acting entities that are horizontally linked."[10] He continues, "My strongest wish for the new [left] Movement is that individuals will find it more and more possible to reconcile, to find common ground, to prefigure another world in the way we relate to each other. That process is the inwardness of nonviolence. What is essential is the wanting and the seeking."[11] Through such seeking, a map began to take shape inside of me, a map of accompaniment. I have not worried that it is sketchy in sections, because it is a map whose contours and multiple places must be co-created with you, my reader, by the work of accompaniment that is unfolding in your own life. Each of us can contribute from our own vantage point what accompaniment looks like on the ground around us, and indeed whether or not seeing through the lens of accompaniment is helpful in a particular context. It is important to me that there is a map, however provisional, because our spirits need reminding at this historical moment that this is a land where we can live and build together public homeplaces and sites of reconciliation that offer freely the support we need from one another.[12] In chapter 7, I differentiate between psychosocial accompaniment and being an ally, an accomplice, or a comrade, as well as explore the common ground of accompaniment.

The practice of accompaniment is embodied, requiring that we move alongside those we are accompanying. At the same time, it draws from deep underground springs of radical imagination and spirituality that enable us to create needed commons. Where division, exclusion, and separation are causes of human misery, in practices of accompaniment we cross over the barriers that have been erected, drawing together what has been sundered.

Mutual Accompaniment and Solidarity

Mutuality is much more than right relations between friends, lovers, or colleagues. Mutuality is the *creative basis* of our lives, the world, and God. It is the dynamic of our life together in the world insofar as we are fostering justice and compassion. Moreover, it is the constant wellspring of our power to make justice-love.

By "relation" I am speaking of the radical connectedness of all reality, in which all parts are mutually interactive. . . . We need to help one another learn how to participate in building a world in which the radically mutual basis of our life together will be noticed and desired, struggled for, and celebrated. Ethically, the struggle for mutual relation becomes our life-commitment.

—Carter Heyward[13]

I have directly experienced in my own life and in the lives of my students many of the mysterious ways in which deep involvement in accompanying others transforms the accompanier and ultimately can lead to a breakdown of the initial seemingly unidirectional nature of accompaniment. Accompaniment of one by another gives way to mutual or reciprocal accompaniment and to a profound reorientation to our interdependency. We are struck by the appearance of feelings of belonging and even joy in the most abject circumstances when this yielding occurs: in a prison, in a refugee camp, in the midst of a disaster.

For those with social and economic privileges that have afforded them distance from much direct psychosocial suffering, accompaniment can be seen as a part of a long pilgrimage of repair. It is an essential ingredient to a process of metabolizing five centuries of colonialism and capitalism that have deformed our relationships with one another and the natural world.

Throughout this book, I stress the importance of the mutuality of accompaniment. Those who want to identify themselves as selfless in what they see as other people's struggles sidestep the necessary task of claiming their own positionality and how they may be implicated in the very generation of the conditions in which people struggle. They fail to grasp the interdependency of their own well-being with that of others. Those they attempt to partner with often see through them as "disaster tourists," "poverty voyeurs," self-appointed "helpers" and "saviors."

Through long-term commitment with others through accompaniment, our interdependence with one another can be experienced at a visceral level. In time it yields to the insight that our liberations are codependent and coarising. The Aboriginal Activist Group in Queensland, Australia, expressed it beautifully in the 1970s:

> If you have come here to help me, you are wasting your time.
> But if you have come because your liberation is bound up with
>   mine,
> then let us work together.

TWO

Creating Social Democracy Through Mutual Accompaniment

The Social Settlement Movement

If we believe that the individual struggle for life may widen into a struggle for the lives of all, surely the demand of the individual for decency and comfort, for a chance to work and obtain the fullness of life may be widened until it gradually embraces all the members of the community and rises into a sense of the common weal.

—Jane Addams, *Democracy and Social Ethics*

To "Settle" In and "Cooperate" with Neighbors Across Economic and Ethnic Divides

At the turn of the twentieth century, mutual accompaniment was practiced in a variety of experimental places called social settlements. Social settlement movements preceded the emergence of the welfare state and the birth of competing and fracturing social services in a capitalist economy. Before social work and psychological work were split into rivaling approaches, before the development of an individual and the development of a neighborhood were conceived separately, and before the social and political were strained from the psychological, settlement members addressed individual and community well-being in a holistic manner. They practiced psychosocial accompaniment in neighborhoods challenged by social and economic inequality. Unfortunately, in the United States, this chapter of history is rarely taught or discussed. As we currently seek to create sites of reconciliation and public homeplaces for the twenty-first century, there is much to learn from these earlier successful experiments in accompaniment.

In 1884, Samuel and Henrietta Barnett founded the first university settlement, Toynbee Hall, in a poor neighborhood in East London. Henrietta Barnett brought to her union with her Anglican priest husband her experience working with Octavia Hill, a developer of social (or affordable) housing and of open spaces for working-class families. Hill simply and forthrightly proposed that we need "places to sit in, places to play in, and places to spend a day in."[1] She joined with others to make such places available to those living in crowded industrial neighborhoods.

Inspired by Hill, the Barnetts also became concerned with poverty, economic inequality, and the stark division between the social classes in England. They decided to encourage university students to live with them in neighborhoods where people had little economic privilege so that they and the students could learn firsthand about inequality and find ways to make some contribution to its alleviation. Samuel Barnett argued that social reform must be "rooted in direct and daily encounters in which lives became intertwined and from which a shared commitment to the common good" is nourished.[2]

The residents of Toynbee Hall pursued three goals: scientific research on poverty, enhancing educational opportunities in the neighborhood, and encouraging local civic leadership.[3] Samuel Barnett had hoped that once vocational education needs were met, a "working man's university" could be developed—a dream that never came about but that has inspired many others' efforts. Henrietta Barnett turned her attention to the welfare of working-class women and girls in her district, including a large number of sex workers.

In 1889, they welcomed to Toynbee Hall a young visitor from the U.S. Midwest: Jane Addams. After college, Addams had entered medical school but had to withdraw for health reasons. She entered a period of personal uncertainty and felt unmoored, as she searched for her life purpose during a historical time when this was narrowly defined as marriage for white women with some economic means. She began a set of European travels after the sudden and premature death of her father, whose character provided her with a strong role-model of civic engagement. During these years of travel, she was often sick and emotionally dispirited. While attempting to follow in the footsteps of her stepmother's aesthetic approach to life, visiting museums and bullfights, Addams hungered for an existence that felt more meaningful. Later in her life, she described the sexism that contributed to her feeling—and that of many young women like her—that there was little consequential use to be made of her faculties and life.

She described a "simple plan" beginning to develop in her mind before her second trip to Europe:

> I gradually became convinced that it would be a good thing to rent a house in a part of the city where many primitive and actual needs are found, in which young women who had been given over too exclusively to study might restore a balance of activity along traditional lines and learn of life from life itself; where they might try out some of the things they had been taught and put truth to the "ultimate test of the conduct it dictates or inspires."[4]

She was concerned that the sheltering and pampering form of education she and other young women of privilege had received had caused them a significant loss of the capacity to respond to the presence of suffering around them. She privately nursed her idea of creating such a house. Then, she wrote,

> It was suddenly made quite clear to me that I was lulling my conscience by a dreamer's scheme, that a mere paper reform had become a defense for continued idleness, and that I was making it a raison d'etre for going on indefinitely with study and travel. It is easy to become the dupe of a deferred purpose, of the promise the future can never keep, and I had fallen into the meanest type of self-deception in making myself believe that all this was in preparation for great things to come.[5]

She made up her mind the next day that she would begin to carry out the plan. Her first action was to share it with her trusted friend Ellen Starr, knowing the importance of moving it from a personal fantasy to a shared intention. She hoped that Starr would join her in embodying her fledgling vision. A month later, in June 1888, Addams turned her listless and aimless traveling to the service of her emergent plan and growing sense of purpose. She traveled to Toynbee Hall to learn all she could about this initiative that bore some resemblance to her vision.

> Five years after my first visit in East London, I found myself at Toynbee Hall equipped not only with a letter of introduction from Canon Fremantle but with high expectations and a certain belief that whatever perplexities and discouragement concerning the life of the poor were in store for me, I should at least know something at first hand and have the solace of daily activity. I had confidence that although life itself might contain many difficulties, the period of mere passive receptivity had come to an end, and I had at last finished with the ever-lasting "preparation for life," however ill-prepared I might be. It was not until years afterward that I came upon Tolstoy's phrase "the snare of preparation," which he insists we spread before the feet of young people, hopelessly entangling them.[6]

After her visit to Toynbee Hall, Addams had a clearer vision of what she and Starr should do.

While Toynbee Hall had inspired Addams to think more concretely about creating a settlement house, Addams and Starr sought to create something that was quite different from Toynbee Hall. They wanted it to be graced with female leadership, more egalitarian, and not religiously aligned.[7] In 1889, Addams, Starr, and their colleagues created a "settlement" in a poor area of Chicago. They settled in the neighborhood not to gentrify it but to join in solidarity with their new neighbors, sharing in the life around them and working to create cross-class and cross-ethnic relationships that were reciprocal and mutual. Their neighbors were primarily immigrants suffering far from their home countries amid industrial and urban abuses, including unfair wages, lack of representation, child labor, lack of safety standards, unregulated hours, and failures in neighborhood infrastructure. They were beset by poverty, poor sanitation, disease, and lack of access to education.

Addams felt that time justified the residents' "early contention that the mere foothold of a house, easily accessible, ample in space, hospitable and tolerant in spirit, situated in the midst of the large foreign colonies which so easily isolate themselves in American cities, would be in itself a serviceable thing for Chicago." The women brought their own treasured possessions, taking delight in creating a home that was at the same time to be shared as a public space. Addams remarked, "Probably no young ma-tron ever placed her own things in her own house with more pleasure than that with which we first furnished Hull-House."[8]

She freely and honestly admitted her own ignorance of conditions she herself had not lived in and understood that it is the people who live in these conditions who understand the most about them. Newcomers like herself needed to be students of their immigrant neighbors in order to de-velop "sympathetic" understanding and knowledge. She and the other set-tlers turned to working-class women neighbors for their own education. It is important to remember that both women and immigrants found them-selves on the margins of a white, male-dominated society in the United States.[9]

The Hull-House settlers did not think that immigrants should be pressured to accommodate to and become assimilated into mainstream American culture. They believed that immigrants should, if they wanted, conserve their culture, practice its arts, and have the opportunity to place their own culture into conversation with that of their American neighbors.

Mutual Education for Social Democracy

Addams's dislike of class hierarchy also influenced her views on education. She believed that education was crucial for democracy, but not an educa-tion of the disenfranchised by the privileged as she had witnessed in so many places, including other settlement houses. She believed the purpose of education was mutual education, where all members—settlers and immigrants—shared their knowledge in an atmosphere of respect for each other's dignity and knowledge. Impulses toward charity needed to be transformed into shared and mutual social education and action: "It has to be diffused in a social atmosphere, information must be held in solution, in a medium of fellowship and good will. Intellectual life requires for its expansion and manifestation the influences and assimilation of the interests and affections of others."[10]

Through exploring different educational formats, Hull-House soon found that "a combination of a social atmosphere with serious study" was the most popular for the adults. The children joined in educational opportunities that were not available in the crowded public schools. Elders were honored by gathering them to share their life experiences and methods of overcoming early hardships. In every instance, the vision that guided the educational efforts was different from that of an elite academy or college that hopes to set its learners apart from the larger society. "On the contrary," noted Addams, education should "connect him with all sorts of people by his ability to understand them as well as by his power to supplement their present surroundings with the historic background." "A Settlement," she wrote, "is a protest against a restricted view of education." It is "held together in that soundest of all social bonds, the companionship of mutual interests."[11]

Daycare, nursery school, kindergarten, afterschool boys and girls clubs, adult education, summer school, college extension classes, a branch of the public library, lectures, and community discussions were all hosted at Hull-House. Addams described it as "constantly filling and refilling with groups of people. The little children who came to the kindergarten in the morning were followed by the afternoon clubs of older children, and those in turn made way for the educational and social organizations of adults, occupying every room in the house every evening. All one's habits of living had to be readjusted."[12]

The scale of operations at Hull-House is hard to imagine. Nine thousand people joined in weekly activities, and the effects on each individual

were multiple. One young man, reflecting on what Hull-House had meant
to him, shared,

> It was the first house I had ever been in where books and maga-
> zines just lay around as if there were plenty of them in the world.
> Don't you remember how much I used to read at that little
> round table at the back of the library? To have people regard
> reading as a reasonable occupation changed the whole aspect of
> life to me and I began to have confidence in what I could do.[13]

For Addams, education was essential to democracy. It was a "form of
liberation and deliverance."[14] She never restricted education to book learning. Indeed, the settlement house was imagined as a place for the exchange
of knowledge and for the deepening of dialogue through which people
could better understand each other and develop what she called "sympathetic knowledge." It is via this mutual understanding that people can come
to care about one another and construct lives and actions that contribute to
"lateral progress." In contradistinction to progress being defined by the advancement of elites, Addams understood democracy to require inclusive
progress for all people.

Addams's democratic vision saw relationships between immigrants
and longer-term residents not as seeking the former to take on the culture
and values of the latter but rather for their shared democracy to be a place
where different cultures could thrive in relationship to one another. This
meant that the immigrant had as much to teach the citizen as the citizen the
immigrant, radically disrupting the usual hierarchical relations between
them.

Addams was committed to helping create educational pathways for
people locked out of the academy. Hull-House became a vibrant educational center for lifelong learning, welcoming key intellectual figures of the
day like John Dewey, Peter Kropotkin, and George Herbert Mead. The University of Chicago put considerable pressure on Hull-House to become an
extension of the school's sociology department and to use the neighborhood as a site for scientific study. Addams resisted this pressure and rejected

having Hull-House act as a laboratory or her neighbors as objects of others' study: "I have always objected to the phrase 'sociological laboratory' applied to us, because Settlements should be something much more human and spontaneous than such a phrase connotes, and yet it is inevitable that the residents should know their own neighborhoods more thoroughly than any other, and that their experience there should affect their convictions."[15]

This reluctance to link with the University of Chicago did not mean that sociological studies were not performed by Hull-House residents and their neighbors, but the studies emerged from the expressed needs of those in the neighborhood and were conducted in a cooperative manner, anticipating what is now called participatory action research. One of the finest pieces of research to emerge from Hull-House, *Hull-House Maps and Papers,* was authored by "The Residents of Hull-House." The residents were not seeking to build their individual research records but to attune themselves to mutual interests with their neighbors and to explore how they could work with them to aid in the issue at hand.[16] It was this spirit of cooperation that distinguished the women's endeavors from academic work that is done in a spirit of professional competition and self-aggrandizement. The settlers and neighbors understood "cooperation" as a method facilitating social reform and as an important antidote to the competitive liberalism and social Darwinism of the day.[17] Importantly and reflective of her philosophy, Addams never understood the work done at Hull-House as her own but as arising from the intersection of communities as neighbors listen respectfully to one another.

From Charity to Justice and Mutual Accompaniment

Industrialization and immigration at the end of the nineteenth century continued to increase social and economic class divisions. The existing charity and philanthropy of the time sought to relieve some of the misery resulting from these divisions but did so without questioning their structural causes. In contrast, Addams was adamant in rejecting traditional ideas of charity and the hierarchical and demeaning forms of relationships that purported to "help" poor "clients." While doing things for instead of with others, those with privilege believed they were acquiring merit, while too often looking down on the objects of their actions and judgments. Addams refused the "unconscious division of the world into the philanthropist and those to be helped . . . the assumption of two classes."[18] The philanthropist and the charity worker blamed the victims of unbridled capitalism for being morally weak instead of working to dismantle the structural causes of injustice and its manufactured miseries. Charity visitors sought to instill virtues of frugality and improve the character of the poor through their own supposedly good example. This emphasis on poverty as caused by the moral and character weaknesses of those suffering relieved philanthropists from examining their own role in perpetuating class inequality, excess wealth, and privilege through the exploitation of workers and nature. Indeed, even when the poverty and suffering they saw was the direct product of capitalist exploitative relationships, capitalism itself was not questioned.

In Addams's first autobiographical work, *Twenty Years at Hull-House,* she described what the residents came to understand their settlement was:

> The Settlement then, is an experimental effort to aid in the solution of the social and industrial problems which are engendered by the modern conditions of life in a great city. It insists that these problems are not confined to any one portion of a city. It is an attempt to relieve, at the same time, the over accumulation at one end of society and the destitution at the other; but it assumes that this over accumulation and destitution is most sorely felt in the things that pertain to social and educational privileges.[19]

During the depression that erupted in Chicago during the 1890s, Addams argued that instead of focusing on what should be done about the unemployed, "we ought to come together and regard [the situation of unemployment] as a common trouble, and we should consider not what we shall do but what we and the unemployed do together, that we may as brothers grow out into a wider and better citizenship than we have ever known."[20] She struggled with whether or not to reverse Hull-House's policy to refrain from direct relief work but ultimately felt she could not stand by without organizing relief as families were increasingly deprived of necessary resources. Speaking of the compromise she reached, she said, "the painful condition of administering charity is the inevitable discomfort of a transition into more democratic relations." She was deeply disturbed by the fact that "there was plenty of charity, too little justice."[21]

Approaching poverty as an individual's problem, charities of the day sent middle-class women visitors out into the neighborhood homes of the poor to encourage middle-class values and address the "problems of character" that the visitors thought caused poverty. Settlement houses were much more likely to approach the poverty suffered by individuals as a systemic issue in need of social reform. Like her friend and colleague educational philosopher John Dewey, Addams understood charity as an attempt to buy off the resentment of those exploited and assuage the consciences of those perpetuating social and economic injustice. Dewey, a frequent guest and friend of Hull-House, commended Addams for the way in which she tore "away the armor-plate of prejudice, of convention, and isolation that keeps one from sharing to the full in the larger and even the more unfamiliar and alien ranges of the possibilities of human life and experience."[22]

The "Subjective" Needs of the Settler and Mutual Accompaniment

Addams stressed the reciprocal nature of the relationship between settlers and their neighbors. The settlement house aimed to further the education of immigrant neighbors as well as to address the educational needs of the resident women and of those living outside the neighborhood who came to visit, learn, and teach at Hull-House. Addams was strikingly clear that the settlement house meet both the "objective" and "subjective" needs of the settlement residents.

By "subjective needs," she was referring to her own needs and the needs of the settler women with whom she lived. These women rejected the narrow roles assigned to them as women at the turn of the century, disenfranchised and consigned to the domestic sphere. They did not reject what were seen as the feminine values of care and nurture, but they sought to extend them and the realm of "housekeeping" into the public sphere. They argued that the industrial city was spawning pollution, disease, poverty, and a lack of sanitation. For a woman, living in a settlement helped her satisfy familial and social claims at the same time. In Addams's case, she remained unmarried and without children in the biological sense. Her life, however, was filled with children and family-like relations to both other settlers ("residents") and to neighbors. She extended her care beyond the borders of normative nuclear family life as she transposed traditional female roles from the nuclear family to the wider community and city.

Addams knew firsthand how her "privilege" had also created ignorance of the conditions of those around her and their cultures. Moving into the settlement made Addams more complete herself and gifted her and the other women with a way of expanding their knowledge and understanding of the wider world in which they lived. She felt an intense need for relationships that were outside the constricting circles of privilege she had been born into. As the Hull-House women deepened into their relationships with immigrant neighbors, they became keenly aware of how much other Americans had to learn about caring and providing for members of the community. Addams believed that if citizens could learn the virtues of social solidarity, democracy would be enhanced.[23] While some described the Hull-House residents as self-sacrificing in their service to others, Addams objected, asserting that living at Hull-House fulfilled a subjective need and provided an opportunity in which one receives as much as one gives.

Addams's experiences at Hull-House deepened her criticism of the education of young women of privilege. On the one hand, they were exposed by their parents to the reports of returning missionaries about the immense challenges burdening millions of lives; on the other hand, they were not encouraged to take part in addressing social ills but to prepare for a sheltered life in a narrow domestic sphere. Addams claimed these women were deprived of their "active faculties" and restricted to situations that made them feel unduly confined, restless, and useless, where their potential was progressively atrophied. She wrote, "In our attempt then to give a girl pleasure and freedom from care we succeed, for the most part, in making her pitifully miserable. She finds 'life' so different from what she expected it to be. She is besotted with innocent little ambitions, and does not understand this apparent waste of herself, this elaborate preparation, if no work is provided for her." Securing "refinement and cultivation" for oneself, over against others, separates her from the "common intercourse" necessary to a "higher civic life." Furthermore, "To shut one's self away from that half of the race is to shut one's self away from the most vital part of life; it is to live out but half the humanity to which we have been born heir and to use but half our faculties. We have all had longings for a fuller life which should include the use of these faculties."[24]

Speaking from her own experience, Addams described such young women as haunted by their desires for action and their wishes to have some meaningful role in alleviating social wrongs. She saw them as bearing "the brunt of being cultivated into unnourished, oversensitive lives" and of being cast into inactivity "at the very period of life when they are longing to construct the world anew and to conform it to their own ideals." She continued, "They have been shut off from the common labor by which they live which is a great source of moral and physical health. They feel a fatal want of harmony between their theory and their lives, a lack of coordination between thought and action."[25] Addams's own physical, psychological, and spiritual struggle that she endured before her visit to Toynbee Hall was relieved by life at Hull-House. By all accounts, she thrived there.

The residents gave attention to the spirit with which they engaged in their work. Addams noted that too often residents moved "with hurried and ignoble gait." She observed,

> It is always easy for those in pursuit of ends which they consider of overwhelming importance to become themselves thin and impoverished in spirit and temper, to gradually develop a dark mistaken eagerness alternating with fatigue, which supersedes "the great and gracious ways" so much more congruous with worthy aims. Partly because of this universal tendency, partly because a Settlement shares the perplexities of its times and is never too dogmatic concerning the final truth, the residents would be glad to make the daily life at the Settlement "conform to every shape and mode of excellence."[26]

Music, art, literature, conversation, cross-generational relations, life-long education, shared solidarity around social transformation, and friend-ship all enlivened Hull-House, making it a homeplace for both residents and visitors. Not only did Hull-House have a music school but it offered weekly Sunday concerts. It encouraged the songs and music of immigrant groups that frequented Hull-House. Addams remarked, "In the deep tones of the memorial organ erected at Hull-House, we realize that music is per-haps the most potent agent for making the universal appeal and inducing men to forget their differences." She described the conviction of the early Hull-House residents "that whatever of good the Settlement had to offer should be put into positive terms, that we might live with opposition to no man, with recognition of the good in every man, even the most wretched. We had often departed from this principle, but had it not in every case been a confession of weakness, and had we not always found antagonism a fool-ish and unwarrantable expenditure of energy?"[27]

Hull-House provided a living example of the residents' philosophy that mutual support is as important as mutual struggle in achieving social progress. They hoped that their inclusive, collaborative, and democratic deliberations, springing from caring relationships, would be a model for the larger society.[28]

Addams shared that the residents of Hull-House were often criticized for living "where they did not naturally belong." She answered this critique: "I protested that was exactly what we wanted—to be swallowed and di-gested, to disappear into the bulk of the people. Twenty years later I am willing to testify that something of the sort does take place after years of identification with an industrial community."[29]

While the role of women in the larger society has substantially changed in the United States, the problem for children of "privilege" is not so different from what Addams described. Racial, ethnic, and socioeconomic groups are often profoundly separated into different schools and neighborhoods. It is still the case that one must intentionally forge a life that crosses these borders in order to experience a sense of the wider society and to create one's place within it. Hull-House was not conceived as a place for the sake of immigrants alone but as a place where immigrants and citizens could be together, deter-

mining needs and strategies to improve the challenging life situations generated by militarism, capitalism, and industrialism. Through classes and clubs,
thousands of Chicagoans crossed neighborhood boundaries and met their
working-class immigrant neighbors directly, making it possible for them to
live in a fuller sense of their own city and their own potential roles in co-
constructing social democracy. The residents were not interested in limiting
their relationships to those of helping, as is common within the helping professions today. Hull-House residents wished to know their neighbors
"through all the varying conditions of life, to stand by when they are in distress, but by no means to drop intercourse with them when normal prosperity has returned, enabling the relation to become more social and free from
economic disturbance." And, importantly, settlers did not see themselves as
helpers and others as the helped. They learned deep lessons about the practice of mutual aid and an ethic of interdependence from their immigrant
neighbors. During a winter of severe deprivation in Chicago, Addams wrote,

> I became permanently impressed with the kindness of the poor
> to each other; the woman who lives upstairs will willingly share
> her breakfast with the family below because she knows they
> "are hard up"; the man who boarded with them last winter will
> give a month's rent because he knows the father of the family is
> out of work; the baker across the street who is fast being pushed
> to the wall by his downtown competitors, will send across three
> loaves of stale bread because he has seen the children looking
> longingly into his window and suspects they are hungry.[30]

The Hull-House residents learned to be similarly attentive and responsive,
creating a space of accompaniment at Hull-House.

Municipal Housekeeping: Extending the "Domestic Sphere"

There were other dimensions to Hull-House living. Women listened carefully to the concerns of their immigrant neighbors, leading to solidarity
of action on a staggering number of issues: addressing the placing of the

elderly into poor houses; the needs of pregnant youth; the birth and development of cooperatives; the understanding of labor issues; the development of a day nursery, a kindergarten, and a playground; helping women emerging from the sex trade; creating lodging for unemployed women; the creation of multiple forums for education; addressing poor sanitation and associated spikes in disease and early death; creating tenement house codes; and lobbying for child labor laws. Hull-House women argued that it was their living in the neighborhood that made their understanding of these kinds of issues possible, and which then naturally led to their placing their energies alongside their neighbors so that change was possible.

Addams described everyday examples of this. For instance, one Christmas the women residents of Hull-House were surprised that so many children who were visiting with them refused the Christmas candies they offered. Through asking a few questions about something so seemingly small, a window was suddenly opened for them on the daily world of these young children. The women found that the children toiled long hours each day in candy factories. Such an observation led to multiple efforts to create legislation to prevent child labor.

In watching and playing with the children, Addams saw that "one of the most piteous aspects in the life of city children, as I have seen it in the neighborhood of Hull-House, is the constant interruption to their play which is inevitable on the streets, so that it can never have any continuity—the most elaborate 'plan or chart' or 'fragment from their dream of human life' is sure to be rudely destroyed by the passing traffic." Playgrounds and game fields were built, and a kindergarten and day nursery were provided in an attempt to meet the children's need for uninterrupted play. By living in the settlement, Hull-House residents were able to partner and advocate with their neighbors for treatment equal to other areas of the city that addressed the lack of sewerage, sanitation, running water, and lighting infrastructure. Addams continued, "We also quickly discovered that nothing brought us so absolutely into comradeship with our neighbors as mutual and sustained effort such as the paving of a street, the closing of a gambling house, or the restoration of a veteran police sergeant."[31] When there was a need, for instance, of a place to bathe, Hull-House opened bath stalls in its basement but then joined with neighbors to press for the erection of public baths in the neighborhood. In so doing, Hull-House did not become an island but rather functioned as a nucleus or catalyst for broader and deeper community change.

Hull-House evolved during the Progressive era, a remarkable period of social justice movements in the United States. During this era, women social reformers and suffragettes began to link their personal homes with the wider city. They understood that the welfare of their children and their neighbors' children depended on the health of the city around them.[32] They collapsed the distance between their homes and city hall, arguing that the domestic sphere should include the sphere of the city, and that the city requires the energies of women to tend to issues such as sanitation, food safety, child welfare, and poverty.

Addams lauded women's values of nurturance and care in the domestic sphere and wanted to see these qualities extended beyond the front gate of the home. She criticized men for failing to tend to civic housekeeping: "The men of the city have been carelessly indifferent to much of this civic housekeeping, as they have always been indifferent to the details of the household. They have totally disregarded a candidate's capacity to keep the streets clean, preferring to consider him in relation to the national tariff or to the necessity for increasing the national navy."[33] The inclusion of women into the sphere of public policy, she argued, would allow attention to be paid to areas of public life neglected by most men.

Social Democracy and the Structural Violence of Capitalism and Militarism

Addams understood "the duties of family, nation, and humanity" as "concentric circles of obligation."[34] While not denying the importance of governmental institutions, Addams was convinced that inclusive, nonhierarchical, multicultural friendships and collaborations at the level of the neighborhood were the foundation for an emergent social democracy and transnationalism.[35] She considered them essential to developing a lived sense of world citizenship and of appreciation for the importance of inclusivity for the flourishing of democracy.

Addams believed that the development of sympathetic understanding among different communities of people was necessary to the construction of "social democracy." Through sympathetic understanding we can come to learn about one another, creating a foundation for caring and acting in solidarity. Through this term she interlinked democracy with social justice and peace. She explored this up close in her neighborhood as immigrants from many different countries and cultures began to form relationships and pursue education and joint social actions at Hull-House. Indeed, Addams claimed that she learned a lot about international peacebuilding through immersion in the cosmopolitan realities of her immigrant neighborhood.[36]

Addams was critical of U.S. imperialism in general and spoke out against the country's annexation of the Philippines in 1899. She understood that this kind of imperialism was based on both a pernicious ranking of civilizations and an adoption of a paternalistic stance toward those defined and demeaned as inferior to Americans.[37] She contrasted the militarized aggression of the nation with the respectful and egalitarian transnational relationships unfolding all around her in her neighborhood. Addams saw women as having a key role in creating cross-border relationships with women in other nations to address issues such as food politics, and later proposed that this be coordinated by the League of Nations. In so doing, Addams not only extended women's roles but the very foundation of settlement houses—cross-border relations—to the international stage.[38]

Addams's stand, however, as a pacifist during World War I cost her dearly. Many who had placed her on a pedestal in recognition of her settlement house leadership now regarded Addams as naive, "a misguided 'good' woman who was ignorant of war . . . [and guilty of] misleading the American public. . . . Finally, she was decried as a 'menace' to society with her strange ideas of cooperation and dangerous beliefs in equality."[39] One newspaper reporter put it this way: "[Addams] is a silly, vain, impertinent old maid, who may have done good work at Hull-House in Chicago but is now meddling with matters far beyond her capacity."[40] During this period, the majority of the progressive organizations that Addams had helped found were disbanded.

Unfortunately, the entrenched sexism of the time affected not only Addams's treatment around pacifism but also her place in the discipline of sociology and the Department of Sociology at the University of Chicago. Both the discipline and the university had profited deeply from her engaged work. In the post–World War I period, applied sociology and its efforts of social reform were demeaned as bad sociology, that is, biased, nonobjective, the stuff of women's work, not reflective of the male-dominated academy. Her work was derided or forgotten by male sociologists. As they sought status for sociology within the academy, they distanced themselves from Addams and her colleagues' excellent work of applied sociology in distressed neighborhoods. Even more importantly, the male professors' efforts to construct sociology as an objective science entailed deserting Addams's strongly held teloi: economic justice, social justice, participatory work with communities, and the strengthening of democracy through intercultural relationships. At the University of Chicago, as Professors Ernest Burgess and Robert Park shaped sociological study, they both built on Addams's efforts without crediting her. Her work, in effect, was disappeared. It was consigned by the men to social work, despite her own understanding of herself as a sociologist.[41] They derided social work as an inferior, unscientific, and unintellectual profession, a world for women, not men. A few of the other men in the Chicago School of Sociology, such as social psychologist and philosopher John Dewey, stood by Addams, remaining grateful to her for all they had learned being at Hull-House.

As conservative and repressive patriotic fervor built during the first Red Scare (1919–1920), the government targeted Addams and labeled her as the most dangerous woman in America. Her labor movement work, Hull-House's hosting of anarchists and Marxists, and her belief that capitalism and democracy created destructive contradictions made her vulnerable to this assault, despite never being a declared socialist or communist herself. Before a Senate subcommittee, she was named at the top of the list of sixty-two individuals deemed the most dangerous and destructive people in the United States. Senator R. Luck demeaned her for un-American activities.[42]

Had Addams lived to speak with Martin Luther King, Jr., they would have had a lot of notes to compare. It is one thing to extend oneself to poor people and their communities. It is another to denounce the deadly causal roots of structural inequality that afflict the society. By denouncing the "evil triplets" of militarism, capitalism, and racism, King was similarly targeted as a dangerous enemy of the corporate military state.

During the Red Scare, the cooperative-democratic movement that Addams was helping to lead was now held suspect as un-American, as were efforts for social and economic equality. She saw clearly the contradiction between social and economic democracy and capitalism, and challenged the latter as it was being practiced as inadequate to helping create harmonious societies, free of the oppression bred by pernicious hierarchies and their accepted inequalities. Sadly, the degree of censure and ridicule she received corresponded to the degree of radicality of her thought and its divergence from mainstream ideologies. Sociologist Mary Jo Deegan rightly characterizes Addams's approach as critical-emancipatory, deepening the "public consciousness and analyz[ing] concrete repressive conditions in light of ideal ones." Addams struggled for a harmonious society based on cooperation, graced by equality, free speech, and democratic governance. She placed the achievement of humanitarian goals over economic ones. The neighborhoods the residents of Hull-House worked in were themselves multinational and multicultural. Their diversity and cosmopolitanism, Addams thought, strengthened democracy. She defined "radical democracy" as "democratic principles to be carried to their extreme for total social, economic, and political equality. All people were to have a voice in decisions affecting their daily lives and society."[43]

In the post–Great Depression 1930s, those effecting Franklin Roosevelt's New Deal were in need of Addams's expertise and experience. Suddenly, she found herself and her ideas again in favor. In a stunning reversal of public assessment, she went from being scapegoated and derided within the United States to being awarded the Nobel Peace Prize in 1931. Addams helped found the Women's Bureau, the Children's Bureau, the National Association for the Advancement of Colored People, the American Civil Liberties Union, the Women's International League for Peace and Freedom, Social Security, and workers' compensation. She worked to promote women's rights and suffrage, nonviolent approaches to conflict, and racial equality. As the state came to assume some of the functions of the settlement house movement, Addams's understandings and insights were called upon. From living in the neighborhood over decades, she had learned to perceive public institutions from the standpoint of the people they were presumably created to serve.

Addams was a seeker of personal integrity, an integrity of her direct experience, her intellectual understandings, her spirit, and her actions. For Addams to enjoy excess wealth in the face of others' destitution constituted a crisis of personal integrity in a context of unbridled capitalism.[44] She helped to create what scholar Mary Louise Pratt has called a "contact zone," a site where people with different life experiences and access to privilege and resources can meet and grapple with differing histories and realities they intimately contend with.[45] I call her lifework "psychosocial accompaniment" because she was able to live alongside the neighbors she worked with, responding to their situation and seeking structural changes at the same time she offered her friendship and solidarity. Her nephew James Linn remembers his aunt Jane:

> It was obvious that if you went to the House you were welcome; if you called, you were called upon; and if you let the young women know there was anything they could do for you, they did it if they could. Ms. Addams herself washed newborn-babies, and minded children and nursed the sick and prepared the dead for burial, as naturally as any other women of the neighborhood did for her friends. She had more friends. That was all. And some things she would do that other women would not do.[46]

While Jane Addams and Hull-House were largely written out of the history of academic sociology, they became foundational to the profession of social work. Social work, however, took a path toward increasing professionalization as it strived to assume a competitive role among human services in a capitalist service economy. This professionalization intensified after World War II when the profession experienced a gender shift from women to men, as men returned home from war in search of work and many white women were urged to yield their jobs and return to the domestic sphere.

While women had gained suffrage and white women were increasingly enlarging the domestic sphere through their work outside the home, many of the issues of life meaning that Addams experienced as a young woman and so eloquently spoke about were (and are) still pressing. Namely, when you have some degree of relative economic and social privilege, how do you live your life in relationship to those who do not? A generation after Addams, Dorothy Day was to suffer this question and live creatively into a response that gave rise to an international movement of houses of hospitality. She too placed mutual accompaniment at the center of her life and spiritual devotion. Indeed, Staughton Lynd shared, "Miss Addams's successors today are not the career-men and executives of the social work profession, but groups such as the Catholic Workers, who, like Jane Addams, have simply gone to live in the slums, and the participants in the Southern sit-in movement."[47] Chapter 3 turns to Day's and the Catholic Workers' form of radical accompaniment.

African American Social Settlements and Missions

The only thing to be dreaded in the Settlement is that it lose its flexibility,
its power of quick adaptation, its readiness to change its methods as its
environment may demand. It must be open to conviction and must have a deep
and abiding sense of tolerance. It must be hospitable and ready for experiment. It
should demand from its residents a scientific patience in the accumulation of facts
and the steady holding of their sympathies as one of the best instruments for that
accumulation. It must be grounded in a philosophy whose foundation is on the
solidarity of the human race, a philosophy which will not waver when the race
happens to be represented by a drunken woman or an idiot boy.
—Jane Addams[48]

Settlement houses spread quickly in the first decade of the twentieth century. In 1900, a hundred settlements were counted in the United States, and a decade later there were four hundred. In 1911, the National Federation of Settlements was born, naming Jane Addams as its first president.[49] While Addams spoke of the need to ground settlement house activities in "the solidarity of the human race," the settlement house movement largely failed to adequately include African Americans into this "solidarity" as the "great migrations" from the South to the North shifted the largest population of urban newcomers from European immigrants to African Americans. While both African American and white women were involved in promoting social welfare and women's involvement in politics, they largely did this racially segregated from one another.[50] Unlike many settlement house leaders, Addams did speak to the need to partner with African Americans in settlement work and called the circumstances of African Americans "the gravest situation in American life."[51] She supported the development of a biracial settlement on the south side of Chicago, the Frederick Douglass Center.

Racist stereotypes of moral "defects" and "weakness" in the African American family attributed to centuries of servitude deeply curtailed whites' inclusion of African Americans in settlement activities. Even when white settlement workers connected the causes of these presumed "weaknesses" to the social environment of slavery and ongoing poverty, racism, and oppression, resisting biologizing them, these attitudes often still led to paternalistic and moralistic approaches.[52] At the same time, there were white settlement house workers who through their growing association with African American neighbors were able to contest the racist stereotypes and grow into a deeper understanding of the effects of racism and structural violence, and the necessity of challenging and dismantling racism and structural injustice. These individuals came to understand that by creating interracial houses and programs, blacks and whites had an opportunity to experience their commonality and to work together on many shared problems, including racism itself.

Settlement houses tried to clarify whether their allegiance should be to a neighborhood, a geographical area, or to a particular population. If it was immigrants, should the house relocate when the immigrant population moved? Or should the population of the house change as one immigrant group left and another migrating group, such as African Americans, arrived?

Some houses chose to be interracial only to be deserted by white participants who refused to attend events and classes with African Americans.

White workers who made a commitment to integration often found
themselves ostracized and their funding withdrawn. By crossing over racial
lines, they found themselves experiencing a small dose of the social exclusion the African Americans with whom they worked were subjected to daily
by white society. Others resorted to being interracial in name only, offering
segregated activities under the same roof. Some strove to have an interracial
staff while working entirely with African Americans. Mary White Ovington
worked to create a model tenement in New York on Henry Street and to
have two white and two black staff living in apartments on the premises. She
ended up being the only white person who would live there. Having some
white presence often proved helpful in bridging African American and
white communities, increasing whites' awareness of the oppression blacks
were suffering, and importantly, securing badly needed donations from
white donors and greater access to city or town resources.

Many African Americans created centers for community uplift, but
because they were faith-based and denominational, these were not included
in the history of the settlement house movement, a movement in the United
States that prided itself on being nondenominational and secular. Social
historian Elisabeth Lasch-Quinn challenged this exclusion and effectively
connected such religiously affiliated African American cultural centers with
the settlement house movement. In doing so, the rich and varied landscape
of settlement work in both the North and the South is thrown into sharper
relief: "The functions of these community centers often included those of
the 'bona fide' settlement houses: delivering social services; strengthening
the neighborhood; responding to community needs; fostering cooperation
through club work in small groups; providing the means to a more fulfilling
recreational, educational, and social life; studying local social conditions
as the basis for lobbying for policy changes; and agitating for broad social
reforms."[53]

The settlement house movement's belief that its decision to be
secular would lead to more inclusivity was misguided, writes Quinn. Ironically, it ended up being dogmatic and exclusionary. It largely missed the

opportunity to affiliate with African American efforts for social service and civil rights reform, and to enjoy the mutual cross-racial learning that could have resulted. Many white settlement house leaders remained fearful of people using settlement houses for proselytizing. What they did not consider was that people already affiliated with black churches were not being proselytized by the church in which they were already members.

African American churches, a key social institution in African American communities, had a long history of providing the same kind of neighborhood services as settlements did, while focusing—as settlements also did—on the larger issue of righting the inequalities making life so difficult. An important function of many settlement missions in the South was their crucial role in education, a fruit of which was a steady stream of African American educators willing to start schools in rural areas. In the North, mission residents sought to meet the evolving needs of African American migrants from the South. The People's Village School and the White Rose Mission are exemplars of the kinds of accompaniment in African American communities that evolved in the South and the North, respectively. Both were begun by women who had themselves been born into slavery: Georgia Washington and Victoria Earle Matthews.

Georgia Washington and the People's Village School

African Americans who created settlement missions and schools in the South left their own communities and took up residence in places that were in dire need of education and social services. Throughout the South, public school education for African Americans was often limited to the third grade and to three months a year of classes. Georgia Washington exemplified the kind of lifelong accompaniment that helped to create schools and cooperative community initiatives, which included needed land ownership for African Americans. After she graduated from Hampton Normal and Agricultural Institute in Hampton, Virginia, in 1882, she continued to work there and then helped Charlotte Thorn and Mabel Dillingham begin the Calhoun Colored School. After a year she left to start a school in what she said was "some out of the way place where no one else cared to go."[54]

Washington arrived in Mount Meigs, Alabama, in 1898 and rented a twelve-by-thirteen-foot cabin for two dollars a month. She began with four pupils. She enlisted the community to help her create and build the People's Village School. In the first year the enrollment increased to one hundred, and village members bought two acres and built an eighteen-by-thirty-six-foot schoolhouse. By 1900, a church and a three-story building had been built. By 1906, there were seven grades up and running. There was now an assembly hall, rooms for teaching industries to both boys and girls, a teachers' house, a dormitory, and a kitchen on twenty-seven acres of land. The teachers encouraged students to continue their education, and many graduates went on to schools and colleges such as Hampton Institute, Tuskegee Institute, Meharry Medical College, Talladega College, Payne College, Spelman College, and Wilberforce University.

Nevertheless, Washington struggled with the fatalism of many community members that reconciled them to a fate similar to their past.[55] She also dealt with several financial crises due to her minimal access as a black woman working in the South to northern white philanthropists. Despite these challenges, the school community created a community center, a working farm that fed the schoolchildren, a night school, a YMCA, a Sunday school, a society for the care of the elderly, and a burial society.

Most of the African American families in Mount Meigs were tenant farmers, placed perpetually in debt by white landowners and subject to sudden eviction. Through the creation of an African American farmers' union, farmers paid monthly union dues. This money was used to purchase plantations, which were then subdivided so that families could farm their own land, decrease and eliminate their indenture, and build homes. In a similar cooperative spirit, seventy-five men bought and shared in the operation of a cotton gin. Both of these endeavors helped to lift community members out of debt and raw poverty.

Lasch-Quinn describes how the women of Mount Meigs also worked cooperatively, selling the garments made in their sewing classes and the goods from the village farm. They organized a Mother's Conference and sent a delegate to the Tuskegee Women's Conference. The women visited others who lived on distant plantations, helping them to organize clubs. They also helped to care for motherless children on plantations.

The school operated on a cascading model, preparing young people to share their education with others by becoming teachers and to approach their communities with an eye to creating the common good. It struggled financially, without needed resources for improvements and continuous salaries. Washington's accompaniment of the people of Mount Meigs was steadfast over four decades, as she took on a number of roles including community visionary, teacher, farm manager, housekeeper, librarian, and principal. School settlements such as Washington's held out a vision of African Americans being able to remain in the South, not as tenant farmers living on white people's land but as educated landowners themselves, in charge of their own labor and committed to mutual aid. Her educational work was part of a network all over the South, a network in which educated black women generously passed their learning on to children and adult students in communities where white leaders were rarely interested in their education and liberation from peonage.

Victoria Earle Matthews and the White Rose Mission and Industrial Association

Victoria Earle Matthews was born into slavery in 1861 in Fort Valley, Georgia. Her mother escaped at the beginning of the Civil War when Matthews was a child. Her mother traveled back to the South to bring her children north to New York City. To help support her family, Matthews worked briefly as a domestic. She enthusiastically embraced her own self-education. She became a journalist and fiction writer, and helped to establish the "Inquiry Club" in 1882 for African Americans to address the postslavery conditions in which they lived. Her interests were wide, including philosophy and politics. In 1892, she helped to create the National Federation of African-American Women and the Woman's Loyal Union, a civil rights organization addressing racial discrimination and in particular supporting Ida B. Wells's anti-lynching crusade.

After the death of Matthews's young son in 1895, she took a special interest in child welfare and considered moving to the South to teach children.

New York minister Rev. Horace A. Miller asked her, "Why go South, the girls in this City and those coming in need help."[56] He assisted her in visiting the homes in the neighborhood surrounding his church. This helped her to hear his neighbors' concerns and to share her own emerging dream of being of some service to young girls and women. She traveled in the South to determine the needs of young African American girls and young women who were migrating north in ever-greater numbers. Historian Stephen Kramer recounts Matthews's discovery of "a particularly horrifying practice, which had apparently flourished since the Civil War: the recruiting of young southern black women, under false and misleading circumstances, to work in urban areas. She investigated the employment agencies that did the recruiting as well as the 'red-light' districts where many of the unfortunate young women ended up."[57]

A light-skinned African American, Matthews was able to "pass" as white, gaining knowledge about exploitative schemes for hijacking young women's dreams for reputable jobs in New York. Too often people who falsely promised the kinds of jobs the young women had hoped for lured and forced them into prostitution. Far from home, alone, penniless, and with no safe place to stay, they were easily exploited. There were several efforts in New York City attempting to address the needs of these young women, but they were too few given the growing number of migrants at the turn of the century. In light of this insufficiency, Matthews argued that African Americans needed to build an infrastructure of support for their own "daughters."

In 1897, she gave a talk entitled "The Awakening of the African-American Woman" at the Society for Christian Endeavor in San Francisco. She called on her audience to make marriage and divorce laws uniform throughout the United States in order to legalize the "union of mutual affection." She argued that the South's penal institutions needed reform so that men and women were separated in jails, and urged the creation of juvenile reformatories so that children would not be thrown together with hardened criminals. She asserted that women had been even more victimized by slavery than men. Slavery had destroyed "all that a woman holds sacred, all that enables womanhood." Furthermore, "There was no attribute of womanhood which had not been sullied—aye, which had not been despoiled in the crucible of slavery. Virtue, modesty, the joys of maternity, even hope of mortality."[58] In her short story "Aunt Lindy: A Story Founded on Real Life," Matthews reunites an older woman who had her children taken away from her by her slave master after the end of the Civil War. Lauded as a short story about reconciliation, it is equally, if not more, about the inexpressible impact on a mother living in a system that normalizes the stealing of her children from her.[59]

Like Addams, Matthews was extremely sensitive to both the plight of girls and women and also to their "female fortitude." She saw the home as "the most noble, the most sacred" place in the nation and began to envision a welcoming home that could begin to address some of the needs of her new neighbors. She wrote to African American educator and leader Booker T. Washington that she wanted to "secure a good-sized house" with the upper portion being used "as a temporary lodging house for women and girls coming from the South or other parts to New York in search of work." What she called "the mission" would protect them as they created relationships in the house and found work with "church-going families." Volunteers would teach classes in sewing, dressmaking, millinery, and cooking.[60]

Her vision was larger than reaching out to only girls and young women, however. In her mind's eye, she saw "a daily kindergarten and manual training for boys" with "lectures in regard to domestic service for young men and boys."[61] She anticipated having trade and professional courses such as typing, stenography, and bookkeeping as well as a reading room, library, and gymnasium. She went to the Hampton Negro Conference in 1898 and made an appeal for support to create a settlement house that could welcome young African American women migrating from the South:

> The youth of our race . . . will pay with their bright young lives . . . for our ignorance, [and] our sinful negligence in watching over and protecting our struggling working class. . . . Many of the dangers confronting our girls from the South in the great cities of the North are so perfectly planned, so overwhelming in their power to subjugate and destroy, that no woman's daughter is safe away from home. . . . Let women and girls become enlightened, let them begin to think, and stop placing themselves

voluntarily in the power of strangers. . . . Appeal should be made
at this conference . . . in behalf of . . . the long-suffering, cruelly
wronged, sadly unprotected daughters of the entire South.[62]

Her appeal was successful. She continued home visits in New York City to young African American women to learn about the issues they were suffering from: racial discrimination, long work hours, low pay, unemployment, need for medical treatment, poverty, inadequate housing, and the limited kinds of jobs for which they were considered. The mission statement for the White Rose Mission came into focus: "This association is incorporated to establish and maintain a Christian, Industrial, non-sectarian home for Afro-American and Negro working girls and women where they may be educated and trained in the principles of practiced self-help and right-living."[63] This was the first African American settlement in New York.

Once the mission opened its door, it gradually added outings for children and classes and clubs in sight-singing, art, health, woodcarving, racial history, literature, cooking, mandolin, waiter training, and housework. The library had not only books on cooking, laundry work, and domestic science but Matthews's own impressive collection of African American literature, abolition literature, and narratives of ex-slaves for the class on racial history. She strove to support racial pride and confidence in those who came to the White Rose Mission. By 1900, there were ten faithful volunteers helping her sustain the house, many of them working fulltime in addition to their devotion to the White Rose. Four to five hundred people were visiting a month for the classes and club activities.

She and other volunteers met boats coming into New York to try to intercept African American young women before they were lied to by men falsely promising them jobs and safe lodging. Seeing how vulnerable the young women were on first arrival and how disastrous their fate often was if there was no one to meet them and guide them to respectable places to live, she founded a traveler's aid society directed to the needs of African Americans coming to Baltimore, Norfolk, and New York City. In fact, the work of the White Rose Mission predated the founding of the Traveler's Aid Society in 1905.

Box 2.1 Girls Educational and Mentoring Services (GEMS) New York City

If Victoria Earle Matthews was alive today, I predict she would enjoy knowing Rachel Lloyd.[a] Lloyd, herself a survivor of commercial sexual exploitation, founded GEMS in 1998 at her kitchen table with thirty dollars. Today, GEMS is the largest organization in the United States dedicated to helping girls and young women (12–24) who have experienced or are at risk for sexual exploitation and trafficking. It not only provides intensive support to over 350 girls and young women but also offers preventive outreach and education to 1,500 youth and training for more than 1,300 professionals each year.

From listening closely to girls and women in correctional institutions and on the streets, Lloyd developed a holistic sense of how to accompany young girls caught in the cycle of sexual exploitation. She and her colleagues have created an approach that honors the voices of the girls and young women they work with. They seek to encourage survivor leadership. GEMS accompanies young girls and women who want to exit sex trafficking and redirect their lives. It is "committed to ending commercial sexual exploitation and domestic trafficking of children by changing individual lives, transforming public perception, and revolutionizing the systems and policies that impact commercially sexually exploited youth."[b]

GEMS begins with a conviction "that all young women have great beauty and worth, and the potential for future success," that each "is deserving, and needs support and services to treat the trauma and violence she has experienced." At the core of their program's philosophy is a commitment to help empower "survivors to express their experiences, observations, and desires for a better life and world." From listening closely to the girls' needs and interests, GEMS develops its programming, offering "viable opportunities for positive change."[c] These include supportive and transitional housing, transitional independent living, educational opportunities, leadership development, court advocacy, alternatives to incarceration, and short-term and crisis care.

GEMS embodies psychosocial accompaniment as a cornerstone of its practice. First, its members are committed to engaging in empathic and supportive relationships with the young women. These relationships counter the enormous stigma the girls experience from service providers, law enforcement, the courts, their families, and society. Second, the group's understanding extends to the wider contexts of racism, poverty, gender-based

Box 2.1 (continued)

violence, and the criminalization of youth that are generative of sexual exploitation. Third, Lloyd and her colleagues are advocates and have introduced laws with significant implications for these young women. In 2008,
Lloyd ensured the passage of New York State's Safe Harbor for Sexually
Exploited Children Act, the first law in the United States to protect traf-
ficked youth. Thirteen other states have followed suit.[d]

---

a. *Girls Like Us: Fighting for a World Where Girls Are Not for Sale* (New York: Harper, 2012).
b. http://www.gems-girls.org/.
c. Ibid.
d. A documentary film on GEMS's work, *Very Young Girls,* directed by David Schigall and
   Nina Alvarez (2007), exposes the commercial sexual exploitation of vulnerable girls in
   New York. Treated as adult criminals by the police and neglected by ordinary social
   service agencies, the girls are exploited by pimps who sell them on the streets.

In addition to offering a safe, temporary home and helping to find
employment for newly arrived girls and women, the mission developed a
home for working girls on the top floor. For one dollar a year other working
girls and women could become members and use the parlor to receive visitors and entertain, as most did not have space in the crowded accommodations where they lived.

Matthews was an effective spokesperson for the needs of new African
Americans migrating to the North, and the White Rose Mission is credited
with inspiring others' efforts to meet these needs. Nurseries to provide daycare for mothers, kindergartens, and clubs for girls were developed, including those at the Brooklyn YMCA, which Kramer describes as in many ways
another social settlement for African Americans. Matthews died in 1905,
but her work was carried on by Frances Kellor, who organized the Association for the Protection of Negro Women, an organization that attempted to
coordinate the multiple groups in the Northeast that had developed to help
protect African American women from exploitation. Later she helped to
create the National League for the Protection of Colored Women, a national
organization with the same aims. Her work helped to educate the members
of the National Urban League regarding the struggles of African American
women. The White Rose Mission closed in 1984.

Box 2.2   A New Way of Life and All of Us or None
South Los Angeles, CA

Victoria Earle Matthews would greet young African American women at the New York dock when their ships arrived from the South. She was aware of the potential dangers that faced them and offered them safe lodgings until they could establish themselves in employment and housing.

Likewise, Susan Burton greets women as they disembark from buses next to Skid Row in Los Angeles on completion of their prison terms.[a] Each woman's remaining possessions are returned to her by the prison in a cardboard box, and she is given two hundred dollars—from which her bus ticket is paid—before being loaded on to a bus to her destination. Too often there is no one to meet her at the other end. The women are prey to pimps and drug dealers who survey those disembarking, sizing up their fear and desperation. Without a place to turn, the women are abandoned to the streets.

Burton knows the perils of this terrifying transition from prison, not only from the hundreds of women she has accompanied through it but from her own six experiences of attempting reentry from prison. She knows firsthand what it is like to try to succeed with most odds stacked against one: no access to public housing or food stamps, employment discrimination against those with felonies on their record, no or inadequate access to drug and alcohol treatment, and often with no one left to believe that your success is possible.

After a policeman accidentally ran over and killed her five-year-old son, she was consumed by grief. Lacking access to counseling and psychiatric medications, Burton turned to illegal drugs for self-medication and found herself embroiled in a lifestyle that could support their procurement and which led to repeated rounds of incarceration.

After finally accessing drug treatment, counseling, and safe housing herself, Burton became determined to create a network of safe recovery houses for women, likened by prison abolitionist Michelle Alexander to the underground railway. A New Way of Life was born. Here the women both find accompaniment and offer it to one another. With the necessary foundations of available food, safe shelter, and support, they are helped to access counseling and drug and alcohol treatment if needed, twelve-step groups, legal help to expunge their records if possible, assistance with meeting the conditions of parole or probation, employment preparation, educational and career counseling, assistance with reentry education, and help to reconnect with their children and embark on the difficult road to healing

Box 2.2 (continued)

emotional wounds within their families and regaining child custody. This impressive "wrap around" support costs $16,000 a year, in contrast to the $60,000 that a year of incarceration costs tax payers. The recidivism rate for the women in A New Way of Life is 4 percent compared to over 50 percent without these kinds of supports and assistance. Burton shares, "It was my goal to live with unwavering empathy for the women at A New Way of Life. I began to view this as my talent: I could connect with people and feel something. I could see the hope and possibilities in everyone. My job was to value each and every woman, to cast aside my doubt and believe in them—and to teach them to cast aside their own doubt and to hold themselves and others to a standard of accountability, integrity, and respect."[b] Burton is also pivotal in helping the women understand systemically why the deck of opportunity has been stacked against them, lifting some of the weight of feelings of personal failure and inadequacy off their shoulders.

Like Jane Addams, Burton has created a pathway from the accompaniment of individuals to legal and policy efforts to restore basic civil and human rights to formerly incarcerated individuals. Along with others, she has founded All of Us or None.[c] This grassroots organization in solidarity with others has mounted campaigns to "Ban the Box," so that those with felonies do not need to announce this up front on job applications; to restore voting rights to both incarcerated and formerly incarcerated individuals; to have the government extend Pell Grants to prisoners and those formerly imprisoned; and to remove the ban on public housing and the receipt of food stamps to those formerly incarcerated. A central tenet of both All of Us or None and A New Way of Life is the development of leadership capacities by those formerly incarcerated: "Nothing about us without us." "We believe," says Burton, "that the people most directly affected by a problem will have the best solutions, because they lived it."[d]

Burton is a leader in building a human rights movement to restore civil and human rights stripped from the formerly incarcerated. This form of psychosocial accompaniment—that spans from the accompaniment of individuals to the sustained fueling of a human rights movement—has required Burton to not only articulate the challenges facing those formerly incarcerated but to learn the historical context and social and political structures that created these barriers: U.S. racism, the "War on Drugs," discriminatory policies of the Anti-Drug Abuse Act, California's three-strikes law, the power and lucrative growth of the prison-industrial complex, and the school to prison pipeline.[e] She also needed to be able to imagine the situation otherwise, to learn the political system and how to create and institute policy change, to form an organization, to join one's own organization in a network with others, to build community support and leadership from within. Through these steps, the accompaniment of some becomes indissolubly linked to advocacy for many.

---

a. Susan Burton and Cari Lynn, *Becoming Ms. Burton: From Prison to Recovery to Leading the Fight for Incarcerated Women* (New York: New Press, 2017).

b. Ibid., 149.

c. http://www.anewwayoflife.org/all-of-us-or-none/.

d. Burton and Lynn, *Becoming,* 251.

e. Michelle Alexander, *The New Jim Crow: Mass Incarceration in the Age of Color-Blindness* (New York: New Press, 2012).

The Erosion of Mutual Accompaniment in a Capitalist Service Economy

The nature of settlement houses changed as fewer people chose to become residents in them or even to live in the poorer neighborhoods where they were situated. As funding was withdrawn, community centers were more likely to maintain only one or two of the programs they had developed, fragmenting "services" between different agencies and personnel. As the language of charity was increasingly criticized, the language of "service" arose. But was this reframing basically window dressing? Settlement houses increasingly presented themselves as "providing services" to those who needed them, reestablishing an imbalance between the needful recipient and the professional worker. Education theorists Keith Morton and John Saltmarsh trace the emergence of "service" language, its roots, and its ongoing legacy. They argue that as the industrialized society gave way to the postindustrial service economy, the affluent came to be seen as consumers of services, "enjoying" services. Those lacking in excess economic and social privilege were defined as "needing" services and were "provided" services by the government and the nonprofit sector.[64]

Unfortunately, the paradigm of radical individualism, divorcing individuals from their social and historical contexts, underlay both the language of charity and the discourse of service. Those seen as requiring charity or services were deemed once again to be wanting: morally inferior, indulgent, lazy, unintelligent, possibly intemperate, or drug dependent. These stereo-types constituted the very undemocratic class assumptions Addams had worked so hard to criticize and dispel. They also played into creating rela-tionships that were unbalanced in terms of perceived needfulness and power. Whereas Addams had always argued that she and other settlement house workers needed their relationships with neighbors as much as some neighbors did with them, professionalized workers generally saw them-selves as exclusively "helping" others. Increasingly, those "in need of ser-vices" were also subjected to the burgeoning clinical discourse of psychopathology, and to the hierarchical and disempowering relationships that become possible when we see people through the prism of pathology. While serving to demean the "recipients" of services, the provision of these services was used as moral aggrandizement for their service providers and those who funded their efforts. Addams pointedly remarked that those who distribute charity have a "cruel advantage" that they do not realize.[65]

The model of voluntary residents partnering with neighbors in settle-ment house neighborhoods yielded to a growing professionalization of paid staff and, in particular, a burgeoning of social work staff who were largely uninvolved in addressing structural injustice to transform society to be less plagued by the excesses of capitalism and its destructive erosion of social democracy. Many social workers now worked for the government "instead of becoming its leaders and voices of reason and dissent."[66] As settlement houses began to fade, the dynamic and intertwined mix of activities and advocacies that had lived in dynamic relationship with one another were broken apart into separate services and agencies, most rarely involved with the emphasis on social critique and reform that had marked the efforts of many early settlement houses.

The emergence of the welfare state in the 1930s and 1940s encouraged a stigmatizing of those caught in poverty and a decisive move away from some attempts during the Progressive era to examine and address the struc-tural roots of inequality. Through a depoliticizing of language, manufac-tured class divisions were increasingly seen as poor people's personal failures to satisfy their needs in the marketplace.[67] Morton and Saltmarsh put it succinctly: "Service in the public sector, welfare dependency realm has the seemingly contradictory meaning of reducing social divisions in order to maintain widening inequalities of wealth and income. These are the subtle problems of service in the present. . . . The flourishing of the nonprofit sector makes amends for the invidious carelessness of capitalism." In their historical tracking of the emergence of the concept of "community service" in American culture, Morton and Saltmarsh extend Addams's critique of charity into the present-day world of the nonprofit sector. They argue that community service "is a modern concept emerging out of the collision of capitalism and democracy at the turn of the [twentieth] century."[68]

Psychotherapist David B. Schwartz examines a shadow of the cultural shift to institutionalized care and human "services" in the United States. Unfortunately, the "radical monopoly of institutional care ha[s] eliminated fragile informal capacities to include people that existed prior to these artificial creations." Informal relationships of care in times of need, he argues, are being continually displaced. Following the critique of Ivan Illich, Schwartz sees the vernacular world of homegrown relationships that provide mutual aid displaced by systems from above: "Small scale, personal efforts to help people become human services corporations." Citizens are relieved of responding to the miseries around them; these problems become—literally—the business of others. The result is a lived sense of alienation, of disconnection, of the short-circuiting of the movement within us from basic sympathetic and empathic feelings to responsive action. This vernacular everyday responsiveness is colonized and commodified, sequestered in professional relations. And while we are all aware of the insufficiency of such formalized responsiveness, we also try to believe we are off the hook. Our integrity suffers as a result. When we look at each other individualistically, disregarding our interdependence with one another, we manufacture the lonely disconnected states we suffer from. To the extent that others are supposed to respond and not we ourselves, we find ourselves outside the web of potential human relationships that exist all around us. Addams stressed that one of the gifts of living in the settlement house was the feeling and the reality of being in a community, of being a part of it, woven into the social tissue. Schwartz reflects that this social tissue, what he calls mediating structures, "are being dissolved as if by a potent social solvent." Moreover, he observes, "There is, it is clear, a spirit about relationships of one person to another that has been lost in the displacement of the associational organs of society by a machinery of caring systems. This spirit might be called by the old name hospitality."[69]

As mediating structures are eroded and eliminated, people lose the kinds of human relationships that give them a sense of belonging. Meanwhile, the state expands its functions of service delivery. Sociologist Robert A. Nisbet linked this erosion of associations with a strengthening of dependence on the state, a condition that makes totalitarianism more possible.[70] He traced this pattern in the French Revolution, in Stalinist Russia, and in Hitler's Germany, where associational entities were outlawed.

Schwartz contrasts Jewish *shtetl* communities in Eastern Europe with the rise of *xenodocheia* in the fourth century. In the shtetl, strangers who came to religious services were invited home by a family by the end of the evening. Xenodocheia were separate dwellings created under the auspices of the Christian church at the time of Emperor Constantine. Church bishops noted that the hospitality of households had dwindled, creating a need for hostels or hospitals. These were established to offer hospitality in the name of the community. The stranger was no longer in the home of a community member; care was transferred to the church. The creation of xenodocheia spread quickly. Some critics, like Saint Chrysostom, urged the faithful to retrieve hospitality for their own homes, readying a bed of straw, food, and candles for the stranger.[71] During the Middle Ages, xenodocheia assumed care not only for pilgrims and strangers but for the poor and the sick. In the next chapter, we find these places of hospitality an inspiration to Dorothy Day and Peter Maurin as they created lay houses of hospitality and worked to embed radical hospitality once again back into the household.

Schwartz and Ivan Illich are leery of the displacement of hospitality from our homes and hearts into formalized systems of care in places separated from us, like asylums and the various facilities that oversee the care of the elderly, infirm, and those with disabilities. Schwartz urges public administrators, practitioners, and advocacy groups to recognize how their "efforts at reform . . . can unwittingly sterilize the soil of human culture." Illich pointed out that the Greek root in "humanity" and "humaneness" is the same as that in "hospitality," so inextricable is hospitality from being human, one with another.[72] Schwartz calls on us to retrieve "the remnants of ancient traditions of hospitality [that] can often be found in the fragmented life beneath our feet."[73] Since we are social beings, we can attune ourselves to supporting one another, both within the institutions we have built and in the informal life we are part of and that happens all around us. This retrieval of hospitality between us is at the same time a retrieval of our integrity, a healing of our splintered condition. Practices of accompaniment are at the heart of this retrieval.

Radical Hospitality and the Heart of Accompaniment

The greatest challenge of the day is: how to bring about a revolution of the heart, a revolution which has to start with each one of us? When we begin to take the lowest place, to wash the feet of others, to love our brothers with that burning love, that passion, which led to the cross, then we can truly say, "Now I have begun."

—Dorothy Day, *Loaves and Fishes*

"The Duty of Delight"

"Houses of hospitality" are places where those in need of human support, housing, medical care, food, or other assistance find refuge and support. They are places outside the radius of where ordinary citizens spend time and devote their monies and energies. When they exist, houses of hospitality are often located on the edges of cities and neighborhoods and are generally underfunded. Neighbors often unite to challenge the presence of such houses. They fear the inhabitants—the poor, migrants, the mentally ill, the formerly incarcerated, those with disabilities, the developmentally challenged—and argue that their proximity causes property values to decline.

In spite of this inhospitality, houses of hospitality do exist. They not only fill needs for their inhabitants but inspire others to co-create their own houses, forming a long, even if insufficient, chain of open doors in the face of adversity. Dorothy Day and the Catholic Worker Movement, cofounded with Catholic social activist Peter Maurin, is one example of the generativity of radical hospitality.

Lay theologian Jim Forest shares the unfolding of Day's relationship with Maurin. As the devastating impacts of the Great Depression destroyed people's lives in the United States, a thirty-four-year-old journalist from New York, Dorothy Day, went to Washington, D.C., to cover the 1932 Hunger March. While there, she went to the crypt beneath the National Shrine of the Immaculate Conception. Recalling this visit, Day shared, "There I offered up a special prayer, a prayer which came with tears and anguish, that some way would open up for me to use what talents I possessed for my fellow workers, for the poor."[1]

Upon her return to her New York City apartment, she found a fifty-five-year-old French stranger awaiting her: Peter Maurin. He had been referred to Day by the editor of *Commonweal,* a Catholic magazine. In one pocket he carried a text by Saint Francis and in the other a book by Peter Kropotkin, anarchist and author of *Mutual Aid* and *Fields, Factories, and Workshops.* Maurin arrived at Day's door with a unique life history that would find its fulfillment alongside her. Before participating in what was known as the Sillon movement, he lived among the poor and worked with orphans and abandoned children in Paris. Le Sillon (The Furrow) was founded in the 1890s by Marc Sangnier to bring the Catholic church into greater alignment with social needs and values. It created hospices for the homeless and poor and rest homes for the elderly, "eating places, where the poor and their advocates from other segments of the population could come together."[2] After arriving in Canada and then traveling to the United States, Maurin "dug irrigation ditches, quarried stone, harvested wheat, cut lumber, laid railway track, labored in brick yards, steel mills, and coal mines. He had been jailed for vagrancy and for 'riding the rails'—traveling unticketed on freight cars."[3]

Dorothy Day had experienced a spiritual conversion and in its wake became a Catholic. The Frenchman too had experienced a religious awakening that led him back to the Catholic church where he developed a life of voluntary poverty, a life committed to downward mobility and freedom from the constraints of property and wealth. After meeting Day, he proposed to her a three-point program: "founding a newspaper and establishing roundtable discussions for the clarification of thought, promoting houses of hospitality for those in need of food and shelter, and organizing farming communities so that both workers and scholars could return to the land." Maurin wanted to help create a decentralized society "of cooperation rather than coercion, with artisans and craftsmen, with small factories that were worker-owned and worker-run."[4] He understood such communal farms as an alternative to industrial capitalism. He imagined a worker-scholar synthesis where they could work and think together. Later, Day said that she did not think the second two agenda items had anything to do with her. History proved her wrong. Given her journalism background, it was natural for her to be eager to begin a newspaper and so the *Catholic Worker* was born in her kitchen and taken to the streets of Depression-ridden New York City. It enjoyed a success that neither Day nor Maurin had imagined and began to bring in income that could be used for Maurin's other two dreams: houses of hospitality and worker-scholar farming communities.

Maurin was inspired by Saint Basil, who created a "city" near Cappadocia, Turkey, in the fourth century. This xenodocheia included a lodging for the poor, a hospital, and a hospice. Inspired by a second saint, Jerome, who translated the Bible from Hebrew into Latin, Maurin borrowed the idea of creating homes where "Christ" could find hospitality, or *xenia*. The Holy Rule of Saint Benedict prescribed to monasteries that each must have a room for the stranger in need, an embodiment of Christ. Maurin took the further step of urging all Catholics to have a "Christ room," a room in their house for the stranger in need. He sought to retrieve hospitality from the institution of the church, reembedding it in the household. This retrieval also entailed a recognition of the equality of the stranger and the host. A fifth-century Carthaginian Church Council urged "each bishop to have a hospice (or house of hospitality) in connection with every parish— places of welcome and care ready to receive the poor, the sick, the orphaned, the old, the traveler and pilgrim, the needy of every kind."[5] Hospices in the early Christian world were places "where the needy were offered rest, food, clothing, a place to pray and collect oneself."[6] Maurin also drew inspiration from seventh-century Irish religious communities that blended spirituality, scholarship, and manual labor, and from the Danish folk schools of the 1800s. He dreamed of co-creating rural communities where balance was rediscovered between "cult, culture, and cultivation" or "prayer, study, and agriculture."[7] While seeking to incarnate the principles of Jesus into his life, Maurin's mission was to nurse these visionary ideas and bring this tradition alive in the contemporary world. Whereas the church had assumed a role in the provision of hospitality, Maurin urged lay people to open their own doors to the stranger.

Day had read a biography of Rose Hawthorne Lathrop, Nathaniel Hawthorne's daughter. After Lathrop's conversion to Catholicism at the age of forty, she rented a tenement flat on the Lower East Side in New York City where she welcomed the terminally ill who were poor. This led to her helping to found the Dominican Sisters of Hawthorne, whose primary mission was to provide palliative care for those with terminal cancer. This story, Forest says, inspired Day to begin to dream a house of hospitality into existence, and she wrote about this possibility in the *Catholic Worker* newspaper.[8]

In 1933, a woman came to Dorothy Day's door to ask about her house of hospitality. Day admitted that while she had written about this idea in the *Catholic Worker*, she had yet to establish such a house. The woman confided that she and her friend had been living in the subway. Earlier in the day, her friend had become so despondent that she had thrown herself beneath a subway train and died. Day responded with action. "That very afternoon," she said, "we rented our first apartment and named it the Teresa-Joseph Cooperative—Teresa for Teresa of Avila, Joseph after the foster father of Jesus. We moved in some beds and sheltered this unemployed woman."[9] Other people in need followed, and Day began to open additional residences to accommodate and welcome them.

While established to respond to the homeless and destitute, neighbors, students, and others came to offer assistance. In doing so, they discovered their need to be of service, to answer the calls of voluntary simplicity and poverty, to experience community and a sense of belonging, and to live in a place where the spiritual principles of living among those marginalized in society could be embodied. Some came and went quickly; others moved in and stayed for decades. Day confided that it was impossible to know when a person first appeared whether or not the Catholic Worker House would become their permanent home. Day was clear that any of us "can do this work wherever" we are.[10]

Some argue that the provision of shelter, food, clothing, medical care, and companionship for the poor and marginalized is charity and as such fails to challenge the social systems that replicate the structural conditions responsible for generating poverty. However, this critique does not adequately acknowledge the radical social position of standing for and with the poor and marginalized in societies that routinely imprison the mentally ill, criminalize the poor, and cast out the migrant.

Dorothy Day encountered similar criticisms. In 1935, Tom Coddington, associate editor of the *Catholic Worker*, reproached Day for being overly concerned with works of mercy, which, he maintained, left little time for the struggle against systems of injustice. Day argued that the needs of the people must come first. She emphasized that works of mercy—what is done for the most vulnerable in society—are opposite to those of war.[11] In the small acts of the everyday, one could mount a resistance to violence and indifference. She believed in immersing herself "in the local scene." She noted, "If I had to be very brief about what localism means, I would say it means a neighborliness that is both political and spiritual in nature. . . . When my friends want to figure out what we mean by community, I say that community is all of us together, trying to be of help to each other."[12]

Day rejected the charity of the church and instead argued for justice and changing the social order that made charity necessary. In speaking of her twenties, Day remembered, "Our hearts burned with the desire for justice and were revolted at the idea of doled out charity. The word charity had become something to gag over, something to shudder at."[13] She weighed in for efforts that honored people's dignity and worth and what was due to them in the name of justice. Day clearly saw the results of structural inequalities, and as she traveled to speak, she embodied a precious conjunction of existential and psychosocial accompaniment, wedding the works of mercy with incisive societal critique and radical experimentation to create a "cooperative order as opposed to the corporate state."[14] She devoted herself to the causes of farmworkers, nonviolent civil rights activism, and draft resistance during the Vietnam War, all the while helping to sustain the day-today activities of the Catholic Worker Houses that had by that time spread across the United States.

Day believed that it was "in the setting of daily life that we find our true arena for holiness," and that the "test of a life is its everyday moral texture—what one does, finally, with all the hours of the day." She offered that words are not the only acceptable form of prayer: "I believe some people—lots of people—pray through the witness of their lives, through the work they do, the friendships they have, the love they offer people and receive from people."[15]

In his biography of Day, Forest shares that her time in jail for nonviolently protesting with Cesar Chavez and farmworkers provoked her reflection on the desperate need for society to respond differently to those convicted of crimes. Instead of damaging inmates through a wholly punitive system, Day thought,

> Would not much more be accomplished in small, homelike settings in which prisoners were recognized as persons of value and promise? In prison, staff was mainly hired to guard inmates, "not to love them." She envisioned rural centers at which the inmates raised much of their own food, baked their own bread, milked cows, tended chickens, engaged in creative activity and shared responsibility for the institution so that it wasn't a static environment but was, "in its own way, a community." Prison as it exists, she found, was the opposite of community.[16]

Day never regarded herself as above anyone else. In a Catholic Worker House, Day saw herself as one among others. Speaking of the Catholic Worker community, she said, "We are relatives—kinfolk, some would say: those who receive, give; and those who give, receive." Day explained, "The houses of hospitality that we have going now are meant to be of help to some people—we who live in them, and others who come to visit us, and eat with us, and pray with us."[17] Child psychiatrist Robert Coles, a close friend and admirer of Day, described Day and the Catholic workers as "antidotes to indifference."[18] The "Catholic Worker houses of hospitality are meant to be communities in which the so-called helpers merge with those who, in the conventional sense, would be regarded as needing help. During stays in these houses I have felt that the aim is for the workers and the guests to be indistinguishable." In a telling anecdote, Day recounted a day when she was not feeling well. A resident noticed her bad mood, and Day had a realization that "he had noticed all of us—our ups and downs. I thought to myself, He is the one who is trying to be of help to others, and we are the ones who need that help."[19]

She was also aware of the mutual transfiguration between "helpers" and "helped" when she considered the many students who volunteered: "The students know so much, and yet they are learning. The poor who come here feel there is little they have to offer anyone, and yet they have a lot to offer. The giving and the receiving is not only going on in one direction."[20] As she struggled with her own impatience, anger, judgments, and irritation in the course of living with others, she said, "then some such thought as St. John of the Cross would come, 'where there is no love, put love, and you will find love' and makes all right. When it comes down to it, even on the natural plane, it is much happier and more enlivening to love than to be loved."[21]

A close reading of Day's writings about houses of hospitality suggests a phenomenology both of some of the essential ingredients of accompaniment and of the transfiguration of the accompaniers that can occur in the process of accompaniment. Accompaniers are able to pause from the habitual and normative absorption that takes place in mainstream life, where concerns for security and comfort prevail. By participating in the accompaniment of hospitality houses, accompaniers make themselves available and attend to the little things that create connection and support others. They are welcoming and attentive to radical inclusivity. They share the gifts of being able to attune to others and embody what Day called, borrowing from John Ruskin, "the duty of delight."[22] This "duty" leads one to the joy of finding, alongside misery, that people experience those small epiphanies of beauty and vibrant life that sustain us all. Accompaniers stand beside others, sundering and surrendering the hierarchy of conventional, professionalized helping relations. In all interactions, they seek to affirm the dignity of others. Their capacity for self-reflection and for searching for ways to live that manifest integrity aid them in their rupture from the normative.

Day was involved in a fierce moral inquiry about what she should be doing with her life.[23] During the process of accompaniment, accompanists often recognize the incompleteness of their own lives and are thus able to experience the multiple ways in which accompanying gifts them with a sense of purpose and belonging. They become bridges between the isolated islands to which mainstream society exiles many of its members.

Toward the end of her life, while compiling her diary entries, Day decided to borrow Ruskin's words and call the volume *The Duty of Delight*. She wrote reflectively, "I was thinking, how as one gets older, we are tempted to sadness, knowing life as it is here on earth, the suffering, the Cross. And how we must overcome it daily, growing in love, and the joy which goes with loving."[24]

"To Walk in the Balance of Joy and Suffering": L'Arche Communities

The accompanier is there to give support, to reassure, to confirm, and to open new doors. The accompanier is not there to judge us or to tell us what to do, but to reveal what is most beautiful and valuable in us, as well as to point towards the meaning of our inner pain. In this way, an accompanier helps us advance to greater freedom by helping us to be reconciled with our past and to accept ourselves as we are, with our gifts and our limits.

—Jean Vanier[25]

A Canadian teacher of moral philosophy, Jean Vanier discovered the joy in loving that Dorothy Day described. While he appreciated the teaching profession, Vanier felt there was another purpose for his life that he must discover. When he was thirty-five years old, during the Christmas of 1963, he visited a Dominican priest, Rev. Thomas Philippe, to whom his mother had introduced him. Philippe was the chaplain at Val Fleury, an institution in France that housed thirty-two men with intellectual disabilities. He invited Vanier to visit him there. During his stay, Vanier was struck by the men's "childlikeness" and their frank desire for love and friendship. That day he felt called to respond to their desire, to offer them friendship and hospitality—in his own words, "to climb down the ladder."[26] Over the next months, he visited a number of such institutions in an attempt to learn as much as he could.

He was overwhelmed and distressed by what he saw. There was one experience in a south Parisian asylum that touched him particularly. The institution was surrounded by huge cement block walls. Within the walls, cut off from the surrounding community, eighty men lived in dormitories. They passed the entire day walking around in circles only broken by a compulsory siesta from 2–4 p.m. Vanier shared, "There I was struck by the screams and atmosphere of sadness, but also by the mysterious presence of God. In that asylum I met Philippe Seux and Raphael Simi for the first time. Both had been placed there following the deaths of their parents."[27]

Vanier was moved to ask the two men if they would like to live with him in Trosly, France. At the time he had no house, but once the men agreed, he was able to raise money to buy a small place in need of many repairs. Vanier wanted to create a community, a sense of family that he and his two new friends could enjoy. He described feeling "open and available":

> Simplicity and poverty characterized *L'Arche* beginnings. The house was poor and had no toilets (we set up a pail in the garden!). There was one tap and one wood-burning stove. . . . Raphael and Philippe helped as well as they could with the different tasks in the house and garden. We began to get to know each other and do things together. We were learning how to live together, care for one another, listen to one another, have fun and pray together.[28]

Like social medicine innovator Paul Farmer, Vanier returns to the Latin meaning of accompaniment, *cum pane,* eating bread together, which, Vanier says, signifies a bond of friendship, a covenant. This Latin root reflects the sharing of the rhythm of life with one another and of the fundamental need and enjoyment of nourishment. The ancient term also points to a deeper mystery and gift: our capacity to "becom[e] bread for others" and to experience the bread that their presence in our lives offers us.[29]

As in the case of Dorothy Day, Vanier's radical hospitality acted as a magnet to the hearts and minds of others. One house became two, two then three. Forty years later, there are 149 L'Arche communities in 39 countries around the world. For Vanier, hospitality entails a welcome not only into one's physical space but within the space of one's heart, a "space for that person to be and to grow; space where the person knows that he or she is accepted just as they are, with their wounds and their gifts."[30] He is keenly aware of how many people with intellectual challenges experience massive rejection and abandonment that darkens their daily lives.

Accompaniers, he has warned, have to be patient for each person to begin to develop trust in another, since that trust has been betrayed and disappointed so many times. Vanier confesses that when he first encouraged others to begin L'Arche communities, he did not understand the degree of accompaniment they and their assistants would need. He understands that such accompaniment of the accompaniers allows each one to have a companion who can support them to "grow in freedom and in the spirit of the community."[31] There are not the accompanying and the accompanied but a web of accompaniment that supports each member, weaving together the whole fabric of the community. This is often not an offering back in return for what has been received but a form of presence particular to the person and the shared situation. The sharing of accompaniment functions in a more diffuse and indirect way, as others outside the immediate situation provide support to those within it who bear a heavy of load of responsibility, practically and emotionally.

Vanier identifies different kinds of accompaniment: spiritual accompaniment, work accompaniment, and community accompaniment: "The essential aspects of these three forms of accompaniment are listening, caring, clarifying, affirming, and challenging. Assistants need to feel that they are listened to, that someone cares for them and clarifies with them work expectations, community expectations, and expectations in their spiritual life; and finally, they need to be challenged and affirmed in their growth and struggle to make choices and efforts. All this rests on a basis of trust."[32]

Community accompaniment is undertaken by someone who is not in the accompanist's work hierarchy. This person can provide support to understand the spirit and traditions of the community, and to provide a space where the assistant can confide his or her struggles and be met with compassion, understanding, and wisdom, rather than judgment.

Vanier appreciates the effect of such communities on the wider context in which they are embedded and function. He notes, "As a community takes root in a neighbourhood and begins to grow, and as its neighbors become involved in it, it will inevitably become aware of social injustices which oppress people and prevent their growth. . . . And so the community might have to take a political stand. It will seek to help people and to modify laws and struggle against injustice."[33]

Vanier puts his faith into creating communities, believing that people who do so can "become the yeast in the dough of society":

> They would not change political structures at first. But they would change the hearts and spirits of the people around them, by offering them a glimpse of a new dimension in human life—that of inwardness, love, contemplation, wonderment and sharing. They would introduce people to a place where the weak and poor, far from being pushed aside, are central to their society. My personal hope is that, if this spirit of community really spreads, structures will change. Structures are—tyrannies excepted—the mirrors of hearts.[34]

Vanier links liberation and accompaniment through his prefigurative living and vision. In other words, we do not liberate ourselves; we become liberated with others. This is the mystery hidden within the heart of accompaniment: the deep realization of our interconnection with others.

My friend and palliative care physician Michael Kearney, who lived as an assistant for a while in one of the communities, shared with me that in the rest of his life, he has never laughed and cried as much as he did at L'Arche.

Box 3.1 Sristi Village
Thazhuthali, Tamil Nadu, India

The founder of Sristi Foundation and Village, psychologist Sristi G. Karthikeyan, grew up in an Indian orphanage that included both children with and without intellectual disabilities. Karthik, as he is known, was saddened to see his friends with disabilities blocked from educational and vocational opportunities. After returning to direct the orphanage in which he grew up for nine years, Karthik dedicated himself to helping adults with intellectual and physical disabilities.

He shares, "'Sristi,' the ancient word derived from the classical language Sanskrit, means 'CREATION.' We want to create a new world for those who are marginalized, especially people with intellectual disabilities; a world that they can call their own, a world where everyone is treated with respect. The main objective of the organization is to establish 'Sristi Village,' a self-sustaining, inclusive and eco-friendly village, which provides a family atmosphere where everyone can reach their full potential regardless of disability, race, gender, etc. Further, people with intellectual disabilities and the marginalized will be equally active contributors."[a]

When I spoke with Karthik, he was unaware of the L'Arche communities, though he seemed to share an angel of inspiration with Jean Vanier: both living to create a home where those with intellectual disabilities could live alongside those without them in equality and dignity. Like Vanier, he was upset by the stigma besetting those with intellectual disabilities, their too frequent abandonment by their families, and their lack of a sense of belonging and worth. He envisioned a farming community based on permaculture principles where those with disabilities and those without them could live together sustainably, while learning farming and other vocational skills that could increase their employability and sense of independence. They began with 8.3 acres, constructing a Kerala-inspired tribal hut where community members live and an organic garden.

As Karthikeyan listened to the region's needs for its members with intellectual disabilities, he responded by creating a small school for children with intellectual and developmental disabilities and a vocational training center for adults. The foundation answers parents' needs by hosting workshops on legal issues for persons with intellectual disabilities, emphasizing a rights-based approach. More recently, the foundation has created the Sristi Farm Academy to help members learn skills for employment and sustainable, self-reliant, and independent living.

Box 3.1 (continued)

    Our paucity of dignified, equitable, and inclusive communities, he believes, create disability out of difference. We must design equitable and dignified communities that are mindful of different forms of physical and intellectual embodiment. We need to design for difference and inclusion.[b]

    Karthikeyan has worked inside and outside of India to create a network of donors, volunteers, and consultants, enlarging the "family" at Sristi Village and educating civil society about its brothers and sisters with intellectual disabilities and their need for accompaniment.

---

a. http://www.sristivillage.org/wp-content/uploads/2015/04/Sristi-Village-1-newsletter.pdf; http://www.sristivillage.org/; https://www.facebook.com/pg/sristifoundation/about/.

b. I am grateful to Samantha Lynne Wilson for introducing me to Karthikeyan and for sharing with me about his philosophy of creating dignified, inclusive, and equitable communities.

Weaving Communities of Hospitality Through Asking

As previously noted, psychologist David Schwartz has analyzed the deterioration of informal hospitality as the government in the United States took on functions of welfare and responded with systems of professionalized care. Inevitably, these systems fall far short of providing those who need care and a sense of belonging to the larger community. His work has been devoted to those with various disabilities, and as he became attuned to their individual needs, he realized that many of them would be best addressed by connection to a caring and responsive person in the community. The situation only required one thing: he needed to ask. The act of asking is almost magical in its healing effects. Many of us would love to be in better relationship with the members of our community from whom we are separated, but there often appears to be no easy access point. The busyness of our lives takes over, and we go on without a sense of interconnection. Schwartz realized that he could be a matchmaker of sorts, linking two or more people together. The person asked is happy to be recognized for qualities or knowledge he or she might have that could be put to use in a relationship. The person who has a particular need or desire often feels alienated and is happy to be placed in contact with another member of the community in an informal and unprofessional way. So, for instance, a young man with a disability that makes job finding difficult could be partnered with another member in his faith community with contacts and sensitivity to the importance of finding work. He experimented with various ways of putting his matchmaking role into motion and advanced the following six "useful actions."

1. Slowing the Destruction of Human Culture
   Slow the "destruction of the cultural matrix upon which humans depend." "No social activity will be permitted that destroys a vernacular cultural practice."
2. Promoting Asking
   Connect strangers who are unlikely to meet. Introduce a person in some kind of difficulty to another whom he or she would be unlikely to meet for their mutual benefit. Schwartz quotes Jean Vanier:

   > For the handicapped person who has felt abandoned, there is only one reality that will bring him back to life: an authentic, tender, and faithful relationship. He must discover that he is loved and important to someone. Only then will his confusion turn into peace. And to love is not to do something for someone; it is to be with him. It is to rejoice in his presence; it is to give him confidence in the value of his being.

3. Stimulating Associational Groups
   "Careful and balanced restoration of decision making to the most local level possible can slow the current suppression of associational activity and thus help mediating structures of all kinds to flourish."
4. Championing "Third Places"
   Third places are spaces where conviviality flourishes, places that make "neighborhoods more supportive of human culture."
5. Preserving Virtuous Professional Healing Traditions

Schwartz cautions us that we need to discern when professional healing approaches are useful to a person and when they are not. He offers some guidelines to those operating as professional healers:

—"Be integral to the culture of a particular place and not be displaced by professionalism or economics."
—"Pursue intervention with the hand of a 'reluctant surgeon.'"
—Constantly ask if it is stimulating native healing capabilities or replacing them.
—Evaluate if it is actually helping.

6. Cherishing Place and Local Economy
   Respect the local economy of a place, its "particular place, soil, way of facing illness, suffering and death intrinsic to that place, a particular culture with particular hospitable traditions."[35]

Schwartz is aware of resistance to these orienting principles from two fronts. First, society members are now convinced that care should be accomplished through systems. Second, professionals whose livelihoods depend on these systems of care are reluctant to sacrifice their professional prestige and income.

Houses of Hospitality Networks

Schwartz emphasizes that when an individual offers his presence and understands the mutuality of the relationship that may evolve, this is so potent an action it "affects not only people in need but an entire expanding informal network of mutual support and caring."[36] This is evident when we widen our gaze to recognize the networks that have evolved from the work of Addams, Matthews, Washington, Day, Maurin, and Vanier. While they gained significant visibility, they were not solitary figures. They each inspired and relied on others, enjoying both the deep and considerable challenges and the daily bread of community life.

In each case, a single house slowly evolved into a network of houses. The network in one domain became linked to similar networks in other places, sharing practices and friendships. Dorothy Day and Jean Vanier both enjoyed a friendship with Mother Teresa, founder of the Missions of Charity and their houses of hospitality for the poor and for those suffering from leprosy. In Calcutta in 1970, Day spoke to Mother Teresa's novices; later, in 1976, Day shared the stage with Mother Teresa at a meeting in Philadelphia to discuss the hungers of the human family. Jean Vanier invited Mother Teresa to spend time in L'Arche communities, where she shared her experience with the dying in Calcutta. In turn, she invited Vanier and L'Arche people to her convents.

Many accompaniers live the life of accompaniment quietly, outside any limelight or public attention. They cleave to the experience itself for their sustenance, finding their place in an intricate network of houses and third spaces of hospitality—that is, outside of ordinary homes and workplaces—that provide potent pathways for sharing ideas, values, practices, commitment, and vision. As I have more deeply studied the life of accompaniment, this lattice began to be visible to me. Some individuals are called to join into accompaniment structures that have already been established. Some choose to accompany in their own personal ways and local settings. In all cases, accompaniers inspire us by living in a way that hears and responds to a call from others. Indeed, their day-to-day lives are transformed by living in deep integrity to this call and response. Those who witness accompaniment perceive striking moral and loving energy, borrowing some essential nourishment for their own lives. They are inspired by the unusual love and unexpected joy they discover and, even briefly, share in.

In 1963, Dorothy Day was traveling to London for the Pax Christi Conference. While in London, she visited the Taena Community, a pacifist community that developed during World War II from a group led by Dom Bede Griffiths. This land-based craft and work community reminded Day of Peter Maurin's dream of agronomic "universities," where scholarship and spirituality were balanced with manual labor on the land. The one thing she most wanted to do was to visit once again with Muriel Lester, the travelling secretary of the International Fellowship for Reconciliation and cofounder, with her sister, Doris, of Kingsley Hall, a community center in London's East End.

Day and Muriel Lester had previously met in the United States and enjoyed a retreat together. Their lives had taken similar paths. They both shared a commitment to voluntary poverty, nonviolence, and pacifism; to the support of labor struggles; and to the works of mercy: feeding the hungry, giving drink to the thirsty, clothing the naked, burying the dead, sheltering the traveler, comforting the sick, and freeing the imprisoned.

Muriel and Doris Lester had grown up with wealth and social privilege, as the daughters of a successful shipbuilder. Their first experience of the poverty that gripped London's East End was as young girls looking through the window of the train. Over time, they began to visit the area to get to know the needs of residents. In 1912, using money from their inheritance, they began what was called the Kingsley Row, named after their brother, who had died young at the age of twenty-six. The sisters established a nursery school that waived tuition for those who could not pay and later a community meeting place for older children. They hoped that these efforts would contribute to the development of the whole person, "the mind, body and spirit—in an environment which brought people together regardless of class, race, and religion."[37]

It was not long before a church, nursery, school, refuge for abused persons, and multiple social and recreational activities evolved. In 1915, the expanded grounds, which included an abandoned church, came to be called Kingsley Hall. It prided itself on being a place where one could always get "a cup of tea and a slice of bread or jam." The old chapel became a "people's house" where friends and neighbors could gather for worship, study, fun, and friendship.

As a pacifist, Muriel Lester was opposed to capitalism and its promotion of militarism, warfare, and imperialism. She gave her support to the suffragettes from the East End. Similar to Dorothy Day, she was an active advocate for equitable and just governmental policies and sought to root out the causes of poverty. She was a close friend to Mahatma Gandhi, embracing his nonviolent approaches to injustice. She became the ambassador-at-large and then the travelling secretary for the International Fellowship of Reconciliation, traveling the world to promote peace and nonviolent conflict resolution and reconciliation. She was nominated twice for the Nobel Peace Prize.

Kingsley Hall remained flexible in meeting the evolving needs of diverse groups. During World War I, it was a center for conscientious objectors; a decade later, it functioned as a shelter and a soup kitchen for workers involved in the 1926 General Strike; and in 1931, it provided a residence for Gandhi during his ten-week visit to London to negotiate with the British over the future of India. Gandhi had refused to stay in a hotel and instead asked for residence with members of the working class. Kingsley Hall was the chosen place to house the Indian leader. As we will see in chapter 5, thirty years later, in 1965, Kingsley Hall was reborn as the Philadelphia Association and carried on in the tradition of a house of hospitality—now for those designated as "mentally ill."

Catholic Worker Houses, the early settlement houses, L'Arche communities, and Kingsley Hall all draw our attention to the use of place as a needed contact zone, a space where each is welcomed, witnessed, affirmed, and supported. In doing so, the initial needs that call the place into existence become superseded by the creation of inclusive, dignified, lively, and loving communities. In such a setting, each member can practice the address-ability and response-ability that are at the core of our subjectivity. Our engaging the possibilities of addressing and responding to those around us, as philosopher Kelly Oliver underlines, is at the root of our subjectivity and is central to our creating loving relations with one another.[38]

Psychosocial Accompaniment

From Liberation Theology to Social Medicine and Liberation Psychology

"To Walk in the Company of Man"

What we want is to walk in the company of man, every man, night and day, for all times.

—Frantz Fanon

On the eve of the Algerian Revolution in the 1950s, Caribbean-born and French-educated psychiatrist Franz Fanon became the medical chief of the French Blida-Joinville Psychiatric Hospital in Algeria. There he intimately encountered the colonial nature of psychiatry and the effects of colonialism on a subjugated population. Each day he struggled to treat both native Algerian resisters of colonialism who suffered from the aftermath of torture and terror at the hands of French forces, and French military and police driven mad by perpetrating torture. The psychiatry he was being asked to perform aimed to patch up psychic wounds incurred in conflicting struggles for liberation and domination, without clarifying and fighting against the system of violent oppression that was producing enormous emotional and social suffering in an occupied people. His conscience demanded that he act to remove the causes of his patients' suffering, which he believed stemmed from the violent and racist colonial domination of native Algerians by French forces. To more directly treat these causes, he resigned his post at the hospital and turned his full attention to revolutionary action. He delivered a searing letter of resignation that denounced the French colonial powers' "abortive attempt to decerebralize a people": "If psychiatry is the medical technique which sets out to enable people to relate to their environment, then I have to state that the Arabs, because they are permanently alienated in their own country, live in a state of total depersonalization."[1] Fanon described that he had tried to reform the hospital, "to render less vicious a system" based on an inhumane foundation. "But what can a man's enthusiasm and concern achieve if everyday reality is a web of lies, of cowardice, of contempt of man? The function of a social structure is to set up institutions to serve man's needs. A society that drives its members to desperate solutions is a non-viable society, a society to be replaced."[2]

Before his untimely death in 1961, he wrote in *The Wretched of the Earth* that "we need a model, schemas, and examples" different from the ones we have inherited from Europe, models that would allow us to join in "projects and collaboration with others on tasks that strengthen man's totality." He urged us to "make a new start, develop a new way of thinking, and endeavor to create a new man." "What we want," he said, "is to walk in the company of man, every man, night and day, for all times"; to claim the "open door" available in our consciousness so that the "possibility of love" can emerge.[3]

When Fanon left Blida-Joinville, he deepened his sociogenetic analysis of the sources of misery native Algerians were experiencing due to a long history of colonialism and brutal repression. Rather than seek individual accommodations to an inhumane societal system, he chose to accompany Algerians in their struggle for independence from the French. This was a decisive shift from a focus on the treatment of individuals to the accompaniment of a group suffering from collective traumas bred by historical and present injustice. This shift was fueled by his developing a psychosocial and historical understanding of the colonial roots of the social and psychological misery he was witnessing among native Algerians. Liberation theology and liberation psychology offer us a language to describe the role that Fanon carved out for himself with respect to the Algerian people: "accompaniment" and "psychosocial accompaniment." Here we seek to further develop an understanding of these, while responding to Fanon's call for models, schemas, and examples that can feed our imagination with regard to how to offer and receive accompaniment outside of colonial forms of relationships.

Accompaniment in Liberation Theology

Accompaniment: to deviate from other pathways for a while (and then forever), to walk with those on the margins, to be with them, to let go. Accompaniment is an idea so radical and difficult for us to comprehend that its power and significance reveal themselves to our Western and Northern minds only slowly and with great difficulty.

—Marie Dennis, Joseph Nangle, Cynthia Moe-Lobeda, and Stuart Taylor[4]

In 1962, at the Second Vatican Council (Vatican II), Pope John XXIII set the stage for the emergence of liberation theology. He rejected the church's traditional practice of alignment with powerful and rich elites, and proclaimed the necessity of working toward a more just world. Six years later, in 1968, as the poor in Latin America continued to struggle in the face of gross economic inequities and repressive and violent governments, the Latin American Episcopal Conference of bishops met in Medellín, Colombia, and drafted the basic outline of liberation theology, emphasizing a political dimension to the Gospels. While the bishops drew on the God of Exodus to emphasize the blessed nature of liberation from oppression, they invoked the Gospels to illustrate Jesus's lived priorities: to minister to the poor, the sick, and the marginalized, those outcast by the dominant society. The bishops announced a preferential option for the poor, withdrawing and redirecting the church's attention and support from elites involved in exploitative and repressive practices to those suffering under colonial regimes and practices. They positioned themselves to defend human rights and to protest the economic dependency of Latin America on the First World.

They rejected a Westernized ideology of development, arguing that what constituted "development" for a few had undermined the development of the many. Instead, they offered the goal of liberation for both oppressors and oppressed, understanding that liberation for one necessitates liberation for all. Oppressors, they argued, require liberation from "social sin" and selfishness that diminish them and those affected by their oppressive practices.

Sin was defined as the absence of brotherhood and love in relationships with others, an absence that manifests in exploitation and domination. The oppressed were seen as needing to create political, social, and economic liberation so that they could develop themselves freely, unchained from crushing poverty. The bishops denounced institutionalized violence and imperialism for creating and maintaining vast inequities in wealth.

Liberation theology advocated for an accompaniment of the "poor" by the "non-poor," for walking alongside and living together, and for political work to change the structures of injustice that distort the poor's daily living. In addition, it nourished mutual accompaniment among those living in poor communities through the establishment of base ecclesial communities. In the late 1960s in Brazil and the Philippines, and then spreading to Africa and Asia, thousands of base communities were formed to support consciousness raising, social support, and direct actions to transform oppressive conditions.

Gustavo Gutiérrez, the "father" of liberation theology, was aware that the non-poor who turn to accompany those suffering poverty, societal oppression, and violence need to develop an understanding of the structural causes of violence. As they do so, they will develop a greater understanding of "unjust social mechanisms." Many require what he called "a conversion": a break with their own social milieu and a commitment to create solidarity with the poor and with those who have suffered oppression: "The conversion will have to be radical enough to bring us into a different world, the world of the poor." Gutiérrez addressed the abstract concept of "the poor": "The solidarity is not with 'the poor' in the abstract but with human beings of flesh and bone. Without love and affection, without—why not say it?—tenderness, there can be no true gesture of solidarity. Where these are lacking there is an impersonality and coldness (however well-intentioned and accompanied by a desire for justice) that the flesh-and-blood poor will not fail to perceive. True love exists only among equals."[5]

Black liberation theologian James Cone speaks of the necessity of conversion for white people. He defines conversion as making the decision to change communities, to move alongside those who have been oppressed and place one's own fate with theirs. He describes this as a "radical movement, a radical reorientation of one's existence in the world." It is only in embracing this conversion, he claims, that the white person can be free. It is impossible to be free while others suffer and one is not at their side. Our "own existence is being limited by [others'] slavery."[6] Freedom is to be discovered in community with others where we can pursue together our co-liberation.

After a long period of the Catholic church's serving the elites in El Salvador, Archbishop Óscar Romero in 1977 began to listen to the suffering of the *campesinos*, the peasant farmers. Seeing from their perspective, he said, transformed him entirely. Instead of focusing on evangelizing the poor, he experienced himself as being evangelized by them.[7] He shared with a friend that it was like a piece of charcoal had been lit inside of him. Once lit, charcoal is long burning and easy to rekindle. Romero urged his fellow priests, who were faced with the prospect of ministering in the midst of a civil war in El Salvador, to take him as an example and to stand next to *campesinos* who were being attacked: "Accompany them. Take the same risks they do."[8] Accompaniment means placing one's life alongside others for the common purpose of addressing injustice. Gutiérrez has clarified that the "poverty of the poor is not a call to generous relief action, but a demand that we go and build a different social order."[9] It is a demand that we stand together, not for "development" but for liberation. The practice of psychosocial accompaniment is inexorably linked to this demand and desire.

Some liberation theologians, like Rubem Alves, interpret liberation theology's intention to aid in the promotion of life as a call not only to meet basic needs but to nurture all that is lively. He created a theopoetics, a theology that turns to the poetic aspects of lived experience, claiming that the goal for all political struggles for justice is to make the world more beautiful: "The origin of my liberation theology is an erotic exuberance for life. We need to struggle to restore this erotic exuberance, to share this with the whole world." He imagines communities of liberation that are filled with "the beauty of the overflowing of love."[10]

Liberation theologian Roberto S. Goizueta argues that one desires the release of others from objectification so that they can be the center of their own world, rather than determined by another's.[11] Accompaniers may come from outside the community or from within it. Referring to outsider accompaniment, Goizueta describes how the accompanier needs to forego his usual safe enclosure apart from those in need: "To 'opt for the poor' is thus to place ourselves there, to accompany the poor person in his or her life, death, and struggle for survival." He continues,

> As a society, we are happy to help and serve the poor, as long as we don't have to walk with them where they walk, that is, as long as we can minister to them from our safe enclosures. The poor can then remain passive objects of our actions, rather than friends, compañeros and compañeras with whom we interact. As long as we can be sure that we will not have to live with them, and thus have interpersonal relationships with them . . . we will try to help "the poor"—but, again, only from a controllable, geographical distance.[12]

Goizueta underlines that accompaniment requires time and commitment, as well as placing oneself alongside the accompanied.

Given the intensely repressive political climate in Latin America in the 1970s, liberation theology had only a brief decade to evolve before the winds of the Vatican turned against it. In 1979, Pope John Paul II at Puebla, Mexico, criticized the bishops involved in liberation theology. He proclaimed that the church should respect the competence of public authorities in political matters for the sake of unity, sending a strong message that clergy should not fight against political elites who were unwilling to share their power and resources. In 1983, John Paul II suspended the vows of priests in Nicaragua who were combating injustice under Anastasio Samoza Debayle.[13]

The seeds of liberation theology had, however, already been sown. Inside of Catholicism, base communities proliferated, using popular pedagogy elaborated by Brazilian pedagogist Paulo Freire. Outside of Catholicism, the key themes of liberation theology found resonance in other regions and religions. Over the last fifty years, we have witnessed the burgeoning of black liberation theology, Jewish liberation theology, Islamic liberation theology, feminist liberation theology, and Engaged Buddhism.[14] Presently, under Pope Francis's leadership, some of the central themes of liberation theology

have reemerged in the Vatican—in particular, understanding the link between rapacious capitalism and the exploitation of the majorities.

After the conference in Medellín, many Catholic clergy influenced by
liberation theology began to reorient themselves away from living within the
security of a church that was aligned with the rich and the powerful to accompaniment, to living and working alongside those suffering extreme poverty, direct and structural violence, and social marginalization. The term
"accompaniment" was borrowed from Latin American liberation theology
by both social medicine and liberation psychology.

Accompaniment as the Foundation of Social Medicine

As long as poverty and inequality persist, as long as people are wounded and
imprisoned and despised, we humans will need accompaniment—practical,
spiritual, intellectual.

—Paul Farmer[15]

As I attempted to theorize the importance of accompaniment in psychological and community work, I was moved to discover "the good company"
I found myself with. Dr. Paul Farmer, cofounder and chief strategist of Partners in Health and internationally renowned innovator of social medicine,
uses the word "accompaniment" to describe his approach to working at the
intersection of global poverty and disease. In advocating for and co-creating
systems of medical care for the poor that have been previously reserved
only for the affluent, he has placed accompaniment as the "cornerstone" of
his practice.

Partners in Health understands and advocates for healthcare as a human right. It has dedicated itself to a preferential option for the poor in
healthcare, arguing that First World healthcare should be available to those
suffering poverty. "The idea that some lives matter less is the root of all that
is wrong with the world," declares Farmer.[16] Poverty is inextricably linked to
social death and premature and unjust physical death.

Beginning in Haiti in 1987, Farmer and his colleagues—Jim Kim, Oph-
elia Dahl, Todd McCormack, and Thomas J. White—dedicated themselves

to creating a community-based program for the treatment of tuberculosis in Haiti. The accompaniment model that was developed through that work is now in force with a network of thirteen thousand people in twelve countries including Malawi, Lesotho, Kazakhstan, Rwanda, Mexico, Peru, as well as in the Navajo Nation and in poor neighborhoods in Boston. It has tackled not only drug-resistant tuberculosis but AIDS, diabetes, and maternal and child healthcare. All of these are complicated by the poor nutrition and lack of clean water, adequate shelter, childcare, transportation, and medical care so common to poor communities. Partners in Health summarizes its mission as follows:

> By establishing long-term relationships with sister organiza-
> tions based in settings of poverty, Partners in Health strives to
> achieve two overarching goals: to bring the benefits of modern
> medical science to those most in need of them and to serve as an
> antidote to despair.
>
> We draw on the resources of the world's leading medical and
> academic institutions and on the lived experience of the world's
> poorest and sickest communities. At its root, our mission is
> both medical and moral. It is based on solidarity, rather than
> charity alone.
>
> When our patients are ill and have no access to care, our
> team of health professionals, scholars, and activists will do
> whatever it takes to make them well—just as we would do if a
> member of our own families or we ourselves were ill.[17]

Farmer stresses that real service to the poor must involve both listening to the poor and developing an understanding of global poverty, that is, a structural analysis derived from and responsive to what is learned from people's experiences of living poverty in a particular context. Distilling Father Gutiérrez's teaching, Farmer offers three points:

> first, that real service to the poor involves understanding global
> poverty. . . . Understanding poverty and inequality requires

multiple disciplines: economics, ethics, law, sociology, anthropology, epidemiology and so forth. Most of all, it requires listening to those most affected by poverty, which is to say the poor
and otherwise marginalized. Listening is also a significant part
of accompaniment and of clinical medicine. Listening is thus
both engagement and research. . . . Second, an understanding
of poverty must be linked to efforts to end it. . . . Third, as science and technology advance, our structural sin deepens. . . .
As the effectiveness of medical interventions grows, our failure
to justly use such interventions widens the outcome gap.[18]

The analysis works from the bottom up and "starts (and ends) with listening to the problems and priorities described by the intended beneficiaries."[19] The understanding that comes from these relationships is needed to
steer and empower efforts to end poverty and create just systems of healthcare in particular contexts.

For Farmer, research divorced from relationships of accompaniment
will fall short of the understandings needed for increased health equity. For
instance, to provide sophisticated medicines to combat pernicious diseases
to those without adequate nutrition or clean drinking water is short-sighted
at best. Partnering with and accompanying those at the local level enables
community members to educate health professionals about what ill community members need to develop and sustain health. Further, in the absence of adequate health facilities in poor communities, those who need
support for their treatment regimens and attention to their evolving states of
health and disease need daily accompaniment. Community members can
be trained to provide this accompaniment, serving several goals at once:
supporting those who are ill to make a recovery, creating a network where
knowledge at the local level can inform those who are helping to develop
and fund needed resources, and bringing money and employment into
communities adversely affected by staggering economic inequalities. In addition to free voluntary testing and counseling and the provision of antiretroviral medicine, food, and social service, daily accompaniment by paid
community health workers has proven to be an indispensable component

to the successful treatment of HIV in settings of extreme poverty. This "wraparound" accompaniment may include such things as transportation to medical appointments, childcare, and nutritional support, while providing the emotional support that is so needed in the face of incurable or intractable diseases. It is important that the work of community-based health workers be paid, both as a sign of valuing them and their offer of accompaniment and as a contribution to the economic health of the community.

In Rwanda, when an *accompagnateur* is able to work with someone infected with HIV, there is a "44.3% reduction in prevalence of depression, more than twice the gains in perceived physical and mental health quality of life, and increased perceived social support in the first year of treatment."[20] This form of community-based accompaniment provides daily home visits by *accompagnateurs* who offer social support and supervision of the taking of antiretroviral medications.

In the aftermath of the 2010 earthquake in Haiti, less than 1 percent of the $2.4 billion of direct aid went to the government: "34 percent was provided to donors' civil and military entities; 30 percent was provided to UN agencies and international NGOs [nongovernmental organizations]; 29 percent was provided to other NGOs and private contractors; 6 percent was provided in-kind to unspecified recipients; and 1 percent was provided to the Haitian government."[21] This meant that the aid delivered went primarily to foreign contractors and NGOs, many of whom have high overhead costs. The aid did not help to rebuild the government infrastructure or to develop the Ministry of Health, and when given to international NGOs, it rarely helped to employ poor and displaced Haitians. Learning from this catastrophe, Partners in Health understands accompaniment from outsiders needs to be devoted to building systems and capacity inside a country and its communities, to finding a new way of accompanying development partners within a country or region: "Sometimes this will include more direct budgetary support for struggling public health and education authorities, more support for local firms, and more local procurement. We are hoping to launch modest projects with some of the big development players, like UNICEF, to show, for example, how child survival projects can save kids' lives while also strengthening local capacity by creating jobs and by procuring more supplies locally."[22] The goal is creating sustainability of health services and increased equity. Therefore, it is imperative that community members learn to deliver services and that trained healthcare providers be remunerated at a level that sustains their local participation and does not contribute to national brain drain, leaving communities without doctors, nurses, and staffed clinics and hospitals.

In partnering to create health equity and equitable development in poor regions, accompaniment is a strategy that is used across all levels of organizations: with governments, ministries, NGOs, communities, and people suffering disease, poverty, and food insecurity. Who are the accompaniers in this model? They are both First World doctors, nurses, and public health specialists and local community members who are trained to be daily accompaniers to support the chronically ill. This accompaniment approach spans economic and health divides. It provides a model of "how to make foreign assistance more needs-based, adaptable, and sustainable in the long-term," and how to implement equitable and effective healthcare for the chronically ill in health "deserts" in the United States.[23]

Economists Jonathan Weigel and Matthew Basilico along with Paul Farmer outline eight principles of accompaniment: (1) "favor institutions that the poor identify as representing their interests"; (2) "fund public institutions to do their job" with accountability and transparency, rather than NGOs that drain the public sector of needed resources; (3) "make job creation a benchmark of success" and contribute to this by (4) buying and hiring locally; (5) "co-invest with governments to build strong civil services"; (6) "work with governments to provide cash to the poorest"; (7) "support regulation of international nonstate service providers" so that their work is not duplicative, inequitable, and unaccountable to the communities they serve; and (8) apply evidence-based standards of care that offer the best outcomes."[24]

Jonathan Weigel differentiates aid from accompaniment. He describes "aid" as a short-term, one-way encounter where one person helps and another is helped. "Accompaniment," he writes, "seeks to abandon the temporal and directional nature of aid; it implies an open-ended commitment to another, a partnership in the deepest sense of the word." Those who accompany take pains not to lead but to listen and respond:

To replace the hubris of traditional frozen assistance with humility, trust, patience, and constancy—to replace aid with accompaniment.

This is not an easy approach. It entails radical availability.[25]

Such availability poses a "physical, mental, and emotional challenge" amid
which most of us are unaccustomed to living.[26]

While Partners in Health is a secular organization, many of its practitioners embrace the corporal works of mercy described in Matthew 25:34:
feed the hungry and thirsty, clothe the naked, shelter the homeless, welcome
the stranger, visit the sick and prisoners, bury the dead. They are clear that
this needs to be accomplished through structural changes for equality that
promote everyone's well-being. Farmer and Gutiérrez have collaborated in
writing and in lectures to educate people about the necessity to shift to a
paradigm of accompaniment in medicine, particularly when gross dispari-
ties of healthcare have been created.

Liberation theology has also influenced the development of a distinctive approach to psychological practice: liberation psychology. Psychosocial accompaniment is its key method in cultural work and participatory
research in communities struggling under an array of collective traumas resulting from systemic violence and injustice.

Psychosocial Accompaniment in Liberation Psychology

ACCOMPANIMENT AS TRANSFORMATIVE PRAXIS: IGNACIO MARTÍN-BARÓ

The choice is between accompanying or not accompanying the oppressed
majorities. . . . This is not a question of whether to abandon psychology; it is a
question of whether psychological knowledge will be placed in the service of
constructing a society where the welfare of the few is not built on the
wretchedness of the many, where the fulfillment of some does not require that
others be deprived, where the interests of the minority do not demand the
dehumanization of all.

—Ignacio Martín-Baró[27]

Ignacio Martín-Baró, a Spanish-born Jesuit and social psychologist, borrowed from the inspiration and example of liberation theology in order to
reorient the practice of psychology toward what he called "liberation psychology." In particular, he embraced liberation theology's emphases on a
preferential option for the poor and on the promotion of life. To turn away
from that which produces death, one needs to study the "historical conditions that give life to people." One has to liberate the structures—first the
social and then the personal—that "maintain a situation of sin," that is, of
greed and the oppression it generates. To promote life, Martín-Baró hoped
that psychology could contribute to creating the conditions for "positive
and joyful modes of interdependence" where "healthy, free, creative minds"
could exist in a "free, dynamic, and just social body," where there are
enough "seeds of life to be able to trust in the possibility of tomorrow."
What we reach for, he said, "is an opening against all closure, flexibility
against everything fixed, elasticity against rigidity, a readiness to act against
all stagnation."[28]

When Martín-Baró worked and lived in El Salvador during the 1970s
and 1980s, he discovered that the psychological training he had received at
the University of Louvain and University of Chicago was inadequate to the
problems the majority suffered in El Salvador. He argued that "to achieve a
psychology of liberation demands first that psychology be liberated." He
defined a reactionary psychology as one whose application lends support
to an unjust society: "What makes a theory reactionary or progressive is not
so much its place of origin as its ability to explain or uncover reality and,
above all, to strengthen or transform the social order."[29] Martín-Baró challenged mental health workers and social scientists to understand that they
are never acting neutrally. If they are not taking a stand on the social issues
from which the majority suffers, then they are serving the interests of the
ruling class.[30]

In analyzing the Eurocentric psychologies he had been trained
in, Martín-Baró critiqued their individualism, arguing that when the individual is taken as the unit of analysis, the social context is disappeared and
thereby not critically questioned. It is naturalized and presented as inevitable: "Psychology offers an alternative solution to social conflicts: it tries

to change the individual while preserving the social order, or, in the best of cases, generating the illusion that, perhaps, as the individual changes, so will the social order—as if society were a summation of individuals." He remembered Salvatore Maddi, his professor at the University of Chicago, arguing that "the healing power of any psychotherapeutic method depends on the dosage of its break with the dominant culture."[31] Martín-Baró saw clearly that the individualistic approach of psychology operated within an ahistorical system of understanding, falsely universalizing its findings to contexts that varied widely. He also questioned the hedonistically oriented telos of much psychotherapy, that is, the pursuit of individual happiness and satisfaction. Working from an interdependent understanding, Martín-Baró questioned the significance of individual happiness as an aim when one is surrounded by human-created suffering. In effect, he argued, most of psychology operates within a homeostatic vision of reality that fails to question and transform oppressive social structures.

Psychology, he said, needs a new horizon, a new epistemology, and a new praxis. Its horizon should address the real problems of the majority. This requires becoming "clear about the intimate relationship between an unalienated personal existence and an unalienated social existence . . . between the liberation of each person and the liberation of a whole people." Psychology's epistemology needs to come "from below, from the people": "This is not a matter of thinking for [the majority] or bringing them our ideas or solving their problems for them; it has to do with thinking and theorizing with them and from them." Psychologists, he argued, need to "relativize [their own] knowledge and critically revise it from the perspective of the popular majority. Only then will the theories and models show their validity or deficiency, their utility or lack thereof, their universality or provincialism. Only then will the techniques we have learned display their liberating potential or their seeds of subjugation."[32]

The new praxis Martín-Baró called for was based in psychosocial accompaniment that assists people in gaining the power to be the protagonists of their own history and to effect changes that create a more just and humane society. He offered a harsh critique to his fellow psychologists:

Generally, psychologists have tried to enter into the social process by way of the powers that be. The attempt at scientific pu-
rity has meant in practice taking the perspective of those in
power and acting from a position of dominance. As educational
psychologists, we have worked from the base of the school, not
of the community. As industrial psychologists we have selected
or trained personnel according to the demands of the owners
and bosses, not according to those of the workers or their
unions. And even as community psychologists we have often
come into the community mounted on the carriage of our plans
and projects, bringing our own know-how and money. It is not
easy to figure out how to place ourselves within the process
alongside the dominated rather than alongside the dominator.
It is not even easy to leave our role of technocratic or professional superiority and to work hand in hand with community
groups. But if we do not embark upon this new type of praxis
that transforms ourselves as well as transforming reality, it will
be hard indeed to develop a Latin American psychology that
will contribute to the liberation of our peoples.[33]

Mental health, he argued, is not only an individual state. It is a problem of social relations among persons and groups. When groups resort to
violence instead of dialogue to solve differences, we can conclude that the
"roots of social coexistence" are deeply damaged. It is crucial that psychologists attend to their relations with the people with whom they are working,
making sure, as best they can, not to reinscribe their society's power differentials, which are themselves a cause of suffering. Indeed, psychologists
should contribute to the creation of new forms of attachment and relationships that are not distorted by centuries of colonial exploitation and racism,
relationships of dialogue where the humanity of each is affirmed. These
relationships must be formed on a solid platform of action to create just and
peaceful conditions.

Martín-Baró used his role as a psychologist to amplify the condition
of the majority in El Salvador in the face of brutal and violent repression of

people and information in the 1980s. Those in power welcomed the prestige of hosting social science research. Because of this, Martín-Baró tried to communicate the realities of the people through research. To do so he created the University Institute of Public Opinion at Central American University in San Salvador. Through his cogent analysis of anonymous surveys, he was able to disseminate information about the political abuses and daily horror that citizens were experiencing and that were too dangerous for individuals to speak about openly. He demonstrated that strategically deployed research can be a means of psychosocial accompaniment, helping to document the situations with which people are struggling, so that civil society can be better mobilized to intervene in and stop ongoing injustices and violence. Here the intimate listening of accompaniment is amplified through research and dissemination strategies. He was aware that this bold work imperiled his life.

A U.S.-trained Salvadoran paramilitary squad entered the residence of Martín-Baró and five other Jesuit fathers in 1989. Members of the Salvadoran Army's Atlacatl Battalion had been tasked with assassinating Father Ignacio Ellacuría, the president of the University of Central America, because he was attempting to negotiate peace between the military and guerilla forces. The priests were labeled as subversives by the oligarchic rulers, and the assassins were ordered to leave no witnesses behind. Fathers Ignacio Martín-Baró, Ignacio Ellacuría, Segundo Montes, Juan Ramon Moreno, Amando Lopez, and Joaquin Lopez-Lopez were killed, along with their housekeeper, Julia Elba Ramos, and her sixteen-year-old daughter, Celina Mariset Ramos.

Martín-Baró concluded his last essay shortly before his assassination with a challenge to psychologists to critically confront the social system within which their work is embedded: "The most radical choice Central American psychologists face today concerns the disjunction between an accommodation to a social system that has benefitted us personally and a critical confrontation with that system." He continued,

> the choice is between accompanying or not accompanying the
> oppressed majorities. . . . This is not a question of whether to

abandon psychology; it is a question of whether psychological knowledge will be placed in the service of constructing a society where the welfare of the few is not built on the wretchedness of the many, where the fulfillment of some does not require that others be deprived, where the interests of the minority do not demand the dehumanization of all.[34]

Before his death, Martín-Baró reflected on the merging of his responsibilities as an academic researcher and as a defender of the poor. In the prologue of one of his many publications, he wrote,

It is possible that the pages that follow may lack the level of objectivity customary in the academic world. By way of explanation, I can only point to the fact that many of these pages have been written in the midst of extreme circumstances—with the police monitoring our home, in the aftermath of a colleague's assassination and the moral impact of a bombing that destroyed our workplace. But we also believe that these experiences have let us enter into the world of the oppressed, to feel more closely the experience of those who carry the weight of years of oppression on their shoulders, and who today are rising up with a new history. There are some truths that one discovers only through suffering or at critical points in extreme situations.[35]

Indeed, in his accompaniment, he experienced directly the violent forces working against the enemies of the oligarchy.

Psychosocial accompanists need to be involved in the process of conscientization. Following the insights of Paulo Freire, Martín-Baró understood the liberating power of dialogue that seeks to help participants understand the social reality that impacts them. Through the development of critical consciousness, participants are able to gather the understanding necessary to transform their reality in solidarity with others. In doing so, the senses of fatalism and impotence have a chance to be disrupted. People are in need of not only food and shelter, Martín-Baró argued, but "for personal development and humanizing relationships, for love and hope in life, for identity and social standing." They need to learn how "to read the surrounding reality," to grasp the mechanisms of oppression and dehumanization, to "write one's history" and work with others to construct a mutually desired future. Through these processes, one is, at the same time, bringing into being more humane ways of being with one another: "Hence concientización does not consist in a simple change of opinion about reality, a change of individual subjectivity that leaves the objective situation intact; concientización supposes that persons change in the process of changing their relations to the surrounding environment and, above all, with other people. . . . The transformative process requires an involvement in the process of transforming human relationships."[36] The accompanist works for peaceful social coexistence where the needs and desires of all are taken into account and where alternatives to violence are found. This also requires the exposure of corruption, lies, and deception.

ACCOMPANIMENT IN THE FACE OF PSYCHOSOCIAL OR COLLECTIVE TRAUMA

Martín-Baró understood that psychologists' critical confrontation with the social system required them to develop an understanding of trauma that exceeded a consideration of its effects on given individuals. He proposed the term "psychosocial trauma" and defined it as "the concrete crystallization in individuals of aberrant and dehumanizing social relations." In doing so, he underscored that trauma can be a normal consequence of a social system's way of functioning:

> Therefore, as psychologists, we cannot be satisfied with treating post-traumatic stress. This is necessary and especially urgent with children. However, the underlying problem is not a matter of individuals but of the traumatogenic social relations that are part of an oppressive system that has led to war. So it is of primary importance that treatment address itself to relationships between social groups which constitute the "normal abnormality" that

dehumanizes the weak and the powerful, the oppressor and the
oppressed, soldier and victim, dominator and dominated alike. If
in the El Salvador of tomorrow we want our people to be able to
raise their voices with dignity and assert their political presence,
we must today contribute toward creating conditions for our children to develop and construct identities without being subjected
to traumatizing and, in short, dehumanizing dilemmas.[37]

We are now more aware of the need to not only address psychological
trauma at an individual level but to recognize the kinds of traumatogenic
sociopolitical, economic, and environmental conditions that beset whole
communities, regions, and even nations of people, and that create conditions that are extraordinary. The terms "collective trauma" and "psychosocial trauma" represent a shift in focus from the extraordinary events that
may happen to an isolated individual to what happens perniciously and too
often chronically to whole groups of people that undermines their health,
psychological vitality, and senses of community and hope. When we think
in a more individualistically oriented way about mental health, trauma is
often defined as the overwhelming psychological effect of an event on an
individual. As we know, psychological trauma can also be experienced in
the face of chronic traumatizing situations and repetitive traumatic events.
When we widen our lens to a more interdependent paradigm of psychological and community well-being, we can see that psychological trauma
can be shared by a group or community (as in the Ninth Ward of New Orleans before, during, and after Hurricane Katrina), and even more widely in
a nation (as in the aftermath of 9/11). Just as a single individual may suffer
post-traumatic stress (PTSD) symptoms in the aftermath of a traumatic
event, finding him- or herself unable to integrate the traumatic experience,
this can happen to groups and communities under the duress of social or
collective trauma: single, chronic, or repetitive. The groups' ordinary coping skills and sources of resilience may be sorely taxed as a sense of trust in
other human beings is shattered or torn.

Psychiatric epidemiological studies reveal the impact of cultural
pathologies on the increased incidence of psychopathology: poverty, the

effects of Western capitalism on Third World countries and the poor and working class within First World countries, urbanization, population mobility, family fragmentation, class inequities, poor and inadequate housing and education, gender inequities, racism, homophobia, torture, rapid social change and social disintegration, war, genocide, unemployment, failures of social and community support structures, and forced migration. The fact that "most mental disorders have their highest prevalence rates in the lowest socioeconomic class," where there is least access to security, resources, adequate food and housing, and healthcare, gives added weight to liberation psychologies' preferential option for the poor.[38]

This approach does not deny a biological basis for some forms of what is designated as mental illness. Instead, it nests the biological paradigm within the more encompassing paradigm of accompaniment. In the case of schizophrenia, for example, outcome is sharply dependent on sociocultural factors that contribute to whether or not one enjoys adequate accompaniment and support (i.e., is one surrounded by family and/or friends, invited to work and contribute, and has access to a safe, supportive place to be during the most challenging periods of one's illness).

As neoliberalism and rapacious forms of capitalism continue to dominate the globe, we see what Brazilian Joao Biehl calls "zones of social abandonment" throughout both the Third and First Worlds.[39] Individuals and groups are left to fend for themselves to cope with war, famine, displacement, inadequate or polluted water, disease, high unemployment, lack of necessary infrastructure, and often violently repressive state security structures.

To live without accompaniment in such situations is—indeed—to be abandoned. Without accompaniment, there is little basis for hope. An essential definition of trauma is that one's usual modes of coping have been shattered by the intensity of the experience. The occurrence of being overwhelmed in the face of trauma is multiplied when one cannot draw on another for support, understanding, and advocacy during the experience and its aftermath. In addition to the original insult, the chronic and pervasive failure of accompaniment consigns one to syndromes of distress that can continue without amelioration. With no witness, no support, and inadequate resources to establish a sense of security and trust, life dwindles or abruptly fails. In the face of collective trauma, accompaniment is critical.

The one who psychosocially accompanies holds the individual's or the community's suffering and well-being in the light of sociocultural, historical, and systemic contexts. Insofar as psychological and community symptoms often memorialize violations that have occurred, the one who accompanies is also a witness. This witnessing is a particularly crucial antidote when the events or conditions suffered have been repressed or denied by those in power and/or the wider society. The creation of opportunities for testimony helps to empower those who have suffered violence and social exclusion to exercise their agency and to bring their experience into the public arena to be acknowledged, witnessed, and redressed, if possible. Opportunities for testimony may help to restore or strengthen self-respect and one's sense of dignity, in addition to educating a wider public about needed changes.

Addressing Frantz Fanon's calls for models, schemas, and examples, the rest of this chapter describes what accompaniment looks like when accompanists work to build liberatory community mental health systems, provide community accompaniment in the face of violence and displacement, and use participatory community research to help achieve community desires for just social change.

INTERNATIONALIST TEAM OF MENTAL HEALTH WORKERS, MEXICO-NICARAGUA: MARIE LANGER

Physician and psychoanalyst Marie Langer learned to move fluidly between the direct service of providing psychotherapeutic accompaniment to refugees fleeing state terror and constructing a national mental health system for a population deeply affected by the losses from a civil war and centuries of colonial exploitation. The former deeply informed the latter.

She was a medical and a psychoanalytic studies student as the political tide turned in what was called "Red Vienna." This period, chronicled by Ellen Danto, was a creative chapter in psychoanalysis in Vienna when social democrats in Austria were in political power. During this early chapter of psychoanalysis, analysts who were members of the international psychoanalytic association either worked a day a week in free clinics or tithed a day a week to support them. This helped psychoanalysis be available to people who needed it but had no resources to pay for it. These analysts created paths between their individual clinical work and work in the wider community. They helped to create kindergartens, experimental schools for children of the poor, school-based treatment centers for children traumatized by war and poverty, the first child guidance clinics, and suicide prevention centers. They worked to establish free reproductive healthcare clinics and made counseling available for women affected by domestic violence. They taught psychology to workers in settlement houses. They consulted with architects to design public housing to enhance community interaction.[40]

Unfortunately, as fascism began to take hold of Vienna before World War II, Jews were no longer allowed to practice in hospitals. Students at the Vienna Psychoanalytic Institute like Langer, a Jew, were required to either refrain from political activity or not speak about it during their sessions.[41] Langer decided to join a medical brigade to support the Spanish Republic during Spain's civil war. After the end of the republic, Langer was forced to take exile and refuge first in Uruguay and then in 1942 in Argentina. There she cofounded the Argentine Psychoanalytic Association and became a human rights leader among mental health professionals in the Southern Cone.[42]

Nancy Caro Hollander, a historian of Latin America and a psychoanalyst, was inspired by Langer and her colleagues and closely studied and wrote about their work. Independently of Martín-Baró, Hollander named the work arising from the conjunction of psychoanalysis and Marxism in Latin America "liberation psychology." She placed Langer at the center of her narrative in *Love in a Time of Hate: Liberation Psychology in Latin America.* Like the liberation theologians' challenge to priests who supported exploitative elites, Langer directly critiqued colleagues in the Argentine Psychoanalytic Association who colluded with a repressive class system, profiting themselves from their treatment of the elite and separating mental health issues from the pernicious psychosocial effects of class struggle. She urged psychoanalysts to use their knowledge to facilitate rather than oppose progressive social movements.[43] Joining together with others, she left the Argentine Psychoanalytic Association to create a revolutionary mental health movement in Argentina in solidarity with others who were protesting economic exploitation and political repression.[44]

Langer was widely considered the most prominent woman psychoanalyst in Latin America, particularly for her feminist and Marxist approaches to women's mental health. Her vocal human rights activism, denunciation of atrocities, and advocacy to democratize mental health care led, however, to her being placed on a death squad list in 1974, causing her to seek asylum in Mexico City. There she treated refugee survivors of the brutal military dictatorships in Central and Latin America and helped to create the Committee on Solidarity with the Argentine People, which helped new refugees with housing, clothes, work, and psychological care while working to document the human rights abuses they had suffered in Argentina. The group's center also welcomed Nicaraguans during brief stays in Mexico, and through her relationships with them, she became attuned to what she called "frozen grief," a state that many of the visiting Nicaraguans suffered. She described this as a marked inability to mourn for one's lost loved ones while participating wholeheartedly in transforming one's society.[45]

In 1981, she joined with twelve other psychologists and medical doctors with psychoanalytic training to form the Internationalist Team of Mental Health Workers, Mexico-Nicaragua. They worked together to accompany Sandinistas in Nicaragua as they created their first national mental health system. Nicaraguan elites had the resources to seek mental health care outside of Nicaragua. But the majority of Nicaraguans had no access to adequate care. The Sandinista government wanted to create a mental health system with universal access and a focus on prevention through the provision of brief problem-focused group therapy for people suffering similar difficulties.[46] Langer and Ignacio Maldonado, co-coordinators of the Internationalist Team, explained the preference for group work: "We work in groups, not only because in a society that desires the integral development of all, individual psychotherapeutic attention is insufficient, but because problems and mental suffering are generated in groups. Group activity is in total accord with Nicaraguan ideology: it strengthens solidarity and teaches people to view their pain in social terms and to alleviate it together."[47] The Nicaraguan Ministry of Health worked to provide psychological assistance through hospitals, community centers, and Centers for Psychosocial Attention, while focusing on primary prevention in the general population.[48] Langer was astute at understanding the relationships between the psychic and the political. She refused to reduce the psychological to the political, carefully training mental health workers to listen to the unconscious at work. She was equally careful not to reduce people's suffering to the psychological as though this was divorced from economics, politics, and culture.

Langer diligently worked through psychoanalytic concepts in the light of on-the-ground needs in Nicaragua to see what terms and practices would be helpful in this particular context. The mental health system needed to attune to the psychological legacy of violence and exploitation. In groups of twos and threes that rotated each month, these twelve professionals managed to teach and train in Nicaragua for ten days each month. The team approach enabled them to provide stable and regular accompaniment until the defeat of the Sandinista government.

PSYCHOSOCIAL ACCOMPANIMENT OF THE
FORCIBLY DISPLACED: SOCIAL BONDS AND
CULTURES OF PEACE

For the past seventeen years, a group of Colombian social, political, and clinical psychologists from Pontifical Javeriana University have been engaged in a project of sustained psychosocial accompaniment, leaving the university to offer their support to people forcibly displaced by paramilitaries from the countryside to the capital of Bogotá. Many of these displaced people have experienced acute and chronic violence and often the loss of family members.[49] For themselves, the accompanists were seeking to construct a daily practice that was consistent with their understanding of social commitment.[50] The members of this group—Social Bonds and Cultures of Peace—committed themselves to resist the trivialization of death and the rampant depersonalization of others that characterized daily reality in their society, one that has been torn apart by armed conflict.

Stella Sacipa-Rodriguez, one of the cofounders, describes her team's perspective on psychosocial accompaniment:

> We conceive psychosocial accompaniment as a way of offering displaced people support and providing spaces for expressing and recognizing the emotional impact these violent events have had on them. Psychosocial spaces are designed to listen compassionately to the victims of forced displacement, spaces aimed at ensuring that these people feel accompanied, in order to provide conditions conducive to their recovery . . .
>
> Psychosocial accompaniment is a process marked by respect, acknowledgment of the human dignity of the person who has suffered displacement, a process which seeks to establish bonds and bridges for the renewal of confidence in a work of successive, respectful rapprochement, aimed at opening up the psychosocial relationship, to reach the heart of others from within oneself, through mutual recognition in everyday dialogue, in active listening and in shared work and play.[51]

Psychosocial accompaniment often includes participatory research and other conscientizing efforts to construct "liberating knowledge," knowledge that will assist in transforming status quo arrangements that undermine the integrity of body and mind, relations between self and other, and between one community and another:

> [It is] a process of offering the displaced person a space to recognize their emotional experience along with the possibility to express their feelings afterward, reflecting on the facts implied by violent acts. We speak of psychosocial process that facilitates recuperation and repair of social and cultural damage. We believe that accompaniment should be directed toward the affirmation of displaced persons as subjects in their own stories and the reconstruction of the social fabric of the community.[52]

Their goal as social psychologists is "to connect not only with the displaced person's logical mind, but also with their affection and spirituality. Informal everyday chats, actively listening, working and teaching [are] the vehicles allowing us to develop open relationships."[53] Through the collection of oral histories, the co-creation of support groups, and the recognition and valuing of community resources that contribute to empowerment and resilience, the participants are able to create a community that gradually connects through ties of developing trust.

The psychologists found that in accompaniment one is often faced with needs about which the accompanist has little knowledge. Together they must learn enough or gather resources to meet these needs. For instance, many of the displaced families wanted it to be clear in public records and memory that their loved ones were falsely assumed to be guerillas. They also wanted to know where their loved ones' remains were so that proper burials could be conducted. Honoring these deep desires, the psychologists needed to become knowledgeable about and effective in interfacing with relevant judicial and public authorities and processes.

This group emphasizes that a fuller recovery from such psychosocial suffering requires societal circumstances that make meaningful work, peace, and a dignified life possible. For the psychosocial reconstruction of a community to be ultimately effective, it must be part of a total approach that includes changes in the social, economic, and political life of the country. For these reasons, at a systems level, the psychologists have also been exploring their possible contributions as psychologists to creating cultures of peace in Colombia. To build peace, they stress the importance of the promotion of principles of tolerance, mutual respect, and solidarity. They embrace UNESCO's call for cultures of peace founded on "solidarity, active nonviolence, pluralism, and an active posture against exclusion and structural violence."[54] Following Martín-Baró, they see political violence as rupturing social relationships, and the healing of post-conflict situations as necessarily dependent on the restoration of trust and relationship. They embrace liberation psychologist Maritza Montero's sense that the "psychologist's role ... is mainly to be an agent of social change engaged with a social project that seeks freedom, justice, equality, democracy, and respect for human rights."[55]

ACCOMPANIMENT THROUGH PARTICIPATORY
ACTION RESEARCH: M. BRINTON LYKES

Of all the forms of psychological research, participatory action research (PAR) is one of the most compatible with the idea of accompaniment. In PAR, a researcher partners with a group or community to offer research support for the questions they are seeking answers to. Instead of participants serving the research agenda of someone outside of their community, the researcher partners to serve the research needs of the community. The researcher may or may not be a member of the community. Community members gain or contribute the skills of formulating research questions, conducting research conversations, analyzing data, and discerning effective ways of disseminating findings that assist in the achievement of shared goals.

Liberation psychologist M. Brinton Lykes's work over decades offers an inspiring example of PAR as accompaniment. Lykes has accompanied Mayan women in Guatemala as they have suffered the effects of genocide, struggled to give human rights testimony, and worked together to make the genocide known in the wider world. Through what she calls an "impassioned scholarship," Lykes says the researcher accompanies over time, "participating and observing while providing resources" and coming to a deeper understanding.[56] During an eight-year process, Lykes collaborated with Ixil and Quiché Mayan women to develop economic development projects, a bilingual educational program for children, and psychosocial creative workshops for women. Women with differing religious and political affiliations, widows of soldiers and guerrillas, and internationalists joined together through a participatory action "photovoice" research process "to create a photo essay that recounts the community's story of war and survival as well as current efforts to rethread social relations and rebuild institutions."[57]

More recently, through the Post-Deportation Human Rights Project, Lykes has been collaborating with human rights lawyers, immigrant community groups in the United States, deportees, and families without immigration documents to explore the effects of current U.S. detention and deportation policies on Salvadoran and Guatemalan families residing in the

Northeast United States. She writes, "A major goal of the [project] is to re-introduce legal predictability, proportionality, compassion, and respect for family unity into the deportation laws in the U.S. through successfully defending individual deportees, thereby setting new precedents and creating a new area of legal representation."[58] Through her longstanding accompaniment of Guatemalans who suffered the genocide, Lykes was intimately aware of the need of many to migrate to the United States, the precarious conditions they suffer without legal documents, the lack of representation most endure when deportation proceedings are initiated, and the family fragmentation that results both from forced migration and forced deportation. She and a team of U.S. graduate students and social scientists have interviewed returning deportees and family members who were separated due to forced migration. She describes the overall project:

> The current interdisciplinary and participatory action research (PAR) project was designed to create collaborative spaces for bridging the growing chasms between citizens and non-citizens and for deepening a shared understanding of and response to injustices that immigrant families (many of which include U.S.-born citizen children) face. PAR is one of several critical approaches to research and seeks to develop collaborative processes that prioritize the voices and actions of those marginalized from power and resources in educational, advocacy, and organizing activities that contribute to knowledge construction and material social change and/or transformation. Through iterative processes, co-researchers, including local community members, members of activist groups, and students and professors from universities or other institutions identify a problem focus, gather information, critically analyze root causes, and press towards redressing the injustice. To realize these aspirations, Fals Borda calls for the activist researcher to assume a moral and humanistic orientation that includes altruism and solidarity. Thus, he describes PAR as a "life project" which includes research and actions.[59]

The interdisciplinary team seeks "to contextualize current risks to families within a socio-historical, sociopolitical and transnational framework," and "to collaboratively respond to current realities through community-based actions, policy development, advocacy and organizing." Many families felt that their traumatic experience of being under siege in Guatemala during the war was reinscribed in the United States in situations where they felt under attack by workplace and home raids, the constant threat of detention and deportation, and the steady assault of racism. The activities of this ongoing research program are multiple: bimonthly support groups; leadership development workshops; periodic meetings to discuss objectives and the research process; community feedback and planning meetings; a series of interorganizational, community-led Know Your Rights workshops that utilize theater and small group discussions. In community feedback sessions, "community members discuss preliminary findings from data analyses, offer alternative interpretations, and engage in debate about, for example, traditional and more contemporary family patterns that constrain or facilitate how undocumented parents face threats posed to their families."[60]

M. Brinton Lykes, Rachel Hershberg, and Kalina Brabeck honestly acknowledge that accompanists who hold societal privilege must question the paradox of personally benefiting from the colonial power they are seeking to disrupt and transform. PAR processes do not escape this paradox and need to be interrogated in each project to examine if practitioners are unwittingly reproducing coloniality, an issue that is pursued in chapter 7.[61]

Lykes, Hershberg, and Brabeck describe how they learned from the experiential knowledge of community members, enabling them to discuss the relevant issues with fellow citizens.[62] This has also been my own experience in being part of a participatory oral history project in Santa Barbara, California, conducted by the immigrant rights group PUEBLO. Aware of the need to build bridges between the Latino immigrant and Anglo communities, I began to regularly attend PUEBLO's meetings, offering my help as requests arose. After more than a year, one of the members, Aidín Castillo, proposed an oral history project that would collect the testimonies of immigrants without documents in Santa Barbara and then organize them into a book that could be used with various community and faith groups, and as part of school curriculum.[63] The goal was to help the wider largely Anglo community understand the experiences and challenges of noncitizen neighbors in Santa Barbara without documents, particularly those from Mexico, our town's largest immigrant source. The hope was to mobilize more people in Santa Barbara to act in solidarity around immigrant concerns.

Trained in participatory research and oral history methodologies, I offered to assist. I was asked to help in various ways throughout the two-year project: contributing to the education of the research volunteers, helping to host sessions that planned the project and crafted the interview questions, assisting in creating a strategy to analyze the interviews with regard to the key themes the group felt would be illuminating for readers, and contributing to efforts to disseminate the findings in ways that stimulated community conversations, particularly between noncitizen immigrant neighbors and citizens. At many points in such a process, the psychologist must make sure she is not usurping others' roles in the research process so it can be a mutually empowering experience, where the knowledge and gifts of each team member can contribute to a successful project. Lykes and liberation psychologist Geraldine Moane describe that such projects require "critical reflexivity and 'just enough trust' to facilitate engagement across differences, in 'spaces' of *choque* [conflict], dialogue and appreciation, wherein we craft solidarity, 'lateral assists' among *nos-otras* [ourselves and others as one], and alliances for a renewed and transformed praxis."[64]

For psychologists used to doing research, the move to accompaniment requires an orientation different from that assumed in positivistic research. They no longer conceive of their projects and questions alone. They no longer take interviews or other data back into the office, offering interpretations that go unexamined by those with whom they have spoken. Instead, the research process is set into motion by the needs of the community because the inquiry is deemed to be of potential value to the community. The process of collaboration allows for the fulfillment of mutually defined and desired goals.

The researcher living out a commitment to accompaniment understands that his or her skills for inquiry can be shared with others so that they can inquire on their own behalf. The accompanier also understands that a community may already have its own approaches to inquiry. Indeed, the movements to recognize Indigenous methodologies are crucially important to disrupting the imposition of Eurocentric approaches to research.[65] While keeping company on the journey, the researcher-accompanier—depending on the needs and desires of those accompanied—may provide individual and community witness and support, solidarity in relevant social movements, assistance with networking, and participation in educating civil society about the difficulties suffered, changes needed, and guiding desires and visions.

Liberation psychologists Irene Edge, Carolyn Kagan, and Angela Stewart draw from the human rights and development fields to characterize the process of accompaniment as involving an invited relationship that becomes close and continuous, based on dialogue. It includes listening, witnessing, and offering specific, flexible, and strategic support. They are clear that accompaniment demands our capacity and willingness to experience the pain and struggle of those we accompany, and that we need to refrain from strategizing on behalf of those accompanied, proposing our solutions to their problems instead of listening intently to their emergent strategies.[66]

The accompanist struggles to help those accompanied have their stories known more widely, if they so desire, and to make sure that these narratives are constructed and positioned to affect public policy and public memory. It is not a practice that is universalizable in a single format but rather demands to be ethically and empathically crafted and situated in specific places according to the needs and desires of particular others.

If we are to honor what we come to understand by listening closely to other human beings and the places they inhabit, then our practices must come to include accompaniment, and the advocacy, witness, solidarity, and critical understanding and action that flow from it. This is not an approach that founds itself first on the positivistic and objectivistic pursuit of knowledge but a way of being with others that bears and responds to the broken heart of our current world.

After the Asylum

Accompaniment in the Context of Mental Illness

WHEN MANY OF US WALK ON the familiar streets of our city or town, past people who are homeless and suffering psychologically, we can feel an uncomfortable admixture of feelings. We feel awkward not knowing a particular person well enough to sense if she or he would welcome conversation or even the informal exchange of a direct salutation. We may feel regret that our towns have not created spaces where we can relate informally with our neighbors who are suffering psychologically so that we can get to know one another. We may experience a deep sadness knowing how few places there are where people with mental health challenges can experience a sense of belonging and mattering, where they feel welcomed, appreciated, useful, and their company enjoyed. And then there is social shame.

A half million people with serious psychiatric illness in the United States now live in our "new asylums": on the streets, subways, riverbeds, underpasses, and in prisons and jails. These "asylums" are hardly new, however. They mirror the treatment of those with mental illness three hundred years ago. Over 125,000 people with psychological difficulties live on the streets, and over 383,000 more are incarcerated due to poverty and lack of appropriate community supports.[1] Many who are incarcerated are placed in solitary confinement, a further frontal assault to psychological integrity. This current state of affairs does not reflect a lack of experience about how people with mental health challenges can thrive. Indeed, there are ample examples of approaches to family, community, and peer accompaniment that are successful in supporting psychological well-being.

In this chapter, we explore how psychosocial accompaniment is creatively and variously embodied to meaningfully partner with individuals and groups of individuals who are crafting their lives in the face of diagnoses of mental illness. As we visit and reflect on diverse inspiring communities and approaches, it becomes clear how accompaniment differs from psychotherapeutic and psychiatric approaches, and how, by adopting accompaniment as a philosophy and practice, we can reimagine living together with our neighbors who face mental health challenges. Accompaniment in these contexts can occur in a variety of settings, ways, and scales. It can occur through the holding function of a small living community, a day community, or a work community, or through the accompaniment by a family—one's own or a "foster" family—or by townspeople. In the next chapter, we turn to both peer accompaniment and, finally, to accompaniment by the other-than-human natural world. All of these forms of accompaniment and the common threads that link them illustrate the difference that a shift from conventional psychotherapy and medical models to accompaniment can make.

Unfortunately, all too often the professions and institutions created to help those with serious mental illness have ended up contributing to their misery. How psychological difficulties are perceived and treated within the mental health, judicial, and social welfare systems affects not only how one perceives oneself and one's peers but how others perceive and treat one. Stereotypes, false ideologies, and misconceptions about psychological "disorders" frequently interfere with everyday human relationships, including those that affect employment, housing, friendship, and intimate partnerships.

While many people have been decisively assisted through their relationships with mental health providers, others have found that the structure of individual psychotherapy does not meet their needs—its limited fifty-minute hour, its location in an office or hospital, its usual separation of the individual from a family or support network, its assumed time-limited nature, its increased reliance on psychopharmaceutical interventions, and its resort to hospitalization if more intensive care is needed. Needs for decent housing, financial stability, support during difficult periods of illness, meaningful employment, leisure activities, and friendships are often ignored to focus exclusively on symptoms.

When therapy occurs in an office in a limited timeframe, it is easier for psychotherapists not to be overwhelmed by the multiplicity of difficulties under which many individuals and families labor. One can maintain the illusion that the need is for a therapeutic relationship and the understandings and changes in behavior and mood it may afford. For psychotherapy to shift toward psychosocial accompaniment, however, has profound implications for the kinds of relationships and interactions that may be needed, and for the range of places where such relationships can unfold. Psychosocial accompaniment also requires that the experienced difficulties be understood within a wider sociocultural, political, and economic frame than that of the family alone. It needs to be inclusive of how this wider context has affected the ways that mental illness is constructed, understood, and treated. In the United States, psychotherapy is decidedly a part of the capitalist economy and system of exchange, with associated corporate brokers of insurance, hospitalization, and psychopharmacology.

Only in seeking to clarify and understand this wider context can we deeply acknowledge how psychological "services" for many have entailed stigma, discrimination, misconceptions, condescension, and disempowerment. Many "psychiatric survivors," "consumers," "peer specialists/providers," and "peer advocates" have perseveringly built and sustained peer networks that have worked to change how they and others are seen and treated. In addition, accompaniers "from the outside" have partnered with those with mental illness to co-create environments in which recovery and everyday living are enriched through a sense of community and more equal access to needed resources for housing, social inclusion, employment, and leisure enjoyment.

All accompaniment of those challenged by psychological difficulties should include a psychosocial dimension, looking at the sociohistorical context in which mental health challenges unfold. Only in doing so does it become clear the kinds of welcoming, acknowledging, and empowering environments and relationships that are needed to counteract the disempowering and isolating environments that make mental health challenges worse. While the kinds of psychosocial accompaniment described here may not be able to "cure" psychological difficulties with largely neurobiological determinants, the severity and course of these difficulties can be radically affected in a positive direction.

I vividly remember my first day working on an adult in-patient psychiatric unit as a mental health worker. I was a shy, reticent, and introverted twenty-one-year-old. I realized that I needed to simply start sitting with or nearby someone and see if he or she wanted to talk. I knew only snippets about each person that I had picked up in morning rounds. For instance, there was a young man in a wheelchair, having suffered double leg amputations after throwing himself in front of a subway train. There was a mother of two young children who came to the hospital after admitting her deep depression prevented her from responding to them adequately, and twenty-two others with life stories that led them to this moment of hospitalization, a moment for me where their lives intersected with mine. I knew I had some anxiety about how to get to know people who wanted to speak with me, but I also knew I was a good enough listener. As a young child, I had grown up enjoying the care and friendship of my uncle Wesley. I was aware of how my learning about his psychiatric hospitalization when I was nine through the whispered conversations of adults had caused me to be afraid of him when nothing had actually changed between us. From my reflections on this experience, I was clear that my anxiety was ill-founded. Once I dove into the waters of relationship on the psychiatric unit, I experienced how both the other person and myself became animated, how speaking began to build a small bridge that could more easily be crossed later in the day or week. I began to feel at home with those designated as "patients." In conversation, people's interests and worries could be shared. Simple recognition of each other, snippets of humor, and nonverbal attention could be exchanged.

At the in-patient unit where I worked, I noticed that some others on the staff seemed to pride themselves on their "advanced psychological standing," in large part due to their level of education and professional role. They often breezed stridently in and out of group meetings and seemed to draw a double yellow line between themselves and the patients. They communicated nonverbally that what others were suffering was not part of a continuum that included them. I did not have this sense, and so their stiff professional-like stance stood out to me. This mode of semi-presence seemed to be trying to substantiate—or perhaps it merely reflected—that they felt as though they had special knowledge warranting their enhanced authority and stature. This was my first job post–college graduation and my source of financial support. But it was not the kind of environment I was most interested in being part of. I was seeking a more egalitarian environment, where mutual learning and development was possible, where the double yellow line was absent or at least seen as a cultural construction and an impediment.

As I had approached college graduation, I had been moved to learn about the Philadelphia Association's bold experiment in Kingsley Hall from 1965 to 1970.

Accompaniment Through Community Living: Kingsley Hall and the Soteria Model

The Philadelphia Association was founded in 1965 by R. D. Laing and his colleagues in an attempt to challenge normative approaches to understanding and treating psychological suffering. The Philadelphia Association opened Kingsley Hall in London as an alternative to hospitalization, creating a therapeutic community where people could explore the meanings of their psychotic experiences and, if desired, find a way through them without medication and hospitalization.

Upon college graduation in 1972, inspired by Kingsley Hall, I volunteered at a "transition house," a "halfway house" for young adults who had been diagnosed as schizophrenic and were moving from psychiatric hospitals to "independent" living. Wellmet Project in Cambridge, Massachusetts, was home to young adults, mixing those with a history of what is designated as "mental illness" with those who, like myself, believed that community living might prove both a means to self-knowledge and an important antidote to the oft-experienced isolation of people struggling psychologically. I was deeply involved in my own "inner" work and psychological development, and saw the project as a potent place to pursue needed psychological understanding for all participants. Indeed, it was. Every person had a role in supporting the functioning of the house, and I assumed the job of being a cook for nightly meals in our community of sixteen persons. There were no paid staff, except for the director, though volunteers like myself received free room and board in exchange for the practical duties we accomplished in the house. It was hoped that such cooperative living would aid in the destigmatization experienced by the residents and in the establishment of equal, respectful, and understanding relationships. At the same time, I worked the night shift at the nearby city hospital and witnessed there the psychiatric treatments of the early 1970s: electroshock, medications, group and individual psychotherapy, and dance therapy.

In his psychiatric training, Laing had also witnessed mainstream approaches to "madness" and came to critique and contest them. Kingsley Hall was an experimental community exploring a different approach to those diagnosed with schizophrenia and those suffering from other forms of mental illness. Neither Wellmet nor Kingsley Hall used the term "accompaniment," but it is an apt expression as residents respectfully lived alongside each other, sharing food, doing chores, and enjoying friendship. Laing understood and summed up the hierarchical power relationships within psychiatric institutions: "You have a key and the patient doesn't." "I, for one," he said, "would have to come off my perch and level out on a man-to-man basis when I meet another human being classified by other people as crazy."[2] At Kingsley Hall, he hoped that people could let go of "playing the parts of patient and psychiatrist" and create an asylum in the original meaning of that word, a safe place where you do not have to feel frightened. Leon Redler, a psychiatrist intimately involved in the houses of the Philadelphia Association, described his own effort to be with a person, caring about them and concerned but also attentive to not be intrusive or offer help that is not desired.[3]

The accompaniment offered at Kingsley Hall was psychosocial, insofar as there was a critical approach to the systems of psychiatric diagnosis and treatment that the residents had participated in prior to their living at Kingsley Hall. There was attention to the social place in which people lived as they navigated their experiences of psychiatric challenges. Laing embraced an abiding belief in the meaning of people's experiences and suffering, and was convinced that if one listens carefully to words and intonations and is present to bodily expression, this meaning could be better understood. This attempt to be fully present helps to restore the humanity to each person, hopefully lessening his or her alienation and anguish. The Philadelphia Association continues to believe that it is best practice to see a person's experience "as a dimension of our common humanity not a disorder that needs to be corrected."[4]

People who chose to ride out periods of psychosis at Kingsley Hall sought an environment free of medication and shock therapy, in an effort to welcome an open exploration of their states of mind and being. Instead of being seen as psychological states that should simply be eliminated, these circumstances were approached as modes of being that give access to realities that can be learned from and valued.[5]

Kingsley Hall announced itself as "a melting pot, a crucible in which many assumptions about normal-abnormal, conformist-deviant, sane-crazy experience and behaviour were dissolved. No person gave another tranquilisers or sedatives. Behaviour was feasible which would have been intolerable elsewhere. It was a place where people could be together and let each other be." The Philadelphia Association called it a "genuine asylum" where people were treated with kindness and respect. In the five years of its operation, during which the "critical psychiatry" or "antipsychiatry" movement began, over 120 people sought its shelter. In its fifty years of existence, the Philadelphia Association has helped create twenty houses such as Kingsley Hall, and presently offers accommodations in two houses in North London for people who have a "desire to change and give meaning to the experiences that have led to their distress." The Philadelphia Association has dedicated itself to four values: "a recognition and respect for the individuality of each person; a belief in the value of ordinary ways of living and being together; a skepticism towards ways of thinking that are too often taken for granted; and, a commitment to conversation as a way of articulating what disturbs people." The accompaniment offered is that of a living community of other people who are often able to provide "a way out of isolation and despair and . . . a way of fostering dignity, responsibility and greater autonomy." Robin

Cooper, who worked closely with Laing and continued the work of the Phil-adelphia Association after Laing stepped down, described the character of therapeutic houses: "The structure of the house is not so much imposed as shaped or opened according to the abiding concerns which its members have. Like an individual, a household evolves a way, a style."[6]

In creating Kingsley Hall with his colleagues, Laing intuited what the Philadelphia Association after fifty years continues to affirm: "that personal crises and seemingly inescapable unhappiness may for many people be trans-formed in households like these. They are places where people can come together to address their difficulties in a situation of shared everyday living."[7]

In the United States, psychiatrist Loren Mosher, the first chief of the Center for Studies of Schizophrenia at the National Institute of Mental Health, took inspiration from Kingsley Hall and began the Soteria Research Project in 1972. For twenty years he researched what I am calling commu-nity-based psychosocial accompaniment as an alternative to psychiatric hospitalization and the use of neuroleptics for those experiencing an initial psychosis.[8] Mosher drew his ideas from a wide array of sources: John Weir Perry's approach to intensive Jungian individual therapy, moral treatment in American psychiatry, Harry Stack Sullivan's interpersonal theory and his milieu treatment designed for people diagnosed as schizophrenic, Thomas Scheff's labeling theory, Frieda Fromm-Reichman's and Harold Searles's approaches to psychoanalytic treatment, and Fairweather Lodges' commu-nity-based treatment.[9] Mosher describes the Soteria method:

> 24 hour a day application of interpersonal phenomenologic in-terventions by a nonprofessional staff, usually without neurolep-tic drug treatment, in the context of a small, homelike, quiet, supportive, protective, and tolerant social environment. The core practice of interpersonal phenomenology focuses on the development of a nonintrusive, noncontrolling but actively em-pathetic relationship with the psychotic person without having to do anything explicitly therapeutic or controlling. In short-hand, it can be characterized as "being with," "standing by at-tentively," "trying to put your feet into the other person's shoes."[10]

The project's accompanists were educated not to see residents and their experiences through the lens of psychopathology, bracketing "preconceptions, labels, categories, judgments or the need 'to do' anything, to change, control, suppress or invalidate the experience of psychosis." Instead, they offered some contextual constraints to create a supportive and predictable social environment:

—do no harm;
—treat everyone, and expect to be treated with dignity and respect;
—guarantee sanctuary, quiet, safety, support, protection, containment and interpersonal validation;
—ensure food and shelter;
—most importantly, the atmosphere must be imbued with hope—that recovery from psychosis is to be expected—without antipsychotic drugs.[11]

Accompanists worked as companions, advocates, and case workers, holding positive expectations of reorganization and reintegration while listening for bridges between life events and a person's emotional states. They strove, says Mosher, to help create "shared meaning and understanding of the subjective experience of 'schizophrenia.'" He further observed,

A primary task of the staff is to understand the immediate circumstances and relevant background that precipitated the crisis necessitating admission. It is anticipated this will lead to a relationship based on shared knowledge that will, in turn, enable staff to put themselves into the client's shoes. Thus, they will share the client's perception of their social context and what needs to change to enable them to return to it. The relative paucity of paperwork allows time for the interaction necessary to form a relationship.[12]

Compared to in-patient hospital staff, Soteria staff was found to be more intuitive, introverted, flexible, and tolerant of altered states of consciousness.

Both Soteria and Emanon, a replication house, were small and homelike with six to eight clients, two staff, and frequent volunteers. The house was run with minimal hierarchy and role definition, with everyone contributing to the day-to-day living. The staff were careful not to engender dependency in the clients and to support the clients' decision-making and sense of autonomy. Clients were free to return for dinner, conversation, and support after moving from the house. Toward the end of their on-average stay of five months, "older" clients supported newer ones.

Despite Mosher's research, which showed the success of the Soteria method compared to psychiatric hospitalization and the use of neuroleptics, it has only been replicated in Anchorage, Alaska; Burlington, Vermont; and Jerusalem, Israel, and with some modifications in Berne, Switzerland. At So- teria Vermont, the focus is on helping accompanists understand how to build relationships to mitigate against the loneliness many undergoing psychosis experience. Staff may be peer specialists or people with social service experi- ence.[13] The same is true in Jerusalem where staff are called "companions."[14]

Mosher analyzed why an approach that does not require profession- als, that does not generate neurological damage from prolonged use of neu- roleptics, that is less costly and more successful with regard to long-term outcome has not been widely adopted:

> Soteria disappeared from the consciousness of American psy- chiatry. Its message was difficult for the field to acknowledge, assimilate, and use. It did not fit into the emerging scientific, descriptive, biomedical character of American psychiatry, and, in fact, called nearly every one of its tenets into question. In par- ticular, it demedicalized, dehospitalized, deprofessionalized, and deneurolepticized what [Thomas] Szasz (1976) has called "psychiatry's sacred cow"—As far as mainstream American psychiatry is concerned, it is, to this day, an experiment that ap- pears to be the object of studied neglect.[15]

Later in this chapter, we see how radical psychiatrist Franco Basaglia and his Italian colleagues confronted the psychiatric establishment and won the deinstitutionalization of patients in Italy. Despite Mosher's research results and his sponsoring Basaglia and some of his colleagues to share their experiences in the United States, a system-wide shift has not been achieved in America. Undoubtedly, however, the many settings in which Mosher shared his ideas and encouraged others to think outside of normative psychiatric practice spawned a number of local initiatives inspired by the kind of accompaniment Mosher found more therapeutic than therapy itself.

Accompaniment and Recovery

After my time living at Wellmet Project I proceeded to graduate school, where I was schooled not to be more capable of living with people in community or joining into the everyday activities of living alongside individuals in different emotional states. Rather I was trained to be increasingly professional and expert in diagnosis, assessment, report writing, and individualized treatment. Rather than live together in the same home with people undergoing psychological difficulties or even to visit in their homes, I was taught to invite people to come into my office space for a highly specific and short period of time each week. It is noteworthy that within my own office, I was comparatively in control and certainly felt less vulnerable. Indeed, the feelings of not being in charge and being vulnerable are too often passed along to those seeking help in an unfamiliar environment.[16]

In 1978, I began my clinical psychology internship at Judge Baker Guidance Center, affiliated with Children's Hospital in Boston. I was "specializing" in the psychological assessment and provision of psychotherapy to young children. My young patients were primarily children of color living in inner-city Boston, in families stressed by poverty and often multiple displacements, in neighborhoods struggling with violence, and in a city known for pernicious racism. They often lacked transportation to get to their sessions, as their parents juggled multiple low-wage jobs or unemployment. The refugee and immigrant children were often brought by older siblings who were not attending school because they were noncitizens without documents and their parents, also without documents, were afraid to enroll them in school. In addition, many of my young friends arrived hungry. The first fifteen minutes of our "sessions" were spent chatting while eating substantial food. While proficient in play therapy, I could not fool myself that our sessions were sufficiently efficacious for these young souls who were struggling with an unpropitious start to their short lives. Psychotherapy, psychological testing, social work with the parent or parents, and even therapeutic schooling at the affiliated Manville School—the "best" coupling of therapeutic services that Harvard Medical School had available—seemed insufficient to surmount the social conditions in which psychological development and distress were unfolding in their young lives.

The other part of my internship day was spent on an in-patient unit for children afflicted with serious psychosomatic diseases that needed careful medical monitoring. Unfortunately, most of their own families were unable to provide this supervision, and many of the children were awaiting placement in foster families and institutions. These children went to a therapeutic school within the hospital, were living in a therapeutic milieu, and receiving both medical and psychological treatment. My formal role was as a psychotherapist and psychological assessor using projective and other tests. But at the end of a long day, I would walk up the single flight of stairs that separated my office from this unit and take up more ordinary activities: read a bedtime story, hear about a worried child's day, listen into fears about what was to happen to a child after leaving the hospital and their family home. Sometimes it meant being in the midst of zany behavior that some children take on as night falls; at other times, I simply sewed a button back on that was needed for the morning. I was more a young aunt or adult friend. Now I understand I was trying in my modest, intuitive way to reinstate vernacular forms of care that are too often sterilized out of institutional care. I struggled to be honest with myself. Despite having already invested five years in studying psychology in graduate school, it was clear to me that these children struggling psychologically with illness needed a loving and competent home with adequate supports for their caretakers, not a psychotherapist, a social worker, and a therapeutic school. Against my strong intuition that this analysis was correct, I countered that perhaps if I became ever more skillful as a therapist, that therapy might indeed be the healing solution for children such as these. In my private life, however, I decided to adopt rather than to bear my own children, a deep personal response to what I felt many of these children needed: a home, not an institution—even a very good one.

In the 1980s, after a decade of work, interest, and study of schizophrenia and other mental health challenges, I was surprised and heartened to learn about the research of Courtenay Harding and her colleagues, who conducted longitudinal studies of people suffering severe mental illness in Vermont.[17] Many of their participants had experienced delusions, hallucinatory voices, disorganized speech, and confused thinking. She tracked 269 patients from one of the first statewide deinstitutionalization programs in the United States. From 1955 to 1965, there was a ten-year rehabilitation program that supported people as they were released from Vermont state institutions. This program maintained continuity of care, helped with housing, provided vocational clinics, offered educational and social supports, and supplied individual treatment planning and social skills training. The participants learned about their disease, the effects of medication, and the how-to's of symptom management. Places with caring people were provided for participants to go when they experienced crises and/or for help with symptom relief. The approach was empowering, helping participants to learn how to access needed health resources and services, housing, and food, in order to gain independence. Programs of self-development and self-enrichment were also available. Through these multiple activities they were able to develop "natural community supports." In fact, their relationships with the professionals involved in the program were often so robust that they continued after the end of the program. Harding found that 62–68 percent of the people hospitalized in the state hospital in Vermont had recovered and showed no signs of schizophrenia. Many were living lives that included work and long-term relationships.

Harding was able to compare these individuals to a similar group of deinstitutionalized people in Maine. The latter group had a lower recovery percentage, 48 percent. Because they were matched so well, Harding believed that the significant variable was the nature of the rehabilitation program and the systematic follow-up that was received to achieve self-sufficiency, rehabilitation, and community integration. Harding spearheaded interviews with people who had experienced recovery and asked them about the important turning points in their recovery. Respondents described two significant turning points. The first was when the individual was able to find and enjoy safe and decent housing rather than having to live on the streets. The second was finding a "mentor" who was trustworthy and caring, and who believed in the patient and his or her possibility of recovery. The Philadelphia Association had melded these, creating a caring community-living environment. In Vermont, they were often not paired but nonetheless were efficacious to recovery.

At the same time, I became aware through the work of psychiatrist, anthropologist, and psychiatric epidemiologist Arthur Kleinman that those diagnosed with schizophrenia in India had a far better chance of recovery than in the United States.[18] In a World Health Organization (WHO) study of remission after an initial psychotic episode, a ten-country follow-up at two years revealed that full remission was 3 percent in America and 54 percent in India.[19] What accounts for the difference in course and prognosis, a difference where people fare better in a less "sophisticated" system of medical care with medications that have often been tossed aside for better ones in the United States? In Europe and America, there is a long history of believing that those with mental illness will fare better if removed from their families.[20] In India, people with psychiatric struggles are not as often excluded from their families, neighborhoods, and employment. The WHO study suggests that the following contribute to the better recovery in developing countries: "better tolerance of the sick role, availability of suitable jobs, supportive family attitudes and extended family networks."[21] People often continue to live with loved ones and work as they are able.

Schizophrenia in India is understood to be an acute disease; in the United States, it has largely been thought to be chronic and lifelong. Indeed, in the absence of supportive accompaniment and a facilitative environment, the person who suffers mental illness is often subjected to a string of traumas that only worsen his or her condition and make recovery seem a remote possibility indeed. Without witnessing the fruits of long-term and facilitative accompaniment of those suffering from mental illness, mental health workers have little idea of what long-term outcomes their former "patients" and "clients" could enjoy.

Through psychiatrist and schizophrenia researcher John Strauss, from the Yale School of Medicine, I was invited to introduce psychiatrists at the National Institute of Mental Health to phenomenological qualitative analysis to be able to more closely study and understand the self-reports of those struggling with serious mental illness. Strauss's research group at Yale decided to learn this mode of analysis in the early 1980s, and we set about studying interviews from sufferers of schizophrenia who had experienced multiple hospitalizations at the Yale Neuropsychiatric Institute. Through examining these conversations with people diagnosed with schizophrenia, conversations about their present lives and their history of hospitalization, it became clear that many preferred not to be admitted to the psychiatric hospital when they began to experience psychotic symptoms. They wished there could be another kind of place, a homelike place, where they could go and be supported at such times, managing their problematic symptoms in the context of everyday life without being subjected to hospitalization.

In the 1990s, Larry Davidson, also a phenomenologically oriented psychologist, began an engaged participatory approach to research with those undergoing multiple rehospitalizations at the Yale Psychiatric Institute. Through participatory research with, rather than on, people, participants are empowered to be active in sharing and understanding their experiences and exploring those implications for how to facilitate recovery.

Davidson, social worker Jaak Rakfeldt, and Strauss articulately addressed the origins and need for a recovery-based model and the changes it requires from mental health practitioners. Instead of believing that people must first recover from their illness and then address how they will engage their lives, the recovery movement underscores that people with mental illness are already engaged in creating their lives and need not be interrupted in doing so by institutionalized treatment unless it is their choice to use it. The recovery model focuses on the unique recovery that is a potential for each person, whether or not symptoms disappear, and respects the ways in which each person manages his or her illness in the context of that person's larger life. Recovery is not to be equated with an end result of cure. It is conceived as an ongoing process nourished by hope, social inclusion, empowerment, and the development of coping skills.[22] Rather than reduce people to their received diagnoses, the recovery model emphasizes the dignity of each person, along with his or her knowledge and capacity for self-determination. Peer movements galvanize peer involvement in assessing mental health systems and in encouraging consumer survivors to be the central voices in visioning and creating the kinds of environments and approaches they need.

What are the implications of this approach for psychosocial accompaniment? The recovery model in most cases is inclusive of both peer accompaniment and accompaniment "from the outside." What are the qualities and actions of such accompaniment that are conducive to the various kinds of support and presence people desire? Davidson, like myself, recognizes in Jane Addams's philosophy and practice, essential ingredients for recovery and well-being. Addams, he says, understood

> that human beings need more than food and shelter in order to live truly human lives, to exist and flourish rather than simply survive. These additional needs include the need for freedom to exercise one's agency and pursue one's own view of happiness; the need for pleasure, enjoyment and a sense of personal meaning and purpose in life; the need for social relationships and to have a sense of belonging to a community and the need for the shared rituals and rhythms of collective life. . . . Addams saw her role as primarily increasing the person's access to the opportunities to undertake those actions [that the person needs to make in order to move ahead in his or her own life] and providing material and social and emotional support for them to do so, when needed.[23]

Respecting people's capabilities, agency, and capacity to envision for their own lives and pursue their interests are essential to both settlement house and recovery efforts.

In both social and psychiatric services, when professionals assume or retreat into a hierarchical model and dictate vision and actions for others, disempowerment, hopelessness, helplessness, and an erosion of basic rights to self-determination too often result. No matter how well-meaning a professional's actions are, if those steps reduce a person to an illness and unwittingly undermine her or his freedom, authority, self-confidence, and self-knowing, the initial disabling by the illness is tragically compounded. Accompaniment within a recovery model begins with a frank underscoring of each person's citizenship and civil rights, rights that have been historically undermined. What I am calling an outside accompanist, according to Davidson and his colleagues, may act as a bridge between the mental health system and the broader community "to allow for easier access of people with mental illnesses to community life and to increase the responsiveness of communities to individual needs."[24]

From their considerable experience, Davidson, Rakfeldt, and Strauss describe the kinds of accompaniment that can be useful both from peers and from outside accompanists. They advocate for a capabilities perspective and underscore the way that this constricts in a positive way the role of accompanists. In the capabilities approach, "the most one party can do for a second party is not to continue to oppress or enslave them, and to offer opportunities to determine their own lives. The second party will then have to take it from there, choosing freely to pursue those activities that they find valuable." The accompanist is constrained to a humble but nevertheless important role in recovery: "to support the person's own choices and pursuits, to be used by him or her as tools for his or her own recovery." Accompanists work to help to dismantle structural barriers and increase access to resources and opportunities for education, employment, housing, and leisure activities that have often been foreclosed due to discrimination. Their role is to clearly see and respect how those they accompany have their own life visions, their own agendas, their own voices to raise for systemic change. At the heart of this approach is clarity about the mutuality of helping and being helped: "A person should not be viewed as being either a person needing help or a helper; rather than being mutually exclusive, people are most often in both roles at once."[25]

Davidson, Rakfeldt, and Strauss use several concepts borrowed from the Russian developmental psychologist Lev Vygotsky to clearly delineate the kinds of accompaniment—both peer and "outside"—that are often needed and appreciated within recovery efforts and settings. Vygotsky was an acute observer of the learning process and appreciated the social dimension of learning, of one person being assisted by another who may be even just a few steps ahead with regard to understanding a particular task. He focused on what he called the "zone of proximal development" in learning. As we learn something, we begin to master the various parts. In the course of that learning, we find that the extent of what we can do and understand based on our own experience and capabilities can be extended if someone who understands the task can see what our next step would be and helps us to accomplish it. If we are asked to do things beyond this zone of proximal development, we often fail and experience a sense of discouragement about the activity involved and our capabilities. If, however, an accompanist acutely observes our capabilities and where our next challenge lies in our learning, the accompanist's efforts can support our success and sense of efficacy, as well as our enjoyment of the activity. The mentor refrains from doing the task for the learner, resisting the temptation to show off his or her own expertise. Rather the mentor's role is a recessive and nonintrusive one, doing just enough so that the learner can accomplish the learning task and feel strengthened in the conviction that she or he can be successful at it alone. The mentor provides supportive scaffolding for the task.

Once the learner has internalized the process, the "scaffolding" is no longer necessary as a supportive structure. Davidson and his colleagues underscore every person's potential to learn if offered sensitive and patient support.[26] This support can be offered by a peer or an outside accompanist but needs to follow the desires and interests of the learner. Whatever the challenges of daily living—whether in the realm of housing, employment, or social relationships—any task can be broken down into its component parts so that one can work at the intersection of one's accomplished learning and the zone of proximal development. In the following sections, we see a variety of contexts that offer variations of support and inclusion that make daily living-in-community fulfilling.

Patricia Deegan, a leader in the recovery movement and a psychiatric survivor, uses the term "accompaniment," referring to Jean Vanier's approach in L'Arche communities. Deegan focuses on the ingredients for creating "hope-filled, humanized environments and relationships" in which recovery is possible. For those working and walking with service users, whether peer or other accompanists, Deegan emphasizes that they need to counter the culturally induced despair associated with mental illness with hope, perseveringly holding "the sanctity of the person as a Thou."[27] She notes,

> So it is not our job to pass judgment on who will and will not recover from mental illness and the spirit breaking effects of poverty, stigma, dehumanization, degradation and learned helplessness. Rather, our job is to participate in a conspiracy of hope. It is our job to form a community of hope which surrounds people with psychiatric disabilities. It is our job to create rehabilitation environments that are charged with opportunities for self-improvement. It is our job to nurture our staff in their special vocations of hope. It is our job to ask people with psychiatric disabilities what it is they want and need in order to grow and then to provide them with good soil in which a new life can secure its roots and grow. And then, finally, it is our job to wait patiently, to sit with, to watch with wonder, and to witness with reverence the unfolding of another person's life.[28]

Those accompanists who have not suffered the experience of being reduced to a psychiatric diagnosis must correct the power imbalance that has been professionally sanctioned. They need to mindfully hand back power to service users so that the latter can exercise their rights to self-determination, to the implementation of personal efficacy and responsibility. Only then, says Deegan, can relationships have the possibility of building common ground and true mutuality. The right to self-determination should not be confused with leaving people in isolation; rather it involves creating and enjoying relationships where all can make choices and learn from them. Self-determination and social connection should not be at odds with one another but coexisting.

Accompaniment Through Family Care and Town Hospitality

In the early twentieth century, as psychiatric care became increasingly institutionalized, professionalized, and medicalized, the hospital replaced home
and homelike settings, removing people from their families. This ended up
being highly detrimental for most who found themselves inmates of large-
scale psychiatric institutions. These institutions offered little treatment that
was efficacious while displacing people from their families, neighborhoods,
and bioregions, and from the prospect of work. In the United States, state
hospitals with over a thousand patients often had only four to eight doctors.
These psychiatrists were usually unable to spend adequate time with individual patients. Patients suffered with little to no accompaniment. They
were separated from the common tasks of daily living, isolated, and deprived of both freedom and arenas to engage their human agency.

One innovative approach to humanizing mental institutions was to
create a replica of a town within the institution. François Tosquelles, a
Catalan psychiatrist and refugee from fascism in Spain, began institutional
psychotherapy. He sought to replicate a small town within the walls of the
French asylum he directed, encouraging patients to begin a newspaper and
a café, to participate in performance groups, and to work—including work
in the garden. Frantz Fanon worked under Tosquelles and took this method
with him to Algeria where he directed the Blida-Joinville asylum. Both men
appreciated that the everyday life of a community is psychologically benefi-
cial in many cultural contexts.[29] One enjoys daily companionship of various
degrees and types, meaningful use of one's energies to contribute to the
community, and the cheer of leisure activities with others. Few institutions
followed Tosquelles's lead, however. Even if they had, people within a
closed institution do not enjoy a full sense of the freedom and social inclusion that values their contributions and the daily exercise of their agency.
The recovery movement came to argue that these qualities should be
understood as necessary for recovery, rather than fruits to be enjoyed after
recovery.

In Algeria, Fanon observed that Tosquelles's model worked well for
European patients, but less well for native Algerians who were suffering

under the multiple collective traumas imposed by colonialism. Improving life in the institution was not efficacious if the life that surrounded the asylum created what Fanon called decerebralization for native Algerians. Fanon resigned his post at Blida-Joinville hospital in 1957, arguing that the struggle for mental health could not be won in a society in which oppression and violence is the norm.

In the United States, the Community Mental Health Act of 1963 began to shift resources from large institutions to community-based mental health centers, igniting the wave of deinstitutionalization that swept the country in the 1970s. Too often insufficient care was offered to help formerly institutionalized people learn the skills they would need to access meaningful work, stable housing, and friendships. Additionally, neighborhoods and families were not adequately prepared to welcome their new members. Had they been, there might have been a different outcome than the one we witness today. The remarkable story of a Belgium village shows what welcome and inclusion can look like.

GEEL MODEL

The need for a home with caring people during a period of psychological crisis or long-term in situations of chronic mental health challenges is readily understandable. In Europe, the town of Geel, Belgium, has a seven-hundred-year history of opening its doors to those with mental illness and creatively integrating them into the life of families and the town itself.[30] The town is dedicated to a saint, an Irish princess who fled her insane father and lived in Geel. Given her experience with her father, she turned her attention to those with mental illness. After her father murdered her, she was named Dymphna and became a patron saint of the mentally ill.

Those with mental illness and other sicknesses came to Geel on pilgrimage in the hopes of healing. Indeed, so many pilgrims arrived that the town built a hospice, a house of hospitality, connected to the church. Some families left their loved ones behind and returned home. In the thirteenth century, these pilgrims would interact with citizens during the day and return to the hospice to sleep at night. While Ivan Illich, as discussed in chapter 3, worried about the effect of the church taking on the responsibilities of the citizen and the family for care, in this instance the citizens stepped forward to amplify and eventually replace the work of the church in providing sanctuary. The farmer-townspeople began to offer shelter and board to some, trading stable housing and family living for farm labor. Many experienced themselves as called by God to open their families and homes to those suffering mental illness. While the history is not without blemishes and abuses, townspeople largely learned to live respectfully with those suffering mental illness.[31] Crucially important, they learned to accept their new family members, regardless of behavior that at times distinguished them from the established social norms.

At its high point in 1930, a quarter of the town's population consisted of 4,000 "boarders" or "guests." This number has decreased today to 330 individuals in 270 foster families. The Belgium government provides small stipends to the hosting families. They are careful not to overfund families to avoid them opening their doors mainly for financial incentives. Indeed, most families note that the recompense is insufficient to cover their expenses.[32] The government also funds an impressive array of supportive and adjunctive services: occupational therapy, in-patient care, medical care, visiting nurses, a day center, job training, arts activities, psychopharmacology when needed, employment workshops, supported employment, activity centers, sports opportunities, and vacations. Ninety-five percent of boarders or clients work. Visitors and researchers have been impressed by how happy people seem and how fully integrated boarders are with their families and with townspeople beyond their families.

Rather than holding a narrow and strict range of acceptable behavior after which people are ostracized, town members have grown up around people who are in and out of various psychological states. There is a quality of acceptance that creates a positive milieu in which individuals do not need to feel badly about non-normative behaviors largely out of their own control. Currently, one-third of the boarders have lived with their families for over fifty years. There are remarkable instances of intergenerational accompaniment, with boarders moving from the home of the older generation of a given family to the home of the next, living with the adult children they have known for decades. Many foster families have offered testimony to the mutuality of the relationships they have enjoyed with their boarders.

> We receive more than we give. John and Allen are an active part of our lives. They lead the family.
>
> Mary is my right-hand person. She keeps me company and gives me so much.[33]
>
> We do it [foster parenting] because that is who we are. We wouldn't feel whole without them.[34]

One foster mother reports that her guests keep her company, that she is never lonely. Together they do chores, enjoy life, and have fun.[35] As foster parents age, the care they generously gave is often given back to them by boarders, who nurse and feed them with love and do extra chores when their "parents" are unable.[36]

The Geel model of family care has spread both in Europe and the United States, and to date can boast of 174 initiatives that are direct or indirect copies of the Geel model. In 2002, the WHO named it a "best practice." Famed neurologist Oliver Sacks commented, "If there can be an effective integration into family and community life (and behind this, a safety net of hospital care, professionals, and medication where warranted), even those who would seem to be incurably afflicted can, potentially, live full, dignified, loved and secure lives." The Geel model reverses mainstream society's fearful withdrawing from and forgetting of those with mental illness. They are acknowledged, accepted as they are, and included in cafés, pubs, sports, and family homes. They enjoy freedom, independence, and inclusion. Eugeen Roosens and Lieve Van De Walle underscore the degree to which people can pursue their own recovery as they like, while enjoying a rare continuity of family care and social inclusion: "A number of key elements of the traditional system have remained intact . . . maximal kin-like inclusion and integration of the patient; the kindness of the broader social context in Geel; the acceptance of a patient's inherent limitations; the strong bond between boarders and foster families; the resilient mutual loyalty; and the entrenched responsibility of the next generation towards the boarders."[37]

FAMILY CARE FOUNDATION, GOTHENBURG, SWEDEN

Family care that resembles what occurs in Geel is happening in Gothenburg, Sweden. Daniel Mackler's documentary film *Healing Homes: Recovery from Psychosis Without Medications*, explores the work of the Family Care Foundation created by Carina Håkansson and her colleagues.[38] This is an alternative care system for people who have been failed by the traditional mental health system. Håkansson and her coworkers provide support to families who welcome individuals into their families. The families are not chosen for their psychiatric expertise; indeed, most are farming families. They are chosen for their stability, compassion, and desire to contribute. The services to the clients are free. As in Geel, usually the family is unaware of the client's diagnosis. By being ignorant of this professionalized dimension, they avoid assuming false expertise about the condition of those who become like family members in their homes. This intentional ignorance releases the individual from the objectification that diagnosis often imposes, and from one's own and others' assumptions of how a given diagnosis limits a person's capabilities.

Håkansson and her colleagues believe that it is most respectful to meet people where they are, without diagnosing or labeling them: "No one likes to be penetrated or analyzed in a way that makes one feel one has lost oneself." They understand psychosis as often resulting from traumas. Their response is to make sure the individual feels welcomed, included, listened to, respected. They do not use the language of "client" or "patient" but of "friend" or simply the name of the person, rejecting the distancing that occurs when one is treated professionally as a victim of trauma or a person with mental illness.

As Mackler interviewed the "friends" and members of the host families, it became clear that each member of the newly composed family "grows" from the experience of sharing life together. One of the therapists says, "We are not just therapists or supervisors, we are human beings sharing." One of the family members says, "I really mean it. We are all people . . . with different problems."

THE OPEN DIALOGUE PROJECT, FINLAND

The Open Dialogue Project in western Lapland, Finland, successfully provides the kinds of supports that families and individuals need during a period of psychosis, supports that enable people to remain within their own home and with their family.

The social work profession has long understood that home visits are often needed, not only to understand family dynamics and living situations but because a family may be functioning under such a heavy set of pressures that timed, regular excursions to a professional's office are not reliably possible. Once in a family's home, the story of a family more easily emerges through its members' distinctive voices, and the actual available resources and needs are often more clearly apparent.

The Open Dialogue Project characterizes its approach as a humanistic way of meeting clients in deep crisis through helping them to trust their own resources and focusing on open dialogue with the members of the person's social network.[39] It has systematically conducted longitudinal studies on its approach to first psychotic episodes. The group offers accompaniment by professional nurses and psychologists, but the manner of their accompaniment is unorthodox in the larger field of psychology and psychiatry. Instead of hospitalizing and medicating early on in a psychosis, a small team of two or three professionals is available to do a home visit within twenty-four hours of being called. They talk both with the person undergoing psychosis and the person's social network—family, friends, coworkers, and so on. They find that such early meetings are important windows that help members of the team and the social network see crucial dynamic themes.[40] They offer what is needed to help the social network support the person during the crisis, including, if desired, having a staff member stay during the night, answering calls for support twenty-four hours a day, or making daily visits when desired. They do not have meetings at the hospital, offering a more mobile and flexible approach. They understand their methods as "democratic," emphasizing the importance of people having their own say about their treatment and of all members meeting on an equal level. Rather than treating a family or social network from the position of experts who arrive on the scene already knowing what to do, they attempt to create a dialogical and mutual connection. They find that they can help to create a sense of security in other ways than taking control of the situation.

Having worked in traditional in-patient settings, these practitioners note how much more open people are to engage in dialogue in their home setting. The team does not see themselves as "treating a patient." To begin with, they do not understand psychosis as something in the brain of a person but rather as residing in the social space between people. While not entering as experts taking control of the situation, staff do bring their own skills, understanding, and knowledge with them while they listen intently and try to understand alongside those with whom they are talking. Attempting to meet as equals, these accompaniers experience their own vulnerability, as well as their own potential to learn. In this way the family remains active, rather than passively surrendering to experts and a preconceived and established mental health system. The family's own resources are not undermined and abandoned but encouraged and relied upon. In addition, team members report feeling inspired by the families they work with, and enjoy and appreciate their relationships.[41]

The results of this straightforward approach are astonishing. Indeed, they are the best reported in the world. Two-thirds of all participants never use neuroleptics and only one-sixth do so continuously. At a five-year follow-up, 81 percent were symptom-free and 85 percent were fully employed. In the region, there has been a 90 percent decline in schizophrenia. The teams believe this is due to the rapid response and the activation of social networks. This enables most to not be hospitalized or treated with neuroleptics. They believe that this increases the likelihood that the initial psychosis will be a transitory situation rather than the beginning of a life-long chronic illness.

Accompaniment in this model involves a commitment to respond promptly, finding ways to support families' needs during active psychosis. While not negating their own knowledge and experience, team members commit to attend to the resources and knowledge of family members and other members of the social network. The manner of relationship is respectful, attentive, listening, and supportive.

Democratic Psychiatry

It all began with a "no."

—Franca Ongaro[42]

We have been able to carry forward a set of practices which demonstrate a certain
set of values for others and have helped spread the possibility of a different
relationship between people.

—Franco Basaglia[43]

Sadly, the psychiatric asylum in Gorizia, Italy, was not unusual for its time.
Unruly patients were placed in cages, while still others were tied to their
beds or chained to benches outside. Few had any prospect of escaping the
locked wards and grounds in their lifetimes.[44] Most were marked by poverty
as well as mental illness. Influenced by phenomenologists (i.e., Martin Hei-
degger, Eugène Minkowski, Maurice Merleau-Ponty), Frantz Fanon, Mi-
chel Foucault, Irving Goffman, Primo Levi, and R. D. Laing, Italian
psychiatrist Franco Basaglia and Franca Ongaro, his wife, began to dismantle the asylum in Gorizia when Basaglia arrived to direct it in 1961.[45] They
were convinced that life in psychiatric asylums was not only noncurative
but detrimental to patients. It constituted a form of social death. Stripped of
their freedom, agency, and human rights, patients' health worsened inside
the asylum. Basaglia admitted that the conditions there were like those of
his own imprisonment during World War II, and that they sickened him.
While a doctor himself, he declared that the institution of the asylum, directed by doctors, had become self-serving and self-perpetuating, serving
the professional, social, and economic interests of mental health professionals rather than the best interests of those it had been created to help.[46]

He and his wife made changes to improve the lives of patients at
Gorizia. They ended the holding of people in restraints, lessened the use of
electro- and insulin shock treatments, and took down walls, opening up
confining wards. They instituted a daily general meeting where all were invited: patients, families, staff, doctors, and interested people from civil society. The patients ran the meetings, which were sometimes chaotic and
sometimes constituted by long silences. Gradually, however, those who had

been silenced by the institution began to speak about issues that mattered to them.[47]

When the nurses from an old-school asylum in Colorno attended a general assembly in Gorizia in 1966, the patients posed them essential questions: What do you do when a patient becomes agitated? Why don't you have a bar? Why do you separate men and women? Why do you tie people up?[48] Onlookers were amazed by these experiments in direct democracy. Basaglia trusted that as the community began to form through democratic dialogue, actions would be imagined and taken that could improve the lives of the asylum's members. Ultimately, however, Basaglia was soon convinced that asylums needed to be destroyed entirely, not reformed. Regardless of the transformations created inside the institution, the power and control still resided with the professionals and not the inhabitants and reinforced the paternalism he felt was so detrimental to the people inside.

When he became the director of the San Giovanni Asylum in Trieste, Basaglia went beyond the changes in Gorizia, ending gender segregation, beginning social cooperatives, welcoming the community and artists inside the asylum walls to attend and create cultural events, and beginning community housing within the old quarters of the hospital. These were preparatory steps to closing San Giovanni and indeed advocating the closure of all asylums in Italy in order to replace them with a community-based system. These initiatives brought civil society into the asylum and began work and living arrangements for the people inside that resembled conditions outside the asylum.

Basaglia argued that mental health personnel had come to focus on symptoms and illnesses, too often forgetting the people in their care. If people could have dignified housing, adequate supportive services, and inclusion in the workforce and the community, he was convinced that those with mental illness could live with fuller dignity, freedom, and human rights outside the walls of the asylum.

The Italian movement for a democratic psychiatry, a psychiatry that destroys segregating structures that breed exclusion and social marginalization, has wide implications. It was clear to Basaglia and to Mario Tommasini, a counselor in Colorno responsible for the psychiatric hospital, that the shift from the coercive, professionalized paternalism of carceral institutions to respectful relationships of accompaniment and inclusion were needed not only by those with mental illness but by all those in similar total institutions of exclusion, such as orphanages; schools for deaf, mute, and blind children; old people's homes; and juvenile prisons. Tommasini shared,

> I used to think that various kinds of health institutions were necessary. The mad in the madhouse, the abandoned kids in the orphanage, the old people in the old people's home. Basaglia taught me everything. I learned how to reject these kinds of solutions, and look for others. I began to understand the real aim of these institutions: to avoid dealing with more serious social problems. Health assistance of this kind was an alibi.[49]

In 1978, Basaglia convinced the Italian Parliament to close all Italian mental hospitals, prohibit building any new ones, and replace them with community-based living and treatment that affirmed rights for those with mental illness. The city of Trieste embraced the challenges the new law created. Basaglia and his supporters assembled a large team to assist in the transition. Law 180, also known as Basaglia's Law,

> mandated the creation and public funding of community-based therapeutic alternatives, affordable living arrangements, sought to restore the human, civil, and social rights of users of mental health services. The restoration of citizenship in its broadest sense—the right to live in and participate in the social life of the community, the right to housing, to form social cooperatives, to participate in unions, political parties, religious, and civil organizations, the right to be mentally different—was central to the process of deinstitutionalization in Trieste.[50]

Mario Colucci, a social psychiatrist from Trieste, says that when you close the doors of mental institutions, you need to engage in hard work to open the doors in the community.[51] The next phase of real work began. Just like the first, it too had conflicts, divisions, missteps, and successes. Through much labor and negotiation, Trieste has succeeded in creating an integrated community-based approach that assists with housing, work, cooperatives and social firms, educational opportunities, emergency beds, twenty-four-hour centers, recreational opportunities (trips, exercise, art and theater workshops, sports), self-help groups, responsive emergency services, and medical care. Slowly the endorsement of community members has been won. This has enabled the development of a welcoming atmosphere, so that those challenged by mental illness feel a sense of belonging, capable of contributing to their community, and able to enjoy leisure activities alongside others. In 1987, the city was designated as the WHO's pilot collaborating center for deinstitutionalization and community mental health care.

For those who accompany those with mental health challenges, there is no room in this model for paternalism and the exercise of coercive medical authority.[52] Genuine relationships that foster a sense of belonging and self-worth are the goal and the gold. Mental health workers need to learn a new form of working, a form I am calling psychosocial accompaniment. Basaglia describes this transition:

> The approach that underlies this work is in no way an attempt to evade the central point of illness. In this new context, however, the conflicts which had previously been regarded as internal to the patient, or at least to the asylum, are thrown back on the wider society from whence they came. . . . For the mental health worker, this means an entirely new role: instead of acting as a go-between in the relationship between patient and hospital, he has to enter into conflicts in the real world—the family, the workplace, or the welfare agencies. Moreover, mental health workers are no longer impartial: they have to face the inequalities of power which engendered these crises, and put themselves whole-heartedly on the side of the weak. Acting outside the asylum situation, they of course lack any established expertise or authority: thus they have to function without any predetermined responses, on the basis of nothing more nor less than their total commitment to the patient.[53]

Mental health workers found that they could only succeed if they engaged each person to get to know him or her—interests, fears, needs, dreams, capabilities. Their role was to elicit and understand what Basaglia called the life project of the person with whom they were speaking. How did the person want to be socially included and what would need to happen to actualize this? The person was released from an isolating daily life of suffering symptoms to imagining with another how his or her life could unfold positively into the future. Now that person had support to mobilize needed resources to actualize life hopes for meaningful activities and relationships.[54]

The task of the mental health worker was no longer to control and manage symptoms but to relate and to respond to the whole person. They needed to learn how to help create opportunities for community inclusion in areas of the person's desire and interest.[55] The workers were often needed to help people emerge from the passivity and limited view of their possibilities, which had been forced upon them by society and the asylum, so they could regain a sense of their own agency and power. The mental health specialists could not use much of their former knowledge that was relevant to life in institutions. They needed to learn alongside the person they were accompanying. Davidson and his colleagues describe the shift that was now required:

> In this case, each person, each issue and each circumstance was unique and required its own unique response. The staff not only had to be adept at recognizing and managing effects of the illness but also had to be socially and instrumentally adept at assisting the person in navigating or negotiating the community terrain, whether this be securing one's disability pension, resolving conflicts with one's family or finding the leverage needed to get a neglectful landlord to repair a leaking sink. It was crucial in all of these circumstances that the staff not take over the situation and resolve it for the person, as this would be to lapse back into the asylum role of caretaker. The staff's role was more that of a mediator, who could help members of the community understand and be responsive to the person with

the mental illness while also helping the person with the mental illness to understand how the world works and what it requires from him or her.[56]

Once this form of accompaniment was understood, it was clear that many others outside of mental health professionals—called "Basagliani"— could also assume the needed roles and relationships that would create a supportive community, one welcoming to a diversity of psychological states. Indeed, as we see in the next chapter, some of the most effective accompaniment is from peers who themselves experience mental illness and its social implications. In evaluating the success in Trieste, it is clear that Italy's provision of a genuine safety net, of healthcare, and of affordable housing were critical.[57]

Basaglia was one of many Italians in the movement for deinstitutionalization who worked to build community resources so that closing asylums could be accomplished not only with a "no!" but with a "yes," with doable ideas for inclusion and relationship. The story of Trieste's groundbreaking achievements demonstrates that the culture of a city can change over the course of a few decades when there is political, social, economic, and interpersonal resolve to reverse processes of social exclusion that have been so profoundly damaging to those suffering mental illness. There must be a commitment to help all residents secure decent housing, healthcare, leisure activities, and employment opportunities. At the heart of these changes is a shift from hierarchical, highly professionalized and distanced relationships geared toward management and containment to relationships of accompaniment that attune to each individual and his or her desire for a dignified, free, and meaningful life among others. Here we can gather a sense of what is possible in our own cities and towns when accompaniment is supported at multiple levels of organization: nation, city, neighborhood, workplace, family, and the "mediation" of a Basagliani-kind of friend.

Beyond Treatment

Peer and Ecological Accompaniment

"Nothing about us without us."
—Disability activists, 1990s

THERE CAN BE A WORLD OF difference between discussing a troubling psychological experience with a peer and discussing it with a mental health provider. For instance, if you share about a voice you are hearing with someone who also hears voices, the encounter is more likely to be normalized, with the sharing of advice won from experience about how to learn from the voice and how to interact with it in a way that minimizes its disruption. The mental health provider is more likely to note the experience of hearing a voice as a symptom of a disease process, schizophrenia, and seek to manage the symptom through drugs and/or distancing the person from the voice. Rather than gain a sense of personal mastery or proficiency in relation to an aspect of one's psychological experience, one is diagnosed, the experience is judged, and the patient treated from above by a person in a hierarchical position of power.

When I worked at Judge Baker Guidance Center, I heard about a retrospective study that assessed how young patients, now adults, had experienced their stays in the psychosomatic in-patient unit when they were children or adolescents. In particular, the researchers wondered what, of the many services experienced, had been helpful in their recovery. Staff were surprised to learn that the most helpful experience reported was patients' relationships with fellow child or adolescent patients, peers who were involved in shared experiences and who offered support and understanding to each other. Indeed, the most therapeutic aspect experienced was friendship itself, accompaniment of one by another, mutual, reciprocal.

The importance of this finding cannot be overemphasized in a world of mental health treatment that is largely based on relationships that are hierarchical, remunerative, and now driven by the biomedically expert. Nor can it be ignored in a societal context that has marginalized those with diagnosed psychiatric illness, too often abandoning them to lonely lives. The "consumer movement" of those "receiving" mental health services has increasingly demanded that the relationships they are part of be between equals, recognizing their dignity, knowledge, and abilities. Shared decision-making is key to nourishing empowerment and self-advocacy.[1] Peer accompaniment takes a variety of informal and formal shapes, the latter including what takes place in so-called Clubhouses, "recovery learning communities," "social firms," "microbusinesses," and "business incubators." In these settings, people with psychiatric disabilities can experience mutual support, camaraderie, and friendship with others who are more likely to share and nonjudgmentally understand some of their experiences.

Richard Warner and James Mandiberg point out that people diagnosed as schizophrenic are often handicapped in their creation of a social network.[2] In societies where independent living outside the family is valued, the eighteen-year-old crosses an invisible threshold where people are encouraged to live on their own even when this leads to greater isolation due to a disability. In addition, government-funded rent subsidies in the United States are conditional on living alone rather than with other people. Emphases on mainstreaming people with disabilities has been blind to the effects of the stigmatization of mental illness that often leave people feeling marginalized, even at work, if work has been offered. Warner and Mandiberg point out that government programs value entrance into competitive employment rather than adequately supporting community-based employment sites that offer both employment and social support.

"Identity communities" are places where people with shared interests, beliefs, experiences, or needs can gather, provide mutual support, enjoy one another's company, and further the interests and dreams of community members. Many members of marginalized communities find such identity communities to be the social centers of their lives, offering the most stable and supportive social networks. They come in many forms.

Social Firms/Social Cooperatives, Business Incubators, and Enclave Communities

One of the successful social experiments in Trieste, Italy, in the 1980s was the development of social cooperatives or social firms. By Italian law, so-called Type B social cooperatives include at least 30 percent members who have a disability or a labor market disadvantage. The cooperative is given tax incentives to have an inclusive workforce. Permanent workers and volunteers assist those with disabilities who need and desire it to integrate into the labor market. All employees are paid a fair-market wage and share the same rights and obligations. In Trieste, social cooperatives have been formed in many sectors, including catering, cleaning, hotel work, restaurants, transportation, building renovation, shopping for the homebound, landscaping, bookbinding, human services, artisans, and a radio station. Instead of government funds being directed toward disempowering handouts, the government encourages and supports inclusion in the workforce and accomplishes much of its own work such as office and street cleaning through the use of such cooperatives. This allows for meaningful participation in the social and economic life of one's town or city and encourages self-sufficiency and relationships. By 2005, there were eight thousand social firms in Europe employing thirty thousand people with psychiatric and other disabilities.[3]

Warner and Mandiberg have closely studied how to develop social firms and cooperatives, working alongside community members in the United States to develop this model. Cooperatives or social firms help those who are disadvantaged in employment due to their disability or due to the stigma and misunderstanding associated with it. These groups may start through a business incubation program, where members are provided with initial support and financial and technical services to begin a small business.

Members can be owners of social cooperatives that enable them to create flexible work conditions where members gain self-sufficiency and succeed economically. For instance, a person might be able to manage the number of hours worked so as not to lose governmental support. Other members might stand in when the demands of an illness interrupt one's usual capacities for work.

Richard Warner draws an analogy between immigrant communities and communities based on a shared disability. Immigrant workers can choose between working in the mainstream, within their own community, or both. Would not many with psychiatric disabilities also enjoy the freedom to work in their own identity communities? Warner questions the universalized value of people working in the mainstream and underscores that some people with disabilities may prefer the mutual support, aid, and friendship of working alongside others with a similar disability.[4]

Mandiberg also turns to the experiences of immigrant communities for a model of how groups considered "other" are able to achieve social and economic inclusion. He argues that "perhaps the route to social inclusion is not the mythic melting pot, but the pluralist notion of a patchwork quilt."[5] For some people, a sense of inclusion may be gained by membership in a subcommunity, which may or may not be a pathway to wider inclusion. In such enclave communities, one enjoys a sense of full inclusion and mutual support that helps offer a buffer from the stigma and avoidance meted out by many outside the enclave. Enclave community members may choose the degree to which they also desire to work and affiliate outside of the enclave, just as refugees and immigrants do. Warner and Mandiberg are aware of the better outcomes enjoyed by those with early psychosis in many poor countries. This is often due to the fact that such individuals still live with the support of their families and neighborhoods. In the United States, where living alone and independently for young adults and mainstreaming of those with disabilities are valorized, those with mental illnesses are often disempowered and socially isolated due to their dispersion. "Living and working," Warner and Mandiberg write, "in proximity with people who do not share one's disability status or life experience makes social interaction difficult."[6] Conversely, affiliation with others who share our life experiences contributes to our sense of identity, acceptance, and inclusion, as well as situating ourselves where mutual aid is more likely.

Mandiberg recounts efforts in the late 1980s and early 1990s to secure housing in three different communities where participants lived within a five-minute walk from others who shared their disabilities. They rented a community gathering place in the geographic center where members could gather. Each of these networks organized themselves to support members in crisis to avert rehospitalization.

Instead of hiring clinical staff, they hired community organizers. These accompanists were not to provide mental health services but to help members organize a mutually supportive residential network. This enabled a differentiation of the functions of treatment and rehabilitation from that of supporting community development, clearly separating issues of illness from those of social inclusion and participation: "Building community also requires a different skill set than what is taught in clinical graduate programs in social work, psychology, psychiatry, and nursing. Community organizing, community development, planning, architecture, social enterprise, and small business development are all skill sets that are needed to facilitate developing mental health communities and economies."[7]

Taking his cue from immigrant enclave communities, Mandiberg observed how enclave communities foster the development of businesses, civic groups, clubs, teams, housing, cultural activities, neighborhood banks, and credit unions. In doing so, they provide valuable resources for their enclave and offer skills that can be used in the broader society, if desired. To explore whether such development was possible within enclaves organized around psychiatric disability, Mandiberg accompanied consumer-survivors and social workers to create several business incubators where members were assisted in envisioning and then starting small businesses, enabling them to enjoy the often-needed flexibilities associated with self-employment.[8]

Such enclaves could also organize credit unions where pooled resources could be more readily available for small loans to start or support businesses. This is particularly important for people who have been unable to establish adequate credit ratings to support borrowing small sums of money. A close analysis of community assets may lead participants to insights about potentially successful businesses. For instance, when Richard Warner and Paul Polak discovered that community members in Boulder were using a high percentage of their modest income on pharmaceuticals, Mandiberg and his colleagues helped members create a mental health pharmacy, adding to the infrastructure of the mental health enclave.

Social firms and Clubhouses, business incubators, shared living arrangements, and clustering of people with shared disabilities in a neighborhood can be pathways to creating supportive and vibrant enclave communities. Here peer accompaniment can more easily thrive, partially or wholly displacing the need for accompaniment by mental health professionals. Bethel House in northern Japan has been an important laboratory for these ideas.

Collaborative Recovery Centers: Fountain House

The Clubhouse Movement is an important part of the story of peer accompaniment, as is the history of Fountain House—the first Clubhouse—whose approach created an amalgam of peer and staff accompaniment. New York City's Fountain House calls itself a "collaborative recovery center."[9] When towns and cities are not oriented around deep hospitality toward those suffering chronic mental illness, places need to be created that stand in their stead and help to provide a bridge to civil society. In 1942, Dr. Hiram Johnson, a psychiatrist at Rockland State Hospital in New York, sought to employ the principles of Alcoholics Anonymous (AA) with his patients. He encouraged friendships among people suffering from similar problems and brought patients together to enjoy each other's company through reading, singing, painting, and discussions. He hoped that on discharge, some of the people in this group, self-named The W. A. N. A. Society (We Are Not Alone), might turn to one another for support. A psychiatric aide, Elizabeth Kerr Schermerhorn, who had studied with Swiss psychiatrist C. G. Jung, was interested in the integration of people diagnosed with mental illness with those without such a diagnosis. She was aware that the kind of mutual support Jung had advised was crucial when he suggested an organization

Box 6.1 Bethel House
Urakawa, Japan

In 1978, a group of people who had been discharged from the local psychiatric hospital in Urakawa in northern Japan began to meet. Two years later, they decided to live together. In 1984, they formed the Bethel House group home and began to welcome others with psychiatric disabilities after their discharge from long-term psychiatric hospitalization. The Bethel set of projects presently comprises 150 "members" and "supporters" who live in eleven group homes and work together in seaweed packaging, fish drying and salting, noodle making, and two Bethel-owned stores. The president and directors are all persons with psychiatric disabilities.

The larger work of this enclave community has been to create a distinctive intentional community that supports independence, freedom, self-determination, and a high degree of individual and group support. Members do not hide their psychological states and are free to be who they are. They want their town of fifteen thousand to lay aside stigma: "We don't ask members to fit themselves to the society. Rather, we ask the society to change itself to become a better place for everyone, including Bethel members, to live in."[a] Bethel spaces are marked by humor, laughter, singing, and a variety of mantra-like phrases.[b] For instance, instead of the norm at many workplaces of "Don't move your lips, move your hands," Bethel members say "Move your lips, don't move your hands!" Conflicts inevitably break out, but there is an overriding sense of warmth and community-feeling.

At Bethel House members are encouraged to engage in "self-directed research." Etsuko Mukaiyachi, one of the founders and a social worker, developed a self-directing workbook to assist with this research. The categories in the workbook help people narrate their experiences and more clearly differentiate between themselves and their "problems." A person is encouraged to create her or his own diagnosis, rather than receive one passively from a medical hierarchy. For instance, "I am Hiroshi who is struggling with the issue of how to stop blowing up even when I don't want to," or "Schizophrenia: Runs-Out-of-Money-by-the-End-of-the-Week Type."[c] This helps members both own their problems and communicate about them to their fellow community members. The self-directed research process encourages people to notice the patterns and processes of their problems and experiment with varying approaches to them. What are their causes? What helps one in relation to them? What hinders? Self-research is periodically presented to community members

Box 6.1 (continued)

who ask questions and offer suggestions. In doing so, other members become aware of the particular challenges each member faces.

Instead of being objects of research, members are the directors. They
develop and test their hypotheses, and often what they learn is incorporated
into Bethel's social skills training workshops and formal research presenta-
tions. Dr. Toshiaki Kawamura, Bethel's chief psychiatrist, comments that
the goal of self-directed research is not to become cured in a conventional
sense. Some members have proposed that Urukawa become a place of self-
study where any or all residents devote themselves to lifelong self-study.

Rather than resorting to medication to eradicate voices, members
are encouraged to be curious about them. A notational system has been
developed to graphically portray the nature and messages of particular figures who speak to the member. Hallucinations are called *Gencho-sans,* or
honorable voices. Negative self-thoughts are called *Okyaku-sans,* or honorable visitors.[d] In meetings, people convey what they are hearing, and
other members may offer advice about how to deal with negative voices.
For instance, sometimes a member is encouraged to use a positive voice to
counter destructive ones. At other times, a person can be reminded that
voices do not always tell the truth.

Each year the community has a contest for the best hallucinations
and delusions: Hallucinations and Delusions Grand Prix. At the annual
Bethel Festival, attended by two thousand visitors, the winning hallucinations and delusions are acted out. This normalization and open acceptance of the kinds of hallucinatory and negative thought experiences
people have enables work and living groups to be places where these experiences can be freely shared. From this, members can develop a sense of
being accepted and understood, often in stark contrast to the stigma they
have endured as a person diagnosed with psychiatric illness. The social
acceptance of a broader range of psychological experience also enables
people to reduce their medications.

In social skills training meetings, members are encouraged to share
and then roleplay everyday social difficulties. Members offer possible solutions drawn from their own experiences. These are acted out, and the
most auspicious are decided on. The person is invited back to report on
how they put one or more of the possible solutions into action and what
the results were, creating a feedback loop to the previous session. Many
other groups are also available including Schizophrenics Anonymous,
gardening, occupational therapy and expressive arts-based groups, house
meetings, groups for couples, and groups for parents.

The psychiatrist who helped found Bethel House, Toshiaki Kawamura, remarks that psychiatrists and other mental health professionals must learn to take a backseat to and privilege the knowledge of members over professional expertise for this kind of communal experience to work. It is joked that while members have diagnosed mental illnesses, staff have undiagnosed ones. Not only do several thousand people visit Bethel House each year to learn about its approaches, but members educate both the general public and mental health professionals through books, talks, and lectures throughout Japan. Japan has a history of lengthy in-patient psychiatric treatment and a high reliance on psychopharmaceuticals. The experiences of Bethel House members have encouraged many communities to rely less on hospitalization and medication. Instead, they encourage communities to lift social stigma and the resulting shame from psychiatric survivors and assist them to build their own communities. Stable housing, support, and work go a long way to establishing the conditions in which people can live meaningful and satisfying lives, graced by warmth, love, acceptance, and humor.

Bethel House is a living testament to the possibility that while a member may experience themselves as mentally ill, they can at the same time be socially well.[e] At Bethel, what I am calling mutual accompaniment is simply part of all daily activities of living, working, self-study, and leisure, reflecting another Bethel mantra: "Don't get well on your own!"

---

a. "What Is Bethel House?" http://bethel-net.jp/bethel-e.html.

b. I am grateful to cultural and visual anthropologist Karen Nakamura's ethnography and films about Bethel House, and I draw on them here for this description: *A Disability of the Soul: An Ethnography of Schizophrenia and Mental Illness in Contemporary Japan* (Ithaca, NY: Cornell University Press, 2013); and documentaries *Bethel: Community and Schizophrenia in Northern Japan,* 2007, and *A Japanese Funeral,* 2007, http://www.disability.jp/soul/films/.

c. Nakamura, *A Disability of the Soul,* 173.

d. Ibid., 12.

e. Erica Rockhold, "Karen Nakamura's *A Disability of the Soul,*" *Somatosphere,* September 12, 2013, http://somatosphere.net/2013/09/karen-nakamuras-a-disability-of-the-soul.html.

such as Alcoholics Anonymous to its founders.[10] After discharge from Rockland, Michael Obelensky, one of the members of Johnson's group, wrote to Schermerhorn and asked her assistance in creating W.A.N.A. outside the hospital. She responded by helping to begin a settlement house with a social club and social and educational programs for people with mental illness. This was to become Fountain House.

In 1948, John Beard, a social worker who had been facilitating activity group therapy at Eloise Hospital outside of Detroit, brought his talents and interests to Fountain House. When he first arrived, he observed Mary Smith, one of the staff, inviting members to help her make lunch. He later recounted that this inclusive act ignited his vision for how to proceed. He called on the members to accomplish needed repairs in the house and be actively involved in meeting every need that arose, including cooking, office work, and outreach. Beard understood that many people who had been living within psychiatric institutions and with societal stigma experienced a sense of personal failure, feelings of inadequacy, a lack of confidence, and a sense of discouragement. Often these feelings intensified their social isolation. Beard discovered that everyday opportunities to assume useful roles could be extremely salutary, increasing a sense of self-efficacy and helping members engage in relationships and shared leadership. Members could experience themselves as useful, needed, and appreciated. Fountain House, the first Clubhouse, began and continues as a "methodology for addressing the social estrangement of its members."[11] Its premise was clear. The members of Fountain House believed that members could succeed at work and in having satisfying social lives despite mental illness. Rather than consign "members" to the role of patients, staff and members work side by side, resisting a medical model. Their mutual and reciprocal relationships are seen as key to the well-being of members and the Fountain House community. While Fountain House acknowledges the mutual nature of relationships, it also adheres to social work ethics that guard against the exploitation of those one works with for the staff member's own needs, growth, and development.

Beard understood the stigma under which patients labored. Their psychiatric difficulties often made relationships and work difficult. Hospitalization further removed them from the community and from experiences where they felt valued, needed, recognized, appreciated, and empowered. Beard wanted to create a place where members could experience being needed, enjoy human relationships, gain a foothold in work, and engage with others in leisure activities. He decided to organize Fountain House around the workday, inviting members to attend from 9 a.m. to 5 p.m. and to freely choose their activities. He found that when members orient to the workday, their focus on symptoms recedes. Work is not seen as an end in itself but as a means of recovery. What I am calling psychosocial accompaniment, Beard named social practice. The intention of social practice is to aid recovery by helping to restore the social networks of members, networks that have been adversely affected by their illnesses and the culture's stigmatization. Social practice has many distinctive aspects that differentiate it from clinical practice and individualized treatment. It is nonhierarchical and committed to shared leadership and consensus decision-making. Consensus processes help to ensure that the community is not divided into winners and losers.[12]

Staff and members collaboratively work and engage in leisure activities side by side in all aspects of the house's activities. There are no separate staff rooms, where staff differentiate themselves from and hide out from members. The outcome of a project is less important than how staff engage in it. One staff role is to invite members to take part in every activity according to their interest and willingness. Staff model activities to support members in learning what is necessary to succeed at tasks if they do not already know. They encourage risk-taking and recognize and appreciate members' achievements and contributions. Throughout any task the staff member is trying to form relationships with members, listening carefully to discover members' interests so that activities and tasks can be offered that intersect with those interests and so that genuine relationships can be built. There is a policy never to hire enough staff to be able to accomplish the work of the house, because the whole point of the work policy is to encourage members' involvement and relationships. Each day members and staff reach out to members who are not present to encourage their participation in an effort to help them overcome social isolation.

In addition, social practice includes getting to know a member well enough so that he or she can be supported to achieve his or her own goals through motivational coaching. Through such relationships with staff and members, each person can feel valued and needed. Alan Doyle and social

worker Fang-pei Chen describe a number of qualities of presence that contribute to the success of social practice: flexibility, spontaneity, enthusiasm,
an optimistic attitude about recovery, a sense of humor, and a positive
spirit.[13] Chen understands what she sees as a professional use of the self to
develop genuine relationships in such a setting: engage members, reduce
the power differential between staff and members, model the management
of relationship boundaries, promote positivity, and develop relationships
that are individualized and founded on each person's particular interests
and ways of being. Part of the flexibility needed by staff is to be open to being taught by members. The normative paradigm of a professional helping
someone who is designated as in need of help is disrupted and seen as potentially disempowering and stigmatizing. It is the member who needs to be
needed, who needs to experience the myriad ways he or she can be of help
to others and the community.

In addition, staff members are discouraged from looking through the
lens of pathology, where ego and cognitive deficits are enumerated and causes
for them sought in the past. This perspective too easily loses sight of the
person who is more than the difficulties and symptoms which beset them.
Instead, accompaniers look for strengths to build on, emergent interests to
encourage, and resiliency in the face of difficulty. This different lens offers
positivity and hope and affirms human dignity. It is moored in the present
and points toward the future. While efforts like those at Kingsley Hall are
attentive to the meanings present in experiences of psychosis, Fountain
House bypasses this in favor of a focus on ego strengths and interpersonal
relationships.

John Beard carefully designed the space at Fountain House to encourage interaction and to offer as many opportunities as possible for contributing to meaningful work. Rather than opt for efficiency of design with respect
to work tasks, his aim was to maximize opportunities for members' work
contributions and relationships. For instance, instead of having an auto-
matic phone system, members staff the phones and interact with callers.

Unlike many Clubhouses, Fountain House does not espouse a sepa-
ratist approach, that is, environments where there are only peer members
and no staff. Indeed, it prides itself on being a community where staff and

members learn from one another, depend on each other, and enjoy relationships with one another. A staffer may learn how to cook from a member, and a member may get some help with a college application from a staffer. In each situation, there is the possibility of providing encouragement and relationship while accomplishing a task. Fountain House combines a case management approach with a self-help model. Work and relationship experiences within the house can provide social experience for members so that they can succeed in work and social relationships outside of the house. Transitional and supportive work programs help members to be successful as they foray into the wider society.

Doyle, Lanoil, and Dudek underscore that Fountain House began as a settlement house, in the tradition of Hull-House, and continues today to reflect that model. Psychiatric epidemiologist Ezra S. Susser says that it "combines the activist and empowerment structures of the consumer and settlement house movements with the recovery intent of humanistic, therapeutic thought."[14] Indeed, one pillar of the latter is milieu therapy, where everyone who comes into contact with a member is prepared to be inclusive, welcoming, and encouraging.

Like a settlement house, Fountain House is responsive to the needs and interests of its members. Housing and employment opportunities are developed alongside wellness activities, culinary work, educational work, and maintenance of every aspect of the house. The gift of a five-hundred-acre farm in northern New Jersey allows interested members and staff to stay during the week at the farm and contribute to growing food and taking care of alpacas.

Importantly, communities like Fountain House are committed to pursuing social justice for their members, just as the original settlement houses were. Staff become advocates alongside members in the larger civil society, as they struggle together for social, political, and economic changes that will improve the lives of members. Just as Partners in Health moves between grassroots and policy-level accompaniment, psychosocial accompaniment at Fountain House and other similar communities includes this crucial role. Instead of blaming the individual who is affected by social injustice, the settlement house worker, the psychosocial accompanier, and the social practitioner attempt to redress the societal conditions that make life more difficult. For instance, Fountain House has worked effectively to gain funding for education, address housing discrimination, develop transitional employment, and win reduced transit fees for people with disabilities.

Realizing that stable housing and employment often present formidable challenges for members, those at Fountain House develop housing opportunities and partner with workplaces to give members greater opportunities. Presently five hundred members live in Fountain House residences. In addition, Fountain House includes an art gallery where its members can exhibit their creative work, an international training institute for Clubhouses, and varied supportive work projects.

The Fountain House model for recovery has been replicated in hundreds of places throughout the world. It is predicated on the conviction that those suffering with psychological difficulties can lead productive and meaningful lives in society. It advocates in its practices and in the wider world for those with mental illnesses to enjoy the same rights of self-determination, control, and choice that others have in their lives. Generally speaking, recovery refers to gaining the skills to manage one's illness so that the fullness of one's life is not unduly compromised. Rather than offering an understanding of schizophrenia as an incurable and lifelong disorder, Clubhouses are "built upon the belief that every member has the potential to sufficiently recover from the effects of mental illness to lead a personally satisfying life as an integrated member of society."[15] How recovery is defined and experienced will differ for each person, but it often includes gaining a greater sense of security, hope, social inclusion, empowerment, and meaningful life activities and commitments.

The Clubhouse Movement

Beginning in 1977, Fountain House launched trainings to help others establish Clubhouses. In 1994, the International Center for Clubhouse Development was begun. The Clubhouse model of mutual aid, supported by multiyear grants, has resulted in over three hundred Clubhouses worldwide, including ones in Canada, Denmark, Germany, the Netherlands, Pakistan,

Australia, Japan, Korea, Russia, England, Sweden, and South Africa. These are not necessarily work-day based and many do not include staff.

A remarkable consensual process was created to craft standards of practice:

> Rudyard [Propst] and the training unit at Fountain House set out to involve the entire Clubhouse movement in the creation of Clubhouse Standards. First, twelve very strong Clubhouses were asked to draft standards describing the essentials of a successful Clubhouse community. With these twelve drafts, a group of members and staff from Fountain House and several other strong Clubhouses met for a long weekend to merge, amend, and clarify the twelve drafts. By the end of that weekend, the group reached consensus on a set of draft standards.
>
> At the Fifth International Seminar on the Clubhouse Model, held in St. Louis in 1989, the draft document was distributed to all 600 participants who had the opportunity to discuss and debate the proposed standards. Changes were made to the document based on these discussions, and the revised draft was then sent out to all of the Clubhouses in the directory for comment. Agreement about the proposed 35 standards was virtually universal, and the International Standards for Clubhouse Programs were promulgated at the end of 1989.[16]

These standards serve as a bill of rights and code of ethics, covering membership, relationships, space, work-ordered day, employment, education, functions of the house, government, and administration.[17] Membership is voluntary and open to anyone with a history of mental illness.

Staff are members of the community. Relationships develop among members as they do in other workplaces, with an emphasis on encouragement, seeing and reflecting back strengths and abilities. Staff are sufficient in number to help members engage with activities while not being so numerous that members are not needed to carry out each function of the house. Staff are not there to treat or educate others. There are no separate staff meetings and no particular staff roles. All of the staff have generalist roles in the Clubhouse; they are involved in all of the Clubhouse activities including the daily work duties, evening social and recreational programs, employment programs, reaching out to absent members, supported education, and community support responsibilities. Members and staff share responsibility for the successful operation of the Clubhouse. Working closely together each day, members and staff learn each other's strengths, talents, and abilities. They also develop real and lasting friendships. Because the design of a Clubhouse is much like a typical work or business environment, relationships develop in similar ways. The staff are present to engage with members as colleagues in important work. Clubhouse staff are charged with being encouraging colleagues, workers, talent scouts, and cheerleaders.

Because the philosophy of the work-centered day focuses on "strengths, talents, and abilities," Clubhouses do not take on the treatment functions of a day center, which often includes medications and various individual and group therapies. Following on the needs and interests of their members, Clubhouses can provide a range of support and activities. Clubhouses offer transitional, supportive, and independent employment opportunities. Recognizing the importance of stable and safe housing, some Clubhouses provide assistance for securing housing. Supporting members in their desired education and helping each other access community resources for education are also roles of club members in relationship to one another. Helping individuals connect with community resources, such as medical and psychological services, is also a useful function of the Clubhouse. The opportunity to socialize in a safe setting can be treasured by people who have felt isolated and stigmatized.

Whether or not psychiatric symptoms recede, members can live their lives as fully as possible with friendship, understanding, and supports when needed. Clubhouses foster an egalitarian and democratic atmosphere where decisions are reached through respectful consensus, a place where each member feels valued for his or her contribution in creating the running of the Clubhouse. The choice of the term "Clubhouse" reflects how important membership and senses of belonging and inclusion are, particularly to those who have been deprived of them by virtue of stigmatization and marginalization. Clubhouses value shared ownership and shared responsibilities, making it possible for the space to belong to its members. There is a felt sense that one is always welcome.

The skills, talents, and creative ideas and efforts of each member are needed and encouraged every day. Participation is voluntary, but each member is always invited to participate in work, such as reception, food service, transportation management, outreach, maintenance, research, managing the employment and education programs, and financial services.[18]

Recovery Learning Communities and Fairweather Lodges

In both Clubhouses and recovery learning communities, there is a decisive shift away from seeing those with mental illness as patients in need of treatment to be accomplished by experts. Instead, members are recognized as people who can take charge of their own recovery process, supported by peers in recovery. Recovery learning communities embrace and amplify this shift and orient their work not around symptom management but around recovery. These communities create a partnership between mental health services and consumer-driven communities in order to help people have access to peer support, information, referral, advocacy, and training in recovery concepts and tools. They are not, however, oriented around a workday model, as Clubhouses are.

Recovery learning communities resemble Hull-House and other early settlement houses. Both kinds of communities affirm the dignity and capability of their members. Members decide together what their needs are and the issues they want to pursue. Attention to meeting members' needs, such as creating employment and housing opportunities, can result in members working across levels of organization to find success, engaging local, state, and federal resources and working to create changes in policies and practices that undermine their community's well-being. For example, the Southeast Recovery Learning Community in Hyannis, Massachusetts, announces their values as genuine human relationships, self-determination and personal strength, mutuality, optimism, healing environments, and respect.[19] The importance of social networks is affirmed, alongside a recognition that mutual relationships where both giving and receiving are present help to sustain members and their community. Members are reminded not to act "clinically" with one another. They are not divided into service providers and service recipients, while they may clearly be professional in terms of having been trained to be skillful at peer support. Members should not hold out one's own path of recovery as necessarily helpful to others. Each person should have the space to define recovery and to pursue and embody it on his or her own terms. Nevertheless, some centers offer resources that have been helpful to others, such as participation in the International Hearing Voices Movement, a movement that demedicalizes and destigmatizes the experience of auditory hallucinations and offers approaches to help people understand and manage their relationship to hearing voices. Such centers embrace self-governance and often have a peer advisory board. While not using the word "accompaniment," they emphasize being alongside and together, rather than subject to a hierarchy of expertise in which some people's knowledge is recognized or valued, often at the expense of others' remaining invisible.

One such community was founded in 1963 by psychologist George Fairweather and his colleagues, who explored the power of group and team membership for people with persistent and serious mental illness. At the Veterans Administration Hospital in Palo Alto, he organized psychiatric patients into work teams so they could gain experience in how to relate together to achieve their goals. They worked and ate together, forming relationships, becoming knowledgeable about each person's desires and skills, and developing leadership skills. When the patients were able to work smoothly together as a team, they were assisted to first house together on the grounds of the hospital and then in the community. Then they were supported to begin a business where each person had a meaningful role and a set of responsibilities. These living and working communities were called Fairweather Lodges. In them peers make decisions jointly for living and working. They create their own empowerment through assuming responsibility and sharing leadership. They support each other in their recovery as they share in household management.[20]

Fairweather advocated for creating new participative social statuses and roles, replacing misguided ideas that limited expectations of people's abilities and fates. Within each lodge a small society is co-created, at first with some support from outside but ultimately with fuller or full autonomy. Rather than be left to fit into normative work and living situations that are not conducive to their well-being, members utilize the structure of lodges to support the achievements of the group and individual goals. There are presently over ninety lodges in sixteen U.S. states.

Accompaniment by the Natural World

Once, and that was a few weeks after I came to the woods . . . for an hour, I
doubted if the near neighborhood of man was not essential to a serene and
healthy life. To be alone was something unpleasant. . . . In the midst of a gentle
rain while these thoughts prevailed, I was suddenly sensible of such sweet and
beneficent society in Nature, in the very pattering of the drops, and in every sight
and sound around my house, an infinite and unaccountable friendliness all at
once, like an atmosphere sustaining me, as made the fancied advantages of human
neighborhood insignificant, and I have never thought of them since. Every little
pine-needle expanded and swelled with sympathy and befriended me. I was so
distinctly made aware of the presence of something kindred to me, even in scenes
we are accustomed to call wild and dreary . . . that I thought no place could ever
be strange to me again.

—Henry David Thoreau[21]

I must acknowledge many other authors, including the goats, ducks, geese, dogs,
cats and other animals who have taught me a great deal about the joy and
spontaneity of authentic life free from the pettiness or evilness found sometimes
in the human world. Trees and plants have also been my great friends, especially a
giant oak tree which sheltered me during many difficult years when I felt
oppressed by alien schools and mean children. And the sagebrush-covered hills,
canyons, and the bare rocky desert gorges have also provided shelter, learning,
and the love of Mother Earth.

It is hard to be an Indian in the white world, but it is easy to be an Indian in
nature, because the Earth, the plants, the animals, and the winged creatures
provide companionship, love or just authentic spontaneity unmarred by hate,
jealousy or greed.

—Jack Forbes[22]

Jack Forbes, a Cree Indian, vividly describes how his culture's intimacy with nature provided a healing salve to the sufferings he endured due to racism. As I worked as a psychologist with people who suffered with diagnoses of chronic severe mental illness, I was moved to discover how some had learned in childhood to turn from the cruel circumstances they encountered at human hands to relationships with sheltering trees, freely flying birds, the welcoming water of lakes, and the faithful companionship of dogs. In the face of social exclusion, disparagement, and illness, they had been able to carry forward their childhood attunement to the natural world and find in their relations with it a sense of belonging and acceptance sadly unachieved in any reliable way with their fellow humans.

Feminist psychologist Mary Field Belenky and her colleagues studied how women in the United States come to know what they know. One group they reported on in *Women's Ways of Knowing* was composed of women who had grown up in abusive and strictly hierarchical families, families that taught their daughters to remain silent and undermined the girls' confidence in their capacity to think through ideas on their own. These families did not engage their daughters in dialogue but issued unilateral orders. There was a marked absence of pretend play, which rests on a foundation of dialogue. Women subjected to this kind of childhood often emerged as reticent, lacking in confidence, and not having the skills and experience to dialogically engage their own children. The authors noted exceptions, however. They were struck by how some women with this childhood background had emerged from "silenced knowing" into a capacity for dialogue and a sense of being able to reflect on their own thought process. One such exception was women who reported having had a significant relationship with a pet as they grew up. We know that children speak to their pets, and most experience their pets communicating with them, one way or another. Indeed, the dialogical rhythm one would hope for with a parent appeared possible with a beloved animal.[23]

Long before ecopsychology began in the 1980s, psychoanalyst Harold Searles wrote a path-breaking book, *The Non-Human Environment in Normal Development and in Schizophrenia*. He argued that while psychology and psychiatry devoted themselves to understanding the interpersonal and intrapsychic dimensions of our living, they had largely neglected the fundamental importance to human psychological existence of our relationship to the other-than-human world: "It is my conviction that there is within the human individual a sense, whether at a conscious or an unconscious level, of relatedness to his nonhuman environment, that this relatedness is one of the transcendentally important facts of human living."[24]

He was aware that many cultures and groups maintain and indeed revere and honor relationships with the beings of the natural world, and experience kinship with other-than-human nature. The benefits of being in nature-blessed settings were implicitly acknowledged in Western psychiatry for two hundred years, as many mental institutions built their facilities embedded in natural landscapes, some offering opportunities to garden and visit places of natural beauty.[25]

But for many, institutionalization deprived them not only of their freedom, sense of agency, families, and work possibilities but their neighborhoods, favorite places, and free access to the natural world of plants and animals, mountains, sky, and water. For still others struggling with mental illness, forced displacement from their neighborhoods and bioregions removes needed other-than-human companionship. Psychiatrist and urbanologist Mindy Fullilove accompanied David Jenkins, one of her patients, on a walk in the Philadelphia neighborhood of Elmwood where he spent the first eleven years of his life. By walking the streets of Elmwood with Jenkins, Fullilove became aware of how deeply we compensate for life's difficulties through the web of human and other-than-human relationships provided by the place of our neighborhood. Vicious scapegoating in his family and sexual abuse outside the family left Jenkins's sense of intimacy twisted and stunted. By contrast, the unrestrained love within the tight circle of the neighborhood gave him a sense of optimism that never deserted him. The enormous endowment of love he received from the neighborhood—"everyone tried to give me as much love as they could"— did not undo the curse put on him by his dysfunctional family. But it did create a buffer that prevented the abuse from becoming the entirety of his world. This buffer gave him reason to live while he healed as best he could.[26]

Many years later Jenkins could still point out on a map of his neighborhood where home cooking was to be found, where the roses grew that he

took to his teachers, the nearby marshland where the turtles and other animals he admired lived, and where the particular people were homed who
sustained him as he made his daily path. Jenkins's neighborhood was seized
for urban "renewal" and destroyed, causing the destruction of the natural
places he visited, dispersing across Philadelphia those who had loved him,
and utterly disrupting the nodes of gathering so important to cultural preservation, particularly of a people once enslaved and multiply displaced.[27]

Fullilove's work is a testament to all that is lost when people are required to disperse from the places that hold them:

> Root shock, at the level of the individual is a profound emotional
> upheaval that destroys the working model of the world that had
> existed in the individual's head. Root shock undermines trust,
> increases anxiety about letting loved ones out of one's sight, de-
> stabilizes relationships, destroys social, emotional, and financial
> resources, and increases the risk for every kind of stress-related
> disease, from depression to heart attack. . . . Root shock, at the
> level of the local community, be it neighborhood or something
> else, ruptures bonds, dispersing people to all the directions of
> the compass. Even if they manage to regroup, they are not sure
> what to do with one another. People who were near are too far,
> and people who were far are too near.[28]

We are potentially sheltered and accompanied not only by family, neighbors, and teachers but by rivers, parks, forests, and mountains, by our relations with animals, particularly pets. In these other-than-human relations, we
often discover a sense of belonging, of being part of a greater whole, held by a
web of natural interdependence. We can experience a lack of judgment on us,
indeed even a sense of acceptance and comfort. Although psychologists have
been slow to acknowledge these connections, each of us has significant emotional relationships with places, animals, and natural elements.

British psychoanalyst D. W. Winnicott underscored the importance
of experiencing moments of liveliness that can coalesce into our sense of
wanting to be alive.[29] Upon self-reflection, we can realize that many of these

critical moments are experienced in our relationships with both built and natural environments. This can happen when we experience a sense of aliveness from the beauty, awe, and strength of nature, as well as when we move in the liveliness of a familiar urbanscape. These relationships become partially constitutive to our sense of being alive and to our capacities to survive pain, disappointment, and anxiety.

In researching settlement houses, Catholic Worker houses, communities oriented around those facing intellectual challenges, and those dealing with mental illness, I have found that so many have relied on being situated in natural settings in the countryside. Some placed in the city have developed a rural arm so that community members can enjoy the benefits of rural life. Others have situated themselves there from the beginning. Farming, gardening, and walking in nature are clearly activities that can be conducive to psychological and physical well-being.

One such place is Gould Farm in Monterey, Massachusetts, founded by Will and Agnes Gould in 1913 for individuals suffering mental illness. It was the first therapeutic community in the United States. Will Gould believed that the countryside could contribute to a desire to live and a sense of belonging, particularly if it was interpreted to guests, "showing them where they fit into the scheme of things."[30] More recently in the Netherlands, Care Farms began in 1998 and offer social care for the mentally ill paired with agriculture.[31] Now there are more than 1,020 farms participating and over 10,000 clients.

In the U.S., Warrior Expeditions was founded by Sean Gobin in 2013 after he experienced the therapeutic value of hiking the Appalachian Trail after his return from military deployments to Iraq and Afghanistan. The tradition of veterans hiking the trail began with Earl Shaffer in 1948, who told a friend he was going to "walk off the war." Warrior Expeditions enables veterans to do long hikes on many trails, as well as long-distance paddles and bike trips. In addition to sharing their military experiences with fellow veterans and being greeted by veterans along the way, they are held by and challenged by nature.[32]

With these examples in mind, I want to propose the term "ecopsychosocial accompaniment" as an important corrective to psychological approaches that disregard the essential importance of our relationship to the other-than-human natural world. In chapters 8 and 9, we address mutual accompaniment between humans and other-than-human animals and between humans and the other-than-human natural world.

The Spectra of Accompaniment

When we experience being accompanied, we enjoy the feeling that there is a place for us on this Earth alongside others. This can make a decisive difference. Through the examples in this chapter, we can see that accompaniment occurs across several spectra. Accompaniment can occur between two individuals, within a small group, or among a larger community. The accompanier can be a member of the community where an individual, a group, or the whole community is being accompanied or can be from outside. While some accompaniment preserves a distinction between the helped and the helper, the served and the server—often for funding purposes— other practices of accompaniment live into the radical mutuality of accompaniment. These latter forms of accompaniment do not divide neatly in terms of pro bono or paid roles: some pro bono accompanists may not grasp and embrace the mutuality of accompaniment, while some within professionalized and remunerated roles do.

Across these spectra, psychosocial accompaniment, as I am defining it, is a practice that asserts the dignity, agency, and human rights of each and every participant and seeks to support full social inclusion when that is desired while also respecting that some may prefer to live and work within enclave communities. Psychosocial accompanists know that access to inclusion, human rights, and a diversity of employment and housing opportunities cannot be taken for granted. Indeed, given stigmatization and marginalization of those living with various disabilities, advocacy that includes policy and legislative struggle is necessary. This will prove both more difficult and more important in societies that are not committed to providing an adequate social net, societies that have not determined that all of their residents should have an adequate income, decent housing, and access to community life, healthcare, education, and employment.[33]

SEVEN

Pathways Through Mutual Accompaniment to Solidarity

[Accompaniment] means listening to each other, learning together, supporting each other on steep and rocky paths, rejoicing in community and mutual respect and commitment for a long journey.

It means living with people and sharing their lives and dangerous times. It occurs on many levels, always moving toward stronger solidarity.

—Debbie Grisdale and Wes Maultsaid

BUILDING SOLIDARITY WITH others to create beloved community is a slow, lifelong, and intergenerational process. Beyond simply showing up, it requires fundamental shifts in one's life priorities, values, and the risks one undertakes. It involves continuing education, always informal and sometimes formal. It certainly necessitates apprenticeship to cultural and ecological workers. Accompanists have the additional tasks of reflexively and critically examining their own complex positionality and developing openness and responsiveness to critical feedback they receive that better orients them in their relationships and work. This is particularly true for those accompanying people from communities other than their own, and even more so when they have access to privileges those they accompany do not. This chapter begins with a focus on this topic and then reflects more generally on education and apprenticeship for accompaniment.

Accompaniment from the Outside

Self-reflection is not a turn inward but a turn toward otherness.
—Kelly Oliver[1]

Those of us who have access to excess social and economic privilege have choices. We can segregate ourselves in a small corner of a sadly divided world, working to build our own personal security and happiness, relatively unconcerned with our lives' effects on others. Or we can live in a more inclusive, vibrant, and challenging world where relationships across differences attune us to the lives of others and where we seek to understand the effects of our living and the systems we participate in. In doing so, we can engage the struggle to understand how we can most meaningfully join in solidarity with others to co-create a more just, peaceful, free, and sustainable world. Accompaniment is a potential pathway to this second world. In this chapter, I want to describe some stepping-stones on the pathway from accompaniment to solidarity.

Unfortunately, efforts at accompaniment can easily go awry if the colonial framework of "helping," "charity," and "being of service" are not thematized and deconstructed. Too often, humanitarian, community, and psychosocial work occurs within the same structure of colonial relations that gives rise to a community's suffering in the first place. Hierarchical relations are mindlessly reproduced, ignoring or denigrating the knowledge of already marginalized community members. Interventions from the outside can displace and disable Indigenous approaches better suited to the particular local context. Ameliorative actions can neglect the deeper causes of distress, particularly those of systemic injustice. When this occurs, creative and transformative work that could have emerged from processes of dialogue and collaboration across differences in experience and knowledge is thwarted. Disempowerment of community members prevails, when outsiders' "solutions" are imposed without any knowledge of the particular site they are being applied to. Paulo Freire called this cultural invasion and contrasted it with cultural synthesis. In cultural synthesis, people "do not come to *teach* or *transmit* or *give* anything, but rather to learn, with the people, about the people's world"—there is a synthesis of worlds through efforts of mutual understanding.[2] In culturally invasive approaches, interpretations and interventions are imposed from the outside. Psychosocial accompaniment counters the cultural invasion of exporting diagnoses, treatment interventions, and research agendas to places around the world when they should not be universalized and imposed from positions of falsely presumed cultural supremacy. The orientation of psychosocial accompaniment requires that we be mindful of the power of each individual and group to construct meanings and to transform aspects of their world. The creativity and resilience of those accompanied and their own cultural resources for understanding, healing (if needed), resistance, and struggling for structural change should be honored and supported, not usurped, in accompaniment.

In addition to being collaborative and dialogical, efforts of psychosocial accompaniment must be tentative, systematically open to honest and critical assessment and feedback, and capable of revision. The stepping-stones described below delineate important shifts from colonial toward decolonial practice. They are drawn from experiences and understandings of many of the accompaniers described earlier in this book, my own experiences, my students' efforts in psychosocial accompaniment, and highlights of the work of Mark Potter. In "Solidarity as Spiritual Exercise: Accompanying Migrants at the US/Mexico Border," Potter presents a "spiritual phenomenology" of solidarity that is particularly relevant to accompaniers who enjoy wider societal privileges than those they accompany. As we move through this chapter, I introduce his "five movements of the spiritual exercise of solidarity," which help to cultivate the humility, courage, and honesty required for accompaniment.[3]

SHIFTING ORIENTATION: TURNING TOWARD AND
REVERSE OSMOSIS

The head thinks from where the feet are planted.
—Brazilian proverb

When individuals and communities experience an extremely difficult situation—acute or chronic—some people come to "lend a hand." Others fail to make themselves knowledgeable about the difficulties of the situation. Some know but ignore that knowledge. Others live in a psychic remove that pretends the difficulty does not exist, they are not implicated, and/or they could not do anything about it if they wanted to. Privilege, including white privilege, can operate to foster a remove from both knowing about and responding to the critical social and ecological realities of our time and their impacts on communities.

The initial insult and harm are redoubled by others' absence, and by their failures of acknowledgment and empathic concern. Accompaniment can be a needed—even if insufficient—antidote to the injuries caused by others' passive bystanding or active denial of the human suffering in their midst. While accompaniment cannot wipe away the pain born of traumatic injuries—individual or collective—it can begin to set into motion needed processes of psychic and social restoration through witness, support, and work to change the structural conditions that gave rise to the trauma.

For those born and educated into privilege, accompaniment may require a fundamental reorientation. Turning toward and moving alongside are necessary movements to orient the practice of accompaniment. Horizontality instead of verticality are the needed coordinates. First, to come alongside others expresses an acknowledgment of one's initial ignorance and of the need to learn at the side of others. Second, to position oneself horizontally communicates a desire not to undermine shared leadership from within a group, all too easy when one holds greater privilege and social power.

This reorientation involves developing counter-tropisms: to look at rather than to look away, to listen rather than to speak prematurely, to encourage and respect others' leadership rather than always assuming and asserting one's own. Accompaniers bring their presence to what is difficult, allowing it to affect them, to matter, to alter their course in life. This reverse osmosis, of intentionally moving across boundaries in the opposite direction of normative responses that bystand or move away from others' difficulties, is a clear mark of accompaniment.

A Brazilian proverb teaches, "the head thinks from where the feet are planted." It is also true that the heart feels where the feet are planted. Potter suggests that the "first movement of solidarity as a spiritual exercise" is to physically enter the context of those who request accompaniment. One may be entering "into a broken reality—the reality of suffering, the violence of poverty, the social context that is normative for the vast majority of people in our world."[4] He stresses the importance of moving one's bodily presence so that one can come into contact with those who suffer or are seeking support in the very place they are living their lives or waging their struggle. They are not asked to come to the psychologist's or social worker's office in a different neighborhood; the accompanist goes to them, moves alongside of them, offering his or her "hands."

Often accompaniers with more relative privilege experience themselves as crossing from the familiar and the comfortable into the unfamiliar and the unsettling. They begin to acclimatize themselves. They prepare themselves to respond. Dorothy Day, Jane Addams, and Staughton Lynd took the radical step of choosing to make their own personal homes in the neighborhoods where they were called to accompany. They were ready to answer knocks on their doors that brought neighbors with needs that required assistance. Staughton Lynd underlines that where we choose to live is an important decision. It is in a particular place, where we are already trusted and have ourselves becomes members of the community, that allows us to be of some use in crises.[5] In advising Quakers to live more deeply in the light of liberation theology, the Lynds offered, "If Friends are to address oppression and injustice, Friends need to encounter in a day-to-day manner the life situation of the poor and oppressed. If we can arrange where and how we spend our lives, giving time and energy, that may be more important than giving money. . . . [We] must be willing to go to out-of-the-way places and stay there for long periods of time."[6]

BEING INVITED

Of course, there are exceptions when a community requests that outsiders do not live with or even visit members. Being sensitive to whether or not one is invited and welcome is critical to an ethical practice of accompaniment. If an invitation has been extended, it is important to carefully clarify what it is for. There can easily be a collision between what accompaniers think they have come to do and what is actually desired.

Accompaniers patiently await a clear invitation to be present and remove themselves if this is not forthcoming. This should be non-negotiable. The accompanier must be transparent and honest as to the uses of his or her involvement, as to who will hopefully profit and how. Those extending an invitation should be able to do so in the fullest knowledge possible of who it is who wants to come and what their motives are. The members of the community must be free to participate with the newcomer or not, and free to ask that person to leave. When there is a conflict between the accomplishment of the visitor's goal (such as research) and the well-being of the participants and the community, the latter should be chosen unequivocally. For accompaniers, the accumulation of knowledge is not an end in itself. They ought to be aware that knowledge is for use and they must strive to be conscious about which uses it will be put to, making sure it is for the sake of the community and, possibly, for other similar communities.

For instance, facilitators of Alternatives to Violence Project workshops in prisons and communities require that participants freely choose to participate or not, and that they are not required by any governing body to attend. Accompaniment programs established to companion immigrants without documents in the United States similarly make their presence known to community members, offering their services but awaiting an invitation to accompany any particular person to his or her court proceedings regarding detention and deportation.

STAYING OR RETURNING HOME

There are legitimate reasons for people and communities to refuse accompaniment or to be particular about how and where it is to occur, if at all, and by whom. There are also legitimate reasons for choosing to carry out work of accompaniment right where one is already placed.

There is an ethics to meeting at the "border" to a community if one is from the outside. Zapatista autonomous communities in Chiapas, Mexico, are called *los caracoles*. They appeal to the image of the snail, *el caracol*, to explain the ethics of engagement they have created.[7] The snail has a flexible door-like structure at the mouth of the shell where exchange can happen. The interior of the snail's shell protects the intimate life beyond this doorway. These communities have created their own protective doorways where they are careful about who comes into their communities and for what purposes. Such clarity is not won easily. It grows out of centuries of resistance to colonial domination where others violently intruded into these communities with their own ideas of how people should live, what they should believe in, who they should obey, and whether they should even exist. "*Ya Basta!* Enough is enough," say the Zapatistas.

These Mexicans have learned from the unwanted intrusions of missionaries, anthropologists, paramilitaries, and others that the interior life of the community must be protected so its ongoing cultural life can be supported.[8] Visitors are required to make a formal request for visitation, specifying their reasons. If granted, they are told to stay out of the communities, to reside in carefully specified contact zones for visitors, for an agreed upon amount of time, so that the daily life of the community is not intruded upon.

One summer I was accompanying a human rights youth delegation that was invited for a week to visit several Zapatista autonomous communities in Chiapas. Our group members were educated about the needs of the community and set straight about what was desired of us and what was prohibited. We were asked not to offer any form of help in the communities themselves. We did not get a request to help in the fields, to teach English or computer skills, to assist with the cooking. Instead we were given a floor to sleep on, latrines and makeshift shower, ample beans and rice, language classes, and classes on Zapatismo. Then a mirror was lifted up for us so we could see ourselves through the lens of a single question they offered. Officers of the Buen Gobierno, the Good Government, asked us, "What struggle do you partake in, or will you partake in, having now understood more about how your situation in the U.S. affects ours?" The implication was clear: as U.S. citizens, the site of our struggle must be in "the belly of the beast," because it was our country that was most affecting their lives. Their concerns extended to the activities of the World Bank, the International Monetary Fund, the North American Free Trade Agreement (NAFTA), the bogus international conservation agencies on whose boards representatives from U.S. pharmaceutical companies sit as they make the appropriation of the Montañas Azules rainforest look like ecological safeguarding, and the U.S. Army School of the Americas (now the Western Hemisphere Institute for Security Cooperation) that trained the trainers of the paramilitary forces that attack the Zapatistas' villages. They pointed our attention back home, as though to say, "We have clarified our 'Ya basta!' What is yours? Around what issue or issues are you prepared to say 'Enough!' and then mobilize to change that situation?" There were moments when I felt that being asked to help harvest corn or teach English would have been a great relief!

The educators at the *caracoles* were pointing us back toward the center, but not to reside in its comforts, its repression of history, its sense of the future as a site for personal and corporate acquisition. They pointed us back toward it so that we could engage, interpret, and struggle with it with their communities' needs and concerns in our hearts. Indeed, the educators greeted us on our first day at the language class, saying that we had entered an anti-neoliberal zone, a rebel space where the heart would be opened, where we must learn to embrace our own rebelliousness in order to "make a world," as Freire put it, "in which love is possible."[9]

Community members from a nearby village asked to meet with us. They said they had never met any people from the United States, although many of their family members who had been forced to migrate had. As our day unfolded, they presented us with a specific request for accompaniment. They wanted our names, phone numbers, and addresses so that their relatives who had been forced to migrate to the United States for economic reasons could reach out to us if they were in trouble. This sincere request had a profound impact on me, leading me to reach out and work alongside my noncitizen neighbors in my home community to better understand and work to rewrite the immigration policies that make their lives precarious, and to accompany them in the midst of the threat of deportation.

Members of a group may find me at best irrelevant to their interests and goals. Or worse, they may have had experiences with outsiders that have led their community to fortify its borders in order to accomplish its work. Several years ago, when studying the proliferation of international walls built against those from a neighboring countries or region, I asked a community psychology program in Palestine if I might visit when in the region. Their program was the same age as mine, and I thought interesting collaboration could possibly evolve. An invitation was not forthcoming nor were clear reasons given for the refusal. Speaking to others more familiar with Palestinian struggles and reading the research of psychologists John Dixon, Kevin Durrheim, Philippa Kerr, and Manuela Thomae, I began to understand what might have happened. These scholars found that in places like Palestine, where oppression and injustice is ongoing, dialogue opportunities, while potentially encouraging prejudice reduction, can de-energize resistance and protest by diminishing "the extent to which social injustice is acknowledged, rejected, and challenged" by those affected by it.[10] They warn against the possible deleterious effects of pursuing elements of reconciliation such as prejudice reduction without prior or at least parallel success at achieving increased justice in areas like racism, classism, and sexism. Often the word "reconciliation" is a misnomer, because there has not been an established relationship that can be restored. One is actually building relationships for the first time. When efforts toward building relationships between members of an oppressor group and members of an oppressed group occur, the potential negative effect of such meetings need to be acknowledged and efforts taken to mitigate against this possible downside.

In sum, a person or a group may not be interested in dialogue with another group, or in being accompanied or witnessed. What some people need and want may diverge dramatically from how I have thought about my potential roles. Further, they may feel that their needs and wants may not concern me at all. They may not want to be "in dialogue." While potential accompanists may be aware of what they want to learn, they have not necessarily questioned whether others want to be in relationship and what their experiences have been of having people from outside their community come "to be in dialogue." Contrast this with those who seek witness, accompaniment, and solidarity.

For instance, because racial discrimination has created such severe and enduring economic and social hardship for communities of color in the United States, there is need for whites to become racial allies and help to disrupt racial injustice. Studying history as well as contemporary events, however, makes it clear why persons of color may distrust and exclude or only carefully and cautiously welcome whites. Worries about infiltration stand alongside weariness from "well-meaning" whites' performance of personal innocence and white fragility in the face of injustice.

Foundational Sensibilities and Capacities for Accompaniment

RESISTING UNCRITICAL REPRESENTATIONS, STEREOTYPES, AND PREMATURE IDENTIFICATIONS

Critical race and Indigenous studies scholar Eve Tuck cautions us that spaces where oppression has occurred can become "saturated with the fantasies of outsiders."[11] When we begin to accompany anyone, we bring our misconceptions, projections, and stereotypes, often misreading people and what is happening around us. To responsibly enter into and engage in the spaces of others, we need to enter a process of self-reflection, of psychic and relational *de*colonization. This effort of what Shawn Wilson calls "relational accountability" occurs in a historical time that has been deeply affected by colonialism and ongoing coloniality.[12] It is best not to think that it is possible to fully liberate oneself from the imposition of colonial relationships; rather, maintain a vigilance, an openness to critique, and a commitment to a path of trying to ever more deeply understand the effects of our own seeing and understanding on others. Alongside understanding, however, de-powerment, de-privileging, redistributing one's own resources, and committing to act for social justice are necessary correlates of relational accountability.

How we represent others can distort and narrow what we see and understand. bell hooks gives an example of this in her discussion of dominant cultures' representations of those who are "poor" as lazy, shiftless, and dishonest. In speaking of representations of the poor, hooks cautions us to resist normative representations of others that diminish them before we have even had the chance to meet them.[13]

Mary Annette Pember in "This November, Try Something New: Decolonize Your Mind" describes how many white people who seek her out as an Ojibwe do not want to hear about what she hopes to share with them: "the diversity of Native cultures, the complexity and history of federal policies affecting us, our sophisticated understanding of our relationship to the earth, or the fact that Native peoples embrace popular culture in addition to their own traditions." Instead, they speak of Ojibwe in the past tense and want to know how they can participate in ceremonies, dances, drumming, and spirituality. She writes, "They wanted me to give them Indian names, identify their power animals, and teach them how to be shamans. Mostly they just wanted to play Indian." Her white interlocutors too often stray into defining Ojibwe by their "plight" as seen by many white people. They also unreflectively offer idealizing representations, seeing Indigenous people as "supernatural noble, selfless defenders of the Earth." Pember laments, "Our cultures, traditions, and spirituality have been subsumed into the great buffet of American consumerism; we are food for hipster and New Age appropriation, one in the dizzying blur of passing social memes." Aware of missionaries' critiques of Ojibwe as wasting their time speaking with one another rather than being more productive in a Western sense, she ironically proposes that decolonizing our minds needs to begin with speaking with one another, getting to actually know one another. This would certainly need to include becoming aware of stereotypes, representations, and idealizations.[14]

Nigerian American writer Teju Cole describes the harm that whites can do when they use "helping" to feel good about themselves and neglect engaging needed complex understandings of the situations they are sentimentally addressing. Speaking of Nigeria, Cole critiques whites who focus on "hungry mouths, child soldiers, or raped civilians, [when] there are more complex and widespread problems. There are serious problems of governance, of infrastructure, of democracy, and of law and order. . . . Such problems are both intricate and intensely local." The problems should not be separated from the foreign policies of white U.S. "helpers," and, in particular, from the United States' hunger for Nigerian oil, despite the human cost to Nigerians, other-than-human animals, earth, air, and water. What I am calling psychosocial thinking, Cole names as "constellational thinking," arguing that racial privilege allows whites to deny the constellation of systemic causes in which they are complicit. Instead of indulging a sentimental need to "make a difference," Cole argues for "due diligence": doing no harm, proceeding humbly and with respect for the agency of the people around you. He cautions that activists and humanitarian workers need to become aware of how their actions may play into the hands of people who have more cynical motives. In particular, attention needs to be given to the role humanitarian aid can play in sustaining the status quo by relieving immediate pressure on the need for systemic change.[15]

Jordan Flaherty, in *No More Heroes: Grassroots Challenges to the Savior Mentality*, describes the savior mentality as wanting to help others but not being open to guidance from these very same people. The "savior" believes that others are helped more by him- or herself staying in the lead. The solutions saviors turn to are within the current system, even when that system is the problem, because the current system is the one that supports the privileges they do not want to interrogate. Flaherty counsels, "And, if people from the community you are seeking to support give you negative feedback, if you are a person in a position of privilege and feel 'called out,' don't act defensively. Don't be fragile. Listen, learn, acknowledge, and use the experience as an opportunity to change your approach."[16]

It is necessary for the accompanier to understand how easy it is to introduce both negative and positive distortions into relationships—through negative projections and positive idealizations. In idealizing projections, I experience either my ideal projections on another or choose only those aspects of that person's self-presentation that fit with my need to idealize. I avoid or am blind to the complexity and multifaceted nature of the ones I am idealizing. The latter was brought to my attention by several educators who work inside of prisons and who noted the tendency of some volunteers to valorize all those incarcerated, failing to appreciate the unique complexity of each person with whom they were working. Gay Bradshaw also points outs this potential tendency among trans-species accompanists. For instance, elephants may be valorized as "all-forgiving," when forgiveness is understood from a human experience perspective that may not take into account whether the concept of forgiveness is appropriate to elephant experience.

In accompanying we need to struggle to be aware of the stereotypes, positive and negative, that distort the personhood/being of others and seek these out, attempting to bracket them insofar as this is possible, to understand their history and functions and to refrain from projecting them. In doing so, we open a space to encounter another in his or her difference from the stereotypes we bring to the situation. This seems to be as true for trans-species relationships as for human relations. For instance, the demonization of wolves has led to murderous consequences for them in many locations.

In accompaniment, I try to open a space to encounter others in their difference from myself. I apprentice myself to them. I assume my experience and theirs may be quite different. I allow myself to be curious about these differences and cultivate a sensibility of humility, of interest and curiosity, of openness. I may discern commonalities of experience but check with these individuals to mitigate against assuming incorrectly, against projection.

We may begin a relationship noticing points of similarity, those aspects of another's experience that we identify with, that overlap with our own. This must be joined with a capacity to acknowledge that there is much about another that we do not know or understand, that is, we need to nourish our attentiveness to difference and to bearing not knowing, rather than reducing others to their similarities with ourselves.

One of the greatest psychic challenges is nourishing curiosity about what we experience as abject. Julia Kristeva in *Powers of Horror: An Essay on Abjection* describes abjection as

> an extremely strong feeling which is at once somatic and symbolic, and which is above all a revolt of the person against an external menace from which one wants to keep oneself at a distance, but of which one has the impression that it is not only an external menace but that it may menace us from inside. So it is a desire for separation, for becoming autonomous and also the feeling of an impossibility of doing so.[17]

Kristeva describes this as a situation where the other is experienced with fascination and horror, where their presence threatens not only from without but from within. I am scared by what I see of myself in the other that I find revolting in myself and cannot even recognize within myself. Attempts to remove oneself from what one experiences as abject by demonizing others or writing them off usually backfires. These others may not appear to me as full human beings, with feelings and needs that also require understanding. At times, they may not be admitted to my direct experience at all. At other times, they suffer what Albert Memmi calls "the mark of the plural," where all individuals within a group are attributed the same characteristics by me.[18] We may abject those whom we position as against our interests or values. In doing so, we fail to find common ground and claim our own intimate relations to those we keep at bay.

Philosopher Kelly Oliver importantly argues that "self-reflection is not a turn inward but a turn toward otherness."[19] There is much about ourselves that we can never understand with only an inward turn. We discover ourselves in and through our relationships, and particularly in relationships where we open to difference. At the fragile moments of meeting others and in our efforts to reflect on them, we need to be attentive to what we bring in advance of actually experiencing one another. For here we find ourselves as much—if not more—than we find who we are hoping to know more deeply. In accompanying accompaniers, there needs to be space made for claiming and unpacking these moments.

bell hooks underscores that "awareness is central to the process of love as the practice of freedom."[20] This love bears no resemblance to the sentimental. It is a critical love that identifies blind spots that perpetuate domination. When those we partner with experience us as open to their critical loving eyes, being "called out" can be transformed into being "called in." Indeed, embodying the capacity to accept and learn about oneself and others through critical feedback is necessary to deserving trust in relationships across the differences constructed by injustice and racism. Meeting the challenge of divesting excess privilege and working through the dominance that is an ingredient to coloniality makes it possible to enlarge the circle of the "beloved community."

RECOGNIZING AND UNDERSTANDING ONE'S OWN
POSITIONALITY AND PRIVILEGE

What is your own complex positionality with respect to dimensions such as race, ethnicity, class, gender, sexual orientation, nationality, religion, ableness? How does your positionality contribute to perpetuating structural injustice? How might accompaniment play a role in addressing this? How might your intersectionality create challenges and contradictions in your practice of accompaniment? What is the history and the power dynamics between the groups you belong to and those you may be accompanying? How does it affect attempts to relate to one another and to understand each other?

Martin Luther King, Jr., decried that "one of the great tragedies of man's long trek has been the linking of neighborly concern to tribe, race, class or nation. . . . One does not really mind what happens to the people outside his 'group.' Racial indifference and blindness—far more than racial hostility—form the sturdy foundation for all racial caste systems."[21] Michelle Alexander, author of *The New Jim Crow: Mass Incarceration in the Age of Colorblindness,* argues that it is whites' failure to care across color lines that "lie at the core of this control and every social caste system that has existed in the world."[22] Accompaniment can be an antidote to such caste systems if it is also linked to changes in daily living that question and give up undeserved privileges that continue to de-privilege others.

In her study of both white and African American settlement house workers in the first half of the twentieth century, Elisabeth Lasch-Quinn writes,

> While many of these reformers, regardless of color, began with a sense of superiority over those they were trying to help, the work itself often forced them to acknowledge the extent of racial discrimination and the ravages of racism and to begin to understand more fully the communities in which they worked. Settlement work was often a transforming and galvanizing experience. For those who worked among blacks, it could culminate in a realization that the problems of the neighborhood demanded

more than activities and services, but also agitation for wider change, which could even mean attempting to tear down the barriers of Jim Crow.[23]

The undoing of assumptions and feelings of superiority when they are present is a needed learning in those wishing to engage in accompaniment. Cross-racial and cross-ethnic relationships often help white activists see themselves from others' points of view. Robin DiAngelo describes how many whites exhibit what she calls "white fragility" when confronted about their racism or criticized by people of color. They are quick to take offense, have their feelings hurt, or respond with denial or anger, rather than take in the learning that is being offered about their attitude and/or behavior.[24]

Unfortunately, the often used term "ally" in social justice circles has proven to be a problematic one. It positions the ally as a member of the dominant group who is assisting people from a less privileged out-group. Those who think of themselves as "allies" may maintain positive images of themselves as helpers to those less powerful, while failing to interrogate and redress their own excess privilege. Social justice clinicians Lauren Mizrock and Konjit V. Page argue that the "ally role may designate the individual as an outsider to oppression, reducing the ally's awareness of being implicated in a system of inequality." Some pseudo-allies, they warn, may use their "ally" role to assuage their guilt, garner applause, and continue to assert patterns of dominance that disempower and offend those they are working with.[25] Members of Indigenous Action Media, a group that offers communications and direct action support for Indigenous communities, also offer a powerful critique of "allyship." They describe allies as most often providing only temporary support, too often romanticizing those they wish to "help," creating a dependency, and positioning themselves as saviors. Indigenous Action as an organization prefers to welcome those who are willing to be "accomplices," willing to commit a crime, to place themselves at risk, a person who "has our backs": "Accomplices listen for the range of cultural practices and dynamics that exists within various Indigenous communities. . . . Accomplices are realized through mutual consent and build trust. They don't just have our backs, they are at our side, or in their own spaces confronting and unsettling colonialism. As accomplices, we are compelled to become accountable and responsible to each other, that is the nature of trust."[26] We can also think of accomplices as co-conspirators, remembering that *conspirare* means to breathe the spirit together. The term "accompaniment" when used for outside accompanists is susceptible to many of the critiques of the term "ally." It is crucial that those who engage in accompaniment understand and experience it as *mutual*. The activity of accompaniment is for the accompanier as much as it is for anyone accompanied, because it is the expression of one's own commitment to living in a socially and ecologically just manner and doing one's part in creating a world where justice and caring mutual relationships can prevail.

MAKING ONESELF USEFUL

Psychosocial accompaniers understand that the violence—both direct and structural—and oppression to which people are subjected has torn the connective tissues that bind us together. If they can only offer one thing, it is to treat everyone with respect, reflecting back the preciousness and dignity of their lives. Accompaniment often entails showing up where others fail to come, at times when showing up conveys requested support and solidarity. Hopefully, the accompanier does not disappear or fall out of communication when staying is inconvenient, even dangerous. She or he is one who, once known, is most often invited in. He or she strives to be trustworthy and reliable.

But where do accompaniers begin in a situation that is not their own and about which they are belatedly learning due to their more privileged circumstances? Jane Addams recalled her uncertainty about how to begin and the "fellowship of the deed" that slowly developed as she began to respond to the needs of her neighbors: "From the first it seemed understood that we were ready to perform the humblest neighborhood services. We were asked to wash the new-born babies, and to prepare the dead for burial, to nurse the sick, and to mind the children." She argued that people involved in settlement work "must be content to live quietly side by side with their neighbors, until they grow into a sense of relationship and mutual interests."

Addams appreciated "the companionship" and "the give and take" of her fellow residents at Hull-House who had also moved to this part of Chicago. But, she warned, for relationships to evolve with their neighbors, she and her colleagues needed to be aware of "a constant tendency" to "lose themselves in the cave of their own companionship."[27]

LISTENING, LEARNING, SUPPORTING, WITNESSING

In accompaniment, others invite me to come alongside of them in the face of difficulties. I try as best I can to bear witness to their situation, feelings, thoughts, and realities. I share what access to resources I have that can be used for advocacy on their behalf, if they want me to. I struggle to be aware of possible differences in privilege and power, and seek to understand their historical origins and contemporary effects. I search for the roots of the conditions suffered, so that I can not only understand the psychosocial context but be better prepared to help transform it with others when desirable. I am open to what is needed from me. I may need to learn new skills, such as how to effect policy or help create connections with other groups undergoing similar challenges so as to enhance potential solidarity. I seek to be aware of the possible shadow of the idea and activity of accompaniment, and am open to feedback that contradicts my own impressions.

"Accompaniment" is a musical term. What can we learn from analogizing the extensive experience of musicians who accompany singers, dancers, and other musicians to accompaniment in communities? The musical accompanist must listen astutely and attentively to the unfolding song or melody or carefully watch the movements of the dancers. Usually the accompanist recedes from the limelight, taking a supportive role. He or she often plays in a lower pitch and sometimes does not play in the final performance. The accompanist provides the background for more important parts, supplying harmony and rhythm to the melody. One is successful to the degree that he or she is in alignment with the unfolding music and in good communication with fellow players. One exception to this necessary subordination occurs in what is called dialogue accompaniment, where the accompanier engages in a call and response to the "lead," being silent or providing rhythm as the lead plays, and playing her- or himself when the lead rests, but always playing in relationship to what has come before—not breaking free of the whole unfolding composition but working in concert with the featured musicians to articulate the evolving music.

Barbara Tomlinson and George Lipsitz, in speaking of accompaniment in American studies, import the practices of musical accompaniment into civic and scholarly work:

> [Accompaniment] means augmenting, accenting, or countering one musical voice with another. Harmonic and rhythmic accompaniments enhance melodic lines, but they also produce dialogues between melodies and countermelodies. A musician playing block chords augments the primary melody through a succession of chords that move in the same direction to the same rhythm. Sometimes accompaniment means *saying less so that others can be heard.* A drummer can play sparely and simply to make the bass lines more audible, while compositions played in stop time include breaks that make room for others to play solos. The dull and routine work of accompaniment can play a crucial role in enabling others to shine.[28]

Jane Addams resonated to musical metaphors, as I do with the word "accompaniment." She explained her preference for choral music like the Hallelujah Chorus in Handel's *Messiah* over "the music of isolated voices." She likened it to what a settlement house attempts to do. In both, the individual voices of the chorus "are lost in the unity of purpose . . . and are lifted by a high motive." In the case of the settlement house, the motive is "to develop whatever of social life its neighborhood may afford, to focus and give form to that life. . . . It receives in exchange for the music of isolated voices the volume and strength of the chorus."[29]

The one who accompanies knows how to resist leading when it is important that others do so. She or he values being alongside of others, working together, enjoying the mutual empowerment and greater understanding that arises when all partners are involved in knowledge-making and desired social transformations. This person has practiced holding plans and interpretations lightly, choosing instead to hear into the desires and meanings of others.

She or he resists performing expertism to the exclusion of others. The accompanist does not arrive to step on to the stage as a solo performer nor to deliver knowledge and "expertise" and then leave: to teach, advise, manage, and, perhaps, do research "on" or "about." This person does not assume unquestioningly a position in an imagined hierarchy above others.

When accompanists are not a member of the community in which the work is unfolding, they are not on their own ground. They join others on theirs—even if this is a temporary place such as a refugee camp. The command accompaniers may wordlessly exercise in their own offices, neighborhoods, and classrooms evaporates. They need to attune themselves to those around them, follow their intended melody, and lean into how they might support it.

Any plan we hold—however gingerly—should be subject to the critique of many voices and displacement by other strategies conceived together or conceived by community members without us. The accompanier requires not only an invitation but a practiced and certain humility. She or he develops a faith in what can arise from common efforts, rather than solely through his or her own expertise and efforts. The accompanist accepts the discomfort of critique. This does not mean that he or she has nothing to share, no chords to introduce. But the person needs to always be aware when she or he is joining the work of others to not mindlessly usurp the melody that is already under way.

Accompaniers have questions but also wonder what questions compel others' interest. They bring certain skills, like writing or producing videos, but wonder how others desire to make their experiences known, if indeed they do. An accompanier listens for the images and storylines that reach through and beyond words. He or she searches for the roots of feelings and symptoms, desiring a more complete understanding of the causes of the situations that give rise to suffering. This person makes a point not only to hear into the suffering being experienced but to witness strengths, beauty, and buoyancy, and to take part in and contribute to activities that feed the spirit.

He or she notes the assets, resilience, and creativity of others, as subtly as sensing their vulnerabilities, uncertainties, and needs. Accompanists do not need to position themselves as speaking for anyone, because they know others have their own voices and can request amplification if they need or desire it.

The accompanist is humble because much is unknown, but she is bold for the same reason, wanting to better understand and act with others as needed. For instance, Alice Lynd, like her husband, Staughton, was deeply involved in accompaniment. Rather than shy away from her legal expertise in her work with draft resisters she insisted that there were *two* experts in the room—a musical jam if you will.

Philosopher Kelly Oliver describes how our experiences of addressing and being responded to build our subjectivity. In situations of oppression and violence, we may experience the absence of any response. As a psychosocial accompanist, I listen as deeply as I can to the experiences people may want to share. But some experiences may surpass what I will be able to understand. I allow people's experiences to affect me even if it is disturbing to me, and I take care to reflect back what I experience and what I do not understand in the wake of the sharing. Witnessing, says Oliver, means both observing and testifying to what one observes *and* what one does not observe. She understands subjectivity to be dependent on the process of being witnessed: "Bearing witness to the other in the sense of testifying to that which cannot be known, observed, or completely understood requires a vigilance toward the other and a constant awareness of one's own limitations in recognizing the other. Unlike recognition, which maintains the mastery of the subject over itself and the other by presuming the primacy of the subject, witnessing admits that the other comes first."[30] Accompanists open themselves to the responsibilities and ethics of witnessing and work in solidarity with those with whom they have spoken. Upon hearing the testimonies of others, the accompanist bears the question of what his or her responsibilities are now that he or she better understands what has been experienced and suffered. For instance, are there people or groups who should know (with the permission of those who have shared)? Are there public policies and practices that need to be challenged and changed? Are there things the accompanier needs to learn in order to better address what has been heard and understood?

Shadows and Pathologies of Accompaniment

As we try to better understand what decolonial accompaniment might look like, we have also been describing its potential shadow: intrusion, entitlement, disempowerment, projection, stereotyping, diminishing. It is best to name these pathologies that may carry over from colonial relations. Hopefully, the accompanier realizes that she or he is not the only one doing the looking, the observing. Some of the descriptors applied to would-be accompanists traveling under a first-world passport are "fly-by-night humanitarian workers," "trauma tourists seeking disasters by deserted beaches," "trauma trophy academics," and "industrial white saviors." Some try to rebrand their vacations as generosity.[31] Indigenous Action Media holds up this mirror to would-be allies: "parachuters," "essentially missionaries with more funding," members of the "ally industrial network" or "establishment," "co-opters," "savior allies," and "action junkie tourists." These labels bespeak the harm created by too-frequent failure by would-be accompanists to take the time to deeply enough understand the situation being suffered, to examine their own relationships and the relationships of their country or group to the problem, and to make an enduring commitment to a community under stress. Instead, frameworks and interventions derived from one cultural location are thoughtlessly applied to another location. These phrases also speak to the need for soul-searching about who such work is for, and whether the potentially self-serving nature of it has been disguised.

There is an apocryphal tale told by Subcomandante Marcos of the Zapatista Movement in Chiapas, Mexico. He says he carries in his backpack a single pink high-heeled shoe that was donated to the Zapatistas. For him this is a symbol of how out of touch people can be with the true needs of the Zapatista communities, and how self-serving supposed acts of generosity can be. Cleaning one's closet of useless items stands in for empathic understanding and relevant action in solidarity with others.

Hopefully, accompanists wonder how they are seen and are willing to discover things unimagined about themselves—or only feared. Of course, what privilege they enjoy is not invisible, far from it. By leaving their comfort zones, they may find that what they have taken for granted about themselves and their lives are thrown into question. They may feel shame, guilt, and embarrassment. They risk a rupture of their own certainties.

Etienne Roy Grégoire and Karen Hamilton adopt Foucault's understanding of reflexivity as thought that questions the very ground upon which one thinks, that attempts to discern where one is located within webs of power. Like Foucault they differentiate between arterial and capillary power, between overarching power structures and diffuse relations of power in on-the-ground daily relationships. Following Foucault's analysis of power, they argue that accompanists protecting human rights activists imperiled by state actors are better prepared to understand the large-scale power dynamics, the arterial level, that they are acting within, for example, the Guatemalan government, the international community, and the Inter-American Court of Human Rights. By contrast, when accompanists are involved in more local conflicts, the capillary level of diffuse power relations is difficult to understand. No longer conducted on the stage of state power, accompanists find it hard to read the conflicting and contradictory identities of the people they are living among with regard to past and ongoing violence, and thereby have a limited understanding of how their presence is actually affecting a given situation. Grégoire and Hamilton, following Stanley Cavell, suggest that accompanists take a more agnostic approach to these local situations in which they accompany so that they do not distort and misunderstand them.[32]

Such efforts at reflection and reflexivity do not necessarily end in accompanists' abandoning their protection and going home, though sometimes this may be the case. Rather, they are able to trade an untroubled sense of their own identity and privilege for a more realistic, complex, and nuanced one. This new view better enables them to understand how those they accompany experience their presence and their role. They become clearer about whether or not their potential to reinforce hegemony is outweighed by the immediate protective effects of their presence.

The example in Box 7.1 illustrates how protective accompanists are struggling to use reflexivity and positionality to understand how they are using their privilege, what the contradictions are in such accompaniment work, and how they and the work of accompaniment are understood by those being accompanied.

Box 7.1 International Nonviolent Protective Accompaniment

Your country has sent us dictators and marines, war and oppression. I never imagined that I would see what I saw tonight—a busload of *cheles* [light-skinned people] arriving in Cárdenas just to touch us, to suffer with us, to accompany us in this struggle. Tonight our peoples touched each other as human beings. Whenever you want to bring people such as these to Cárdenas, they are welcome.

—Frente Political Secretary for Cardenas, official Frente Sandinista de Liberación (FSLN) representative in Nicaragua

Without accompaniment, I would not be alive today.

—Amilcar Mendez, Mayan human rights worker, 1990 winner of the Robert F. Kennedy Foundation Human Rights Award

The practice of international protective accompaniment began in the 1980s when members of Witness for Peace and Peace Brigades International offered their presence in Nicaragua to help protect communities in danger from the U.S.-supported war against the Sandinistas. Thousands of church members from the United States joined delegations to travel to Nicaragua to learn firsthand about the Nicaraguans' struggles for peace and justice. When they returned home, they formed part of a powerful lobby against U.S. foreign policy in Central America.

Peace Brigades International began to accompany activists and civil society organizations operating in Guatemala, often under death threat.[a] Since the early 1980s, approximately a thousand volunteers from twelve countries have accompanied human rights activists, refugees being repatriated from Mexico, and victim witnesses. The accompanists hope that by making the local situation known to the international community, the latter will help to deter violence by the threat of imposing sanctions and condemnations. Accompanists help to increase the political action space in which local activists can work while decreasing the impunity of local actors who threaten the activists' work. Accompanists witness and report, making violent actions visible to civil society and the international community. Violent actors—paramilitary or state-sponsored—are usually not looking for witnesses of their atrocities and international condemnation. They tend to back away when there is international presence. Other functions of accompanists include encouragement, solidarity, and the legitimizing of human rights activities.[b] The daily life of accompanists can include "escorting human rights defenders; living in communities of displaced people; meeting with the military or civilian authorities; observing a demonstration, checkpoint, or road-block; launching an international alert; writing a report; or simply cleaning a house."[c]

Subsequent accompaniment teams have worked in El Salvador (1987–1992), Sri Lanka (1989–1998), Colombia (1995–present), Haiti (1995–2000), Indonesia (1999–2010), Mexico (2001–present), and Nepal (2005–present). Since 1993, Christian Peacemaker Teams have been working in Haiti; the same group later established accompaniment teams in Hebron, Palestine; Chiapas, Mexico; and Kurdistan, Iraq.[d] Currently there are twenty-four organizations doing international accompaniment in twelve countries.[e] Thousands of human rights workers, grassroots organizations, and communities have been offered some protection over the last three decades through this grassroots peacebuilding strategy.[f]

For the past twenty years Colombian "peace communities" (also known as "humanitarian zones" and "communities for dignity and life") have been resisting armed struggle and displacement from their land. They have welcomed accompanists from a variety of groups. The presence of international accompanists, particularly from the United States, often deters paramilitary and government-sponsored attacks on human right workers and villages in nonviolent resistance.

Accompanists are careful to establish relationships with their congressional representatives, on whom they rely to help them communicate with generals in charge of a specific geographical location. Once accompanists return to the United States, they are vocal against U.S. policies that support the ongoing violence. Their firsthand knowledge of the grassroots situation in a given country has made them powerful spokespersons for developing solidarity movements.

---

a. Liam Mahony, "The Accompaniment Model in Practice," *Fellowship* 77, nos. 7–12 (Summer 2013): 12–16, http://archives.forusa.org/fellowship/2013/summer/accompaniment-model-practice/12385.

b. Liam Mahony and Luis Enrique Eguren, *Unarmed Bodyguards: International Accompaniment for the Protection of Human Rights* (West Hartford, CT: Kumarian Press, 1997).

c. Mahony, "The Accompaniment Model in Practice."

d. Ibid.

e. Colombia, Guatemala, Honduras, Nicaragua, Mexico, First Nations territory in North America, Palestine, Kurdistan (Iraq), Mindanao (Philippines), Sri Lanka, Nepal, Sudan.

f. Sara Koopman, "Making Space for Peace: International Protective Accompaniment in Colombia," in *Geographies of Peace,* ed. Fiona McConnell, Nick Megoran, and Philippa Williams (New York: I. B. Tauris, 2014), 109–130.

Claiming One's Own Spiritual "Poverty"

Decolonial philosopher Nelson Maldonado-Torres confronts us with the fact that "colonialism creates a reality in which some subjects become privileged givers while others do not even have bread to eat or to give."[33] Working toward a decolonial future requires us to look behind the curtain of this seeming beneficence to understand how the lives of those who have the privilege to give are implicated in the structures that reproduce need and suffering. This necessitates both a historical understanding and a bold attempt to claim one's own spiritual poverty.

Mark Potter draws on the work of Jesuit theologian Jon Sobrino. Sobrino escaped assassination in 1989 when he was away from his residence in El Salvador, the residence where Ignacio Martín-Baró and five other Jesuits, their housekeeper, and the housekeeper's daughter were murdered by a U.S.-trained paramilitary death squad. From his reading of the *Spiritual Exercises* of Saint Ignatius of Loyola, Sobrino believes that solidarity could potentially be a spiritual practice that can engender mutual transformation. Honoring and living into liberation theology's preferential option for the poor, the practice of solidarity is not a selfless act for others characterized as "poor."[34] Rather, the spiritual poverty and indifferent remove of those who live on islands of affluence is challenged, leading to a potential for self-transformation from an isolated "I" to a self-in-solidarity-with-others.

Many accompanists from affluent origins who have grown up amid pervasive individualism, competition, and secularism are struck by the community-minded spirit and love of those they accompany. For instance, noticing the richness of spiritual experience and practice; the integration of music, poetry, and art into daily life; or loving modes of raising children and taking care of elders may provoke a profound sense of shame at the "poverty" in one's life amid affluence. It may also lead to the accompanier's realizing more fully the paradox of "service" and "reverse service": that often it is the people who began hoping to be of some help who are deeply helped themselves.

In addition, enjoying affluence in the midst of other people's pervasive and unsatisfied needs can sow seeds of shame. One way of dealing with this potential experience is to fail to interact with those whose lives are marked by struggling with injustice. Another is to engage feelings of shame, to learn and work with them, allowing them to have a transformative impact on one's life's orientation.

Philosopher, theologian, and priest Ignacio Ellacuría, one of the Jesuits assassinated along with Martín-Baró, rejected embracing "the accumulation of capital as the engine of history, and the possession-enjoyment of wealth as the principle of humanization."[35] He contrasted a competitive and individualistic culture that has as its aim accumulation of capital—a culture marred by arrogance, greed, and a propensity to use violence to achieve and retain power—with cultures of solidarity where the meeting of everyone's basic needs is a primary and foundational goal.

The accompanying relationships developed between the non-poor and the poor in a time of dizzying income divides can be a living protest to the centrifugal processes set into motion by transnational corporate globalization. To place oneself in proximity, alongside those abandoned in what Chris Hedges calls "zones of sacrifice," is to enter into conversation that rejects a vertical ordering of relationship, that seeks to metabolize the feelings of shame that arise through restorative action, and to reorient one's life to honor what one has come to understand.[36] Such a model clarifies how accompaniment can serve the ones who set out to accompany, and by virtue of their encounters with others become clearer about how to seek greater integrity in their lives through committed solidarity. For white people in the United States, such accompaniment should necessarily involve grappling with not only the systemic issue of reparations—to African Americans for the crime of slavery and continuing racial discrimination, and to Native Americans for the crime of genocide and displacement—but also the forging of multiple grassroots reparations.

The Role of Reintegrative Shame: Aligning Our Actions with Our Understandings

Confronting, instead of quickly covering, an experience of shame as revelation of oneself and of society—facing "actual life"—requires an ability to risk, if necessary to endure, disappointment, frustration, and ridicule. Commitment to any position or to any loyalty, like commitment to another person, involves the risk of being wrong and the risk of being ridiculous. It is relatively easy to take even difficult

action if one is sure one is right, that one has grasped the truth of a situation; it is
relatively easy to entertain multiple possibilities of truth and of right action if one
remains a spectator on the sidelines. Far more difficult than either is to give
everything one is in supporting all the truth one can see at any given time, with
full awareness that there are other possibilities and that further knowledge may
enlarge and revise the hypotheses on which one has risked everything.
Engagement with life and with history—self-discovery and further discovery of
the world—has always involved just such risks.

—Helen Merrell Lynd[37]

Accompaniment is a risky endeavor and best undertaken with an acceptance of likely failures and feelings of deserved shame. Shame, however,
can be generative. I distinguish deserved from undeserved shame.[38] Sometimes we are made to feel undeserved shame by things that happen to us,
for instance, being raped, growing up in poverty, being disparaged for our
skin color. At other times, we do or do not do something that causes us
to feel grave disappointment in ourselves. Perhaps we did something with
one intention and find that grievous unintended consequences resulted,
and we are suffused with shame for our inadequate forethought or understanding.

In most Western cultures, people have been taught to avoid feelings of
shame. To do so, many of those who can, segregate themselves from situations that would generate feelings of deserved shame. Throughout the
world, normalized practices of segregation insulate those with relative privilege from feelings of deserved social shame. This insulation increases what
philosopher Christopher LeBron calls "moral disadvantage."[39] For instance, one may—if white—espouse liberal values that uphold the equal
worth of people in the United States at the same time that one's actions
betray a failure to create meaningful relationships and necessary political
solidarity to bring these values into daily reality. Internally, one suffers a lack
of moral integrity that effaces one's existence.

In some Eastern cultures, shame is recognized as a noble emotion and
as a gateway to compassion. It is recognized as a necessary emotion for
helping us live lives of integrity. Feelings of deserved shame, if recognized
and allowed, can be potent messages regarding the reorientation necessary

to rejoin one's life path, that path that expresses an integration of what we know and feel with how we live and how we act.

Potter, building on Sobrino's thought, stresses that through inward attention, the non-poor accompanier may experience a "double humility" that quickens appropriate feelings of shame. The first humility, Potter says, is one of association, where one's proximity to people who live closer to death places one into more intimate relationship with one's own vulnerability and insecurity. The "second humility," he says, "is the realization that one has somehow been responsible for causing or exacerbating the suffering of others," through action or inaction and inattentiveness: "In this sense, the scandal of the poverty and suffering of another—that which threatens their dignity and humanity—indicates a grave deficiency in my own human dignity that I have been complicit in the dehumanization of others. In other words, my encounter with the consequences of sin experienced by others makes me much more aware of my own sin." In the formation of relationships across the border between poor and non-poor, both parties confront the ways in which oppression and domination cut across our experiences. "The sin of one's suffering," says Potter, "is directly related to the sin of another's active complicity or indifference."[40] Potter describes how facing into this understanding can entail a period of profound desolation for the non-poor. Some can be fearful of the wrath of the poor. Indeed, some poor may be understandably angry and resentful regarding the condescension, violence, and greed of the non-poor.

Potter argues that through a combination of the non-poor's willingness to help shoulder the burdens of the poor, the poor's generosity, and grace, a relationship can be born that may bear forgiveness and acceptance:

> The non-poor receive from the poor a new horizon in which to understand their responsibilities to participate in the transformation of the social reality that separates them, and a consciousness of why they so desperately need the humanizing influence of the poor to overcome their own sins. In short, they experience and learn the truth of the phrase, "We need each other," and experience without fear or misunderstanding the truth of the claim that "apart from the poor there is no salvation."[41]

Australian criminologist John Braithwaite introduced the concept of reintegrative shame in 1989. For shame to become reintegrative, first one needs to separate the shameful action from the totality of the person, denouncing the offense but not the offender. Second, one needs to create a focus on a path where the person can change the kind of action that created shameful results. This may include expressions of remorse and apology but also needs to extend to significant shifts in behavior. These may include restitution and reparation. Attention to reintegrative shame enables relationships to take stock of where harm has been created and to relationally change in the future the courses that led to this, reintegrating the offender into a more generative pathway of living.[42]

As Dorothy Day reoriented her life to live with previously homeless people, she was exposed more intensely to her own sense of shame. She shared that she and other Catholic Workers were "constantly overcome with a sense of shame because we have so much more than these others [who come in the morning to eat with us]."[43] It is clear that her ego-ideal was the poverty of Christ. Attention to her shame helped to embolden her stance of voluntary poverty and her commitment to living with and alongside the poor. This choice of voluntary poverty was a pathway to her own sense of integrity, led as she was to live in opposition to the pernicious separations created by capitalism. Jane Addams also rejected living a life shut off from the experiences of people outside her immediate class. She felt that such a wall would separate her from her own abilities and intelligence. Here inner and outer integrity become one.

Helen Merrell Lynd, psychologist and mother of historian-activist Staughton Lynd, emphasized the importance of shame in helping to reveal to us the ideals we hold for our long-term life purposes and goals. These may include not only actions but ways of being. Helen Lynd borrowed from the work of Gerhart Paris to emphasize that feelings of guilt arise when one transgresses a societal boundary, whereas shame suffuses us when we fail to reach a deeply held goal. Shame, she advanced, "confronts one with unrecognized desires of one's own and the inadequacy of society in giving expression to these desires." It thus, she continued, "indicates a real 'shortcoming'": "Shame interrupts any unquestioning, unaware sense of oneself. But it is possible that experiences of shame if confronted full in the face may throw an unexpected light on who one is and point the way toward who one may become. Fully faced, shame may become not primarily something to be covered, but a positive experience of revelation."[44] Lynd was particularly interested in shame that comes in situations where we have fulfilled societal norms and expectations but failed our own conscience and our higher aspirations for living. In these instances, shame reveals crucial insights into our society as well as ourselves.

Psychosocial accompaniment almost inevitably awakens feelings of deserved shame in "outside" accompanists, feelings that when metabolized can become generative. This inevitability issues from what "psychosocial" means. The one who accompanies from the outside in a psychosocial manner has learned to see—to better understand—structurally the social misery they are witnessing. It is clear to them, as Jon Sobrino puts it, that "poverty results from the actions of other human beings."[45] For this reason, psychosocial accompaniment is a gateway to conversion to the accompanier becoming a neighbor.

Mutual or Reciprocal Accompaniment: Co-Liberation

If one is sensitive to learning from others, one will discover our liberations are codependent. With an intentional and practiced generosity, feminist Chicana writer Gloria Anzaldúa has worked against a politics of exclusion and toward a visionary inclusivity. She invites white people in, knowing that in time they will find that they are not "helping," but "following our lead." The accompanier becomes accompanied. Anzaldúa argues that Anglos and Chicanos are "implicated in each other's lives," that they leak into each other, taking on the attributes of one another. "So we are really neither one nor the other; we are really both."[46] She practices what radical relationship coach Mel Mariposa calls "calling in" whenever possible. Calling in holds someone accountable and invites that person to do better. It rejects a reactive dismissal of someone with some shared values but rather encourages active listening to build mutual understanding. By contrast, calling out is a one-sided declaration and critique of others regarding how they have fallen short that offers little hope for their change. It has a performative aspect that can be shaming and outcasting.[47]

When poor and non-poor live and work alongside one another, Mark Potter says, they may codiscover that their "salvation depends upon one another," and that their transformation can occur through relationship with one another.[48] Staughton Lynd arrives at the same conclusion: "What would it do to this discussion to say that we are all accompanying one another on the road to a better society?" He continues, "'Accompaniment' is simply the idea of walking side by side with another on a common journey. The idea is that when a university-trained person undertakes to walk beside someone rich in experience but lacking formal skills, each contributes something vital to the process. 'Accompaniment' thus understood presupposes, not uncritical deference, but equality."[49]

For Lynd—as for Dorothy Day and Jane Addams—accompaniment is understood as a reciprocal process: "I do not organize you. I accompany you, or more precisely, we accompany each other. Implicit in this notion of *'accompanando'* is the assumption that neither of us has a complete map of where our path will lead."[50] The accompanier often feels directly accompanied by members of the community with whom he or she is working. Many times, however, accompaniers also need and request the accompaniment of someone or others outside of the situation. Jean Vanier built this kind of outside group of accompaniers into L'Arche's houses of hospitality. While many groups that provide accompaniment attempt to address self-care, the need for support continues.

It is possible in our meetings to experience the sacredness and dignity of each other. This is not a matter of an idealizing projection but of grace, and it is most often linked with the emergence of love and an attitude of respect and caring.

Education for Accompaniment

Because accompaniment can occur in many different contexts and locations, education and mentorship that supports it will vary accordingly. The education for peacebuilding accompanists, for instance, is different from that for environmental justice advocates. There are, however, some general principles to consider for those who wish to accompany. This section draws together some of the lessons learned in previous chapters, while also reflecting on supportive curriculum, community apprenticeship, and mentorship. Education for accompaniment can occur both in academic institutions and directly in the community from cultural workers. Accompaniment does not require professionalization, though it need not be incompatible with it, as long as the latter does not inculcate colonial patterns of superiority and dominance.

LENSES FOR ACCOMPANIMENT

Historical

Accompanists learn to see the situation they are addressing in its historical context. This is necessary so that symptoms observed in the present can be traced to their structural and historical roots. For instance, by seeing the growth in incarceration of people of color in the United States through the lens of history, Michelle Alexander, author of *The New Jim Crow: Mass Incarceration in the Age of Colorblindness*, was able to understand it as one more expression of a racial caste system present in America from its inception and early embrace of slavery.[51] The growth of the prison industrial complex during the "War on Drugs" was not about containing increasing rates of crime but reflected the use of the criminal justice system for racial control. I accompany a few of those incarcerated via cofacilitation with Alternatives to Violence groups, a program designed by inmates and Quakers in the aftermath of the 1971 Attica Prison uprising. Many of the African American men in these groups were arrested for small amounts of drugs during drug searches in their neighborhoods. Although the prevalence of drug use was equivalent in neighborhoods of color and white neighborhoods, the increased police presence and surveillance of neighborhoods of color resulted in appreciably more arrests there. Many of these men have no record of perpetrating violence, although many have suffered state and prison violence. Knowing the history of racialized incarceration in the United States enables me not to see the men coming to such a program as necessarily dealing with their own history of perpetrating violence, though some clearly are, but of trying to learn strategies for resisting the violence of prison. Many are also committed to passing on tools for nonviolent relationships to their children, with whom they struggle to remain in contact despite the many obstacles in their way.

After two decades of teaching liberation psychology in a graduate psychology setting, I am a firm believer that to responsibly teach psychology, counseling psychology, and social work, we must engage our students in a study of history. This allows us to understand the difficulties of the present in their wider sociocultural context and to think critically about the particular discipline we are working within. As we endeavor to create and embody decolonial psychosocial and ecopsychological practices, we must ground ourselves in an understanding of the history of colonialism and its present-day embodiment in neoliberal power and practices. Students need to develop an understanding of psychology's complicity with colonial relations and practices. U.S. students need to understand the five hundred years of worldwide colonialism that have brought us to this historical moment, while learning in detail about settler colonialism and slavery in America, the effects of U.S. imperialism, and the development of internal colonies throughout the United States. This historical understanding clarifies the relative failure of psychology to deviate from individualism as its rooting paradigm, and thus its failure to conceive of the individual within a fully delineated historical, psychosocial, and environmental context.

Ameliorative and Transformative Lenses

Without understanding the wider historical context of the difficulties we witness, much of the work of helping professions consigns itself to ameliorative approaches. Critical community psychologists Isaac Prilleltensky and Geoffrey Nelson have clarified differences between ameliorative and transformative approaches.[52] While both are concerned with promoting well-being, they often do so differently. The ameliorative approach, as they define it, focuses on various interventions at the personal and relational levels, emphasizing values of holism, care, and compassion. The transformative approach engages people in a collective level of analysis, seeking to understand

and affect the root causes of affliction. It focuses on eliminating oppression and unjust power differentials while embodying and enacting values of social justice, interdependence, collaboration, egalitarianism, and solidarity. The transformative approach strives for collective and systemic change through collaborative partnerships and community participation. In Prilleltensky and Nelson's intervention processes, these partnerships aim for "conscientization, power-sharing, mutual learning, resistance, participation, supportive and egalitarian relationships, and resource mobilization."[53]

When enhanced well-being is understood through the lens of power, possible outcomes delineated by Nelson and Prilleltensky include "increased control, choice, self-esteem, competence, independence, political awareness, political rights and a positive identity; enhanced socially supportive relationships and participation in social, community, and political life; the acquisition of valued resources, such as employment, income, education and housing; and freedom from abuse, violence and exploitation. Outcomes at multiple levels of analysis that emphasize power-sharing and equity are in the foreground."[54]

Psychosocial accompaniment includes both attention at the individual and relational levels but, like transformative approaches, seeks to understand and address systemic causes of suffering. Through seeing with a wider historical lens, psychosocial accompanists do not reduce the difficulties a person faces to the individual level of analysis but neither do they neglect the needs of individuals and communities who are presently afflicted. Refugee communities, for instance, may seek accompaniment to get help meeting immediate needs. At the same time, such accompanists may be involved in advocating at policy and legislative levels for refugee rights while engaging in interventions that could affect the need for forced migration. The examples offered in this book point to a spiral pathway between individual and community care and transformative efforts to affect the systems that cause unjust sufferings. Each of the accompanists focused on in these pages gave attention to individual and relational well-being but also struggled to learn about the systemic causes of the difficulties people suffered, entering into collaborative partnerships to change or introduce laws, policies, and alternative practices that could create a more just system.

In mentoring students in their cultural and ecological work, it is important to challenge them to see the issues they are working with at various levels of organization. Each student may have a level of organization that principally informs their work and at which they feel personally comfortable working. Nevertheless, that level can be informed through an analysis of the problem at various other levels. Such analysis often catalyzes more effective action that seeks long-term transformative change.

For example, I am working with several groups who accompany immigrant families caught in the United States' deportation pipeline. A family member may have a pressing need for a forensic psychological evaluation to help a lawyer show to the immigration judge the extreme hardship this person's deportation would cause to family members who are citizens. Such evaluations are steeped in individualistic and medical model thinking. Yet reports like these can make use of such a format to convey the human dimensions of an immigrant's story. In the course of our conversations to accomplish such an evaluation, we see the need for psychological support, as each family member suffers in his or her own way the precarity of the family situation. Their narratives point to wider and shared issues such as unjust working conditions, U.S. racism and xenophobia, and poverty. Seen in historical perspective, the United States has a tragic history of exploiting foreign workers without sufficiently offering legal status, equitable wages, and dependable workplace safety. This creates an always expendable underclass that contributes more than they receive from the society. The provision of support through accompaniment—and possibly sanctuary—in cases of imminent deportation are inextricable from needed advocacy for immigration reform and work toward the achievement of fundamental human rights.

Using a Freirean model of analysis, community fieldwork students and cultural workers can clarify the work that needs to be done at each level of analysis around the issue they are attending to in order to achieve both amelioration and transformation: the psychological, familial, school, neighborhood, town/city, bioregional, national, international. Such an analysis facilitates strategic networking with those working on the same issue at different levels of organization. Accompanying a single person facing deportation can be linked to family accompaniment, work to end detention facilities and the criminalization of immigrants, broad national immigration reform, international efforts to increase capacity for care of forced migrants, and multiple approaches to addressing the issues that cause forced migration from particular locations.

Strength-Based Versus Damage- and Deficit-Centered Lenses

Unfortunately, human services agencies and providers have too frequently peddled damage- and deficit-centered narratives of the people and communities with whom they work. In addition to the racism that can be an ingredient to such narratives, there also may be self-serving and self-perpetuating motives, conscious and unconscious. As they are currently configured, "helping" professions are dependent on addressing the "needs" of their clients. Seeing others principally through their needs is a highly distorting lens. Such a lens constructs the other in a disempowering light, even if the stated goal is empowerment. "Helping" unwittingly becomes complicit with harming.

In reflecting psychologically on community and ecopsychological accompaniment, we need to become clearer about the effects of lenses we are using to represent others and ourselves. For instance, critical race and Indigenous studies scholar and Aleut Eve Tuck urges us to become aware of the long-term effects of damage-centered research on marginalized populations. While such studies, she says, have been used in the hope of obtaining needed reparations and political or material gain, it is time to consider the long-term consequences of communities thinking of themselves as broken and being presented to others unidimensionally in this light.[55] Damage-centered studies reduce those studied to speaking of their pain, deprivation, and wounds. When the colonial context of these wounds is not clearly articulated, those who have suffered the wounds are themselves seen through a pathologizing lens, neglecting a focus on the cultural and individual pathologies of the perpetrators. As feminist liberation psychologist Geraldine Moane underscores, the strengths born of oppressive conditions, such as generosity, courage, perseverance, ingenuity, and solidarity, are too infrequently and adequately acknowledged and witnessed.[56]

Tuck contrasts the pathologizing consequences of a damage-centered paradigm to the empowering and affirmative aspects of a paradigm focused through the lens of desire. While not denying the loss and despair wrought by colonization and ongoing racism, a focus on a community's desire points members toward the future they hope is possible and the efforts under way to achieve that future. It creates a space for vision and hard-won wisdom. Tuck concedes that there is a role for damage-centered inquiry to document the harms suffered, but communities are so much more than the damage they have had to endure.

APPRENTICESHIP TO CULTURAL AND ECOLOGICAL WORKERS

People trained in universities often have the most to learn from people who have been working for decades within their own communities and by the light of their own cultural traditions. Most often those who emerge from the academy with advanced degrees have been taught to imagine themselves as experts, worthy of larger than average salaries and expectant that others will judge them by their capacities to lead and command projects of varying degrees of complexity. An education for accompaniment is paradoxical, indeed, urging humility and careful listening to others as basic to all work.

One thing is clear: being helpful is not the application of one's arsenal of expertise regardless of the particularities of a given situation. Mary Pipher, a psychologist living in a city with a large influx of refugees, slowly realized that usual psychotherapy sessions were not what was most helpful to her new refugee neighbors.[57] Sure, many had suffered trauma and needed someone attentive to this. But attention to this did not require psychiatric diagnosis but being a reliable and caring human being in the face of the egregious wrongs committed by other humans against this particular person and his or her group. Moreover, many refugees are in more immediate need of learning how to navigate in their new environment so they can gain a foothold of security and familiarity. Rather than apply a lens of trauma to every refugee, accompaniers need to listen closely to where each person is and what it is they may need assistance with. People's needs and desires can be surprising, and often they do not neatly fit the skill sets we have developed. The Colombian psychologists who worked with internally displaced Colombians in Bogotá, described in chapter 4, realized that they needed to learn some things about the judicial process in order to help their new neighbors clear the names of their relatives killed by paramilitary squads.

Too often students are unleashed on community groups with the message that the students should practice what they have learned. When this learning is not based principally in dialogue, collaboration, listening, and learning from others, the stage is set for disrespectful and uninformed encounters that are a costly waste of time for the community group. Regardless of our age or professional experience, psychosocial accompaniment relies on learning from and with community members, recognizing their years of experience and knowledge about the challenges they are working on. One is never too experienced oneself to undergo the humility of apprenticeship to knowledgeable and experienced cultural and ecological workers. It may be evident in time how one can best, most precisely be of assistance given one's own skills and knowledge, but initially offering to assist with the work at hand is a more potentially successful way to build relationships and establish oneself as trustworthy and capable of solidarity.

Transdisciplinarity and Epistemic Disobedience

> Decoloniality requires epistemic disobedience, for border thinking is by definition thinking in exteriority, in the spaces and time that the self-narrative of modernity invented as its outside to legitimize its own logic of coloniality.
> —Walter Mignolo[58]

Western psychology competed for academic recognition largely by positioning itself as a natural science, segregating the psychological from the social and historical, embracing the dominant ideology of radical individualism and too often failing to interrogate its own embodiment of normative ideological values that are not conducive to individual and community well-being. A decolonial psychology must reach toward transdisciplinarity to understand the social, political, economic, environmental, and historical contexts of the urgent crises individuals and communities labor under in neoliberalism.

Ecopsychosocial accompaniment requires fidelity to the situation one is trying to understand, rather than to a particular discipline. A lot of professional work goes into fortifying and gaining power for one's discipline or for a particular approach within that discipline. In doing so, the purported purpose of the work of that discipline is weakened. While one may begin within a particular discipline, the requirements of the situation one is addressing with others may well necessitate going far afield and sometimes into paradigms that directly conflict with the epistemic dictates of one's earlier training.

Engagement in ecopsychosocial accompaniment may require not only transdisciplinarity but at times counterdisciplinarity. Insofar as conforming to disciplinary borders distracts us or impedes us in the work of accompaniment at hand, we would do best to leave them behind. Accompaniment asks that we attend to the needs of a particular situation with particular people. Rather than apply a disciplinary approach to a situation, those in that situation need the freedom to make use of what is helpful in the achievement of their shared desires. This may or may not conform to normative disciplinary approaches. Zapatistas announce *Preguntando caminamos!* We walk asking questions. Rather than pursue a predetermined and fixed destination, we listen, ask, listen, question, sensing our way with others.

Reflecting on my decades of working toward psychologies of liberation, decolonial theorist Walter Mignolo's term "epistemic disobedience" has gathered force in my mind. I tell prospective students that psychology is not a discipline that can simply be learned and practiced. It is a discipline with a troubling history of colonialism and coloniality, with defining chapters of complicity with racism, capitalism, sexism, militarism, and homophobia. As liberation psychologist Ignacio Martín-Baró urged us to see, psychology itself is in continuing need of liberation, of critical deconstruction. Its basic goals must be radically questioned and supplanted with those that would more surely create individual and community well-being. Following Martín-Baró's advice, we need to replace the homeostatic work of psychology—changing the individual while keeping the social structure in place—with the transformative work of changing the social structures that create human misery, radically repositioning the psychologist as a cultural worker among other cultural workers.

At the least, scholar-activist–cultural workers and accompanists involved in this task will suffer academic and/or professional wounds: struggles for publication, employment, and tenure. In too many departments, those involved in the deconstruction of psychology will find their colleagues at odds with them, leading to marginalization. To gain academic space for liberatory theories and projects may involve years of dedication to the institution, hard administrative work so that one can gain the curricular space to open up a new set of decolonial vistas for those who are psychologically minded.

In my experience, this requires breaking through the borders of psychology, counseling, or social work itself, so that the psychological is placed within its necessary context: history, social struggles, and prefigurative imagining and living from below. In such an approach to the psychological, students will recognize the deeper sacrifices made by some of the key theorists they study: exile, ostracism, voluntary poverty, early death, assassination.

Students who have grown up in communities suffering and confronting racism, poverty, and social exclusion will not be surprised by these possible consequences of liberatory psychological work. Those who have grown up with societal privilege undertake an often painful excavation of their positionality as they learn critical community, Indigenous, and eco-liberation psychologies. Their conscientizing education will include their reckoning with what Santiago Castro-Gomez calls "the hubris of the zero point" by decentering themselves and their own knowledge, learning depowerment instead of professional expertism, and practicing solidarity instead of professionalized leadership.[59] Students' repositioning can be a source of their own liberation from further generating the oppressive structures that they were born into. For them, the deployment of the terms "epistemic privilege" and "epistemic disobedience" can be extremely helpful. Instead of being surprised by and personalizing the uphill trajectory of their work, embracing epistemic disobedience and being in solidarity with those who have painfully discovered the devaluation of their own knowledge provides an opening to life paths with greater integrity, that is, of congruence between our understanding of what causes human misery and our own daily living.

Mignolo describes Maori anthropologist Linda Tuhiwai Smith, author of *Decolonizing Methodologies: Research and Indigenous Peoples,* as using anthropology to advance the cause of Maoris, rather than to study them and advance the discipline of anthropology.[60] Similarly, Mignolo portrays how Aymara sociologist from Bolivia Félix Patxi Paco inverts his role in sociology. "Instead of listening to the dictates of sociology, he uses sociology to communicate and organize his argument," which is derived from the knowledge and memories of Indigenous people themselves.[61] In a similar way, Frantz Fanon also created a border epistemology, using the concepts of psychoanalysis to introduce his analysis of the psychic effects of colonialism on the dispossessed of Algeria and Martinique.

This shift is pertinent to "psychology" and to "community psychology," as we use the theoretical and practical tools of both to advance environmental and social justice, peace built on justice, environmental sustainability, and a lived ethic of compassionate interdependence, rather than for the fortification of our academic discipline. I place psychology and community psychology in quotation marks, however, because there is a problem with their stated singularity. Epistemic disobedience and the delinking from coloniality it calls for requires that those of us at the "zero point" shift our location and redefine it as one among many, our iteration of "community psychology" as one possible embodiment located in a particular place and time, capable of being in dialogue with those from other places but dedicated to disrupting the evangelization of European American approaches. When our students do community and ecopsychological practicums or fieldwork in other countries, usually in the global South, we ask them to see what they can learn of approaches there that could be useful in their home communities in the United States, rather than being purveyors of U.S. community psychology. This does not mean that there cannot be fruitful dialogue and mutual learning but that the "hubris of the zero point" must be seen through and discarded.

In sum, I am proposing that a central tenet of accompaniment and of critical community psychologies be epistemic disobedience. Rather than operating as an epistemically obedient professional in an obedient discipline, one, as Mignolo says, that trains "new (epistemic obedient) members and control[s] . . . who enters and what knowledge-making is allowed, disavowed, devalued or celebrated," we should embody decolonial intentions and offer ourselves and our work as bridges beyond us.[62]

"Negative Work"

Psychosocial accompaniers would do well to embrace their vocation as "negative workers," giving away what may be useful and working for *buen vivir*[63] and well-being rather than disciplinary power.[64] The radical Italian psychiatrist Franco Basaglia described "negative workers" as professionals who give their allegiance not to bourgeois institutions but to those who most need their help. As we saw in chapter 5, Basaglia honestly and courageously faced how psychology and psychiatry were harming those they had set out to support through the carceral institutional places and practices of psychiatric asylums.

Nancy Scheper-Hughes, as she argues for accompaniment within anthropology, offers, "The negative worker is a species of class traitor—a doctor, a teacher, a lawyer, psychologist, a social worker, a manager, a social scientist, even—who colludes with the powerless to identify their needs against the interests of the bourgeois institution: the university, the hospital, the factory."[65] Likewise, Merrill Singer and Hans Baer describe negative workers as creating "'openings' in mainstream institutions that allow for critical" practice.[66] If accompaniment is to be a role with integrity, it must not feed off those who suffer from the collective traumas of our time but be genuinely committed to changing the conditions that sow the seeds of these difficulties, thus painstakingly undoing the need for the role. Whatever psychological knowledge is useful should be made available to those who express a desire for it, instead of being hoarded to make one's expertise more valuable.

Conceiving of ourselves as negative workers entails devoted partnerships with cultural workers and committed labor with those suffering socially created disadvantages. It means a focus on cascading models of training where participants gain knowledge and skills to teach what they have learned in their own communities, eliminating the need for outsiders to do so. These shifts require embracing more collaborative forms of practice with lay people and disidentification with expertism. They require an acute awareness of others' disempowerment that can flow from our identification with being the expert. It also requires, in the case of psychology, increased mindfulness about professional psychology's relation to affluence, an affluence that has often been cultivated and preserved in a capitalist world that is sickened by sharp income divides and differential access to needed resources for living.

Accompanying Accompaniers

During fieldwork practicums on community and ecological work where the student is involved in accompaniment, the fieldwork mentor is, in effect, accompanying the accompanist. As we have seen from the work of Jean Vanier in chapter 3, the need for accompaniment may continue well past the initial stages of work. For this reason, many humanitarian organizations try to provide some accompaniment for their staff and volunteers, aware that spaces need to be created to reflect on the work one is doing, one's relationship to it, and the challenges it poses not only in the practicalities of accomplishing it but with regard to the emotional terrain that is constellated for the accompanist. Indeed, there is a fine balance between reflection on the intersection of the work with one's own life and meeting the needs within the work itself. One strives to avoid both the paralysis of excess introversion and the blindness of reflective action.

Each of the issues a student or fledgling accompanist takes on has a history, approaches that have already been tried, scholarship, community knowledge, and praxis surrounding it, and the need for creative and informed approaches in the present. Mentees use their intimate connections to the issue to fuel their exploration of these facets, liaison with others who have common interests, find groups or communities that are working around the issue, or begin what we have called a convened community to do so. From the beginning, we have sought to see through and reject "missionary-like" approaches, ones that determine the problem and the answer in advance of immersion in a community and dialogue with those who constitute it. Through community and ecological fieldwork and research, students work in the area of their calling while deepening their ethical discernment, reflecting on their own positionality, widening their repertoire of dialogue and arts-based approaches, and gathering the theoretical insight and practical skills needed to join with others in the work at hand.

Building Your Skillset, Preparing Your Backpack

Staughton Lynd, a Quaker deeply influenced by liberation theology, has long reflected on El Salvadoran Archbishop Oscar Romero's call to accompany the poor. Lynd, trained as a historian, used oral history to help working-class and poor people tell their histories, particularly their important history of labor organizing. He called his form of oral history with others "guerilla history," describing this writing history "from below" as a form of accompaniment. By "below" he referred to communities that have few resources to meet their needs and little access to mainstream political power. He called for a "partnership between academics, or committed religious, on the one hand, and workers, peasants, or prisoners on the other, such that neither denigrates itself or reflexively defers to the other, but both, together develop a vision of a better world."[67] He understood this as "reciprocal accompaniment."

As he struggled to understand how he might best embody accompaniment, he realized he needed a skillset that was useful to poor and working people. Although already a historian, Lynd chose law as his "helpful skill." He advised others interested in accompaniment: "Armed with such a skill, just behave as a moderately decent person and 'accompaniment' will be a piece of cake. People will need you, and over time as you offer a useful service, trust and friendship will emerge of themselves."[68] I do not experience accompaniment as a "piece of cake"! But I respect Lynd's commitment to retooling himself in light of the needs of the community where he lives.

Accompaniment can take place in many spheres of life and does not necessarily require professionalization. However, to take it seriously within psychology and social work, graduate training requires a reimagining of curriculum and practicums. The spheres in which students are preparing to undertake accompaniment need to directly influence the curricular offerings.

For instance, those seeking to work with communities recovering from violence will need not only an understanding of individual and collective trauma and varied approaches to individual and community healing. They will also need to understand the long history of the conflict in the particular region in which they are working and the present psychosocial needs of the community. In their "backpack" or "toolbox" they will want to understand what contributes to cycles of violence, how communities have influenced these factors, and how to build dynamic and sustainable peace-building. Students will need to have experiences, through community and ecopsychological fieldwork, of joining into the work of a community, of learning to deeply listen and be nimble in being of assistance, often outside of the categories imagined for oneself. It will be helpful to understand how to undertake participatory research in case this is needed, and how to evaluate the results of programs that may be instituted in concert with community members to assess their actual effectiveness. A holistic understanding of how to move between interdependent levels of organization (individual, family, interpersonal, community, regional, national, global) is necessary to an understanding of psychosocial and ecological accompaniment, as is a knowledgeable openness to addressing policy and legislation that may impact a given situation. In addition, students must undergo a continuing exploration of their own subjectivity for remnants of coloniality and examine the intersection of their families' history with historical and ongoing injustice and exploitation.[69]

Normative schooling often fails to adequately educate students in collaboration, dialogue, consensus-building, conscientization, crafting generative questions, appreciative inquiry, community visioning, antiracist and antidiscriminatory discernment and opposition, and attention to community ritual. For psychologically oriented accompaniers, their backpack for accompanying can include these skills. For instance, in the doctoral specialization in community psychology, liberation psychology, Indigenous psychologies, and ecopsychology at Pacifica Graduate Institute where I teach, students learn about a variety of approaches to small- and large-group dialogues: council; appreciative inquiry; Theater of the Oppressed; CAPACITAR, a popular education approach to the somatic sequelae of trauma; Public Conversation; clearness committees; community dream work and visioning; and Alternatives to Violence.[70] Similarly, Helene Lorenz and Susan James facilitate Students of Color and Racial Justice Allies groups to help students understand and counter racist microaggressions in the classroom and in their communities and workplaces.[71] Approaches to addressing collective trauma, engaging in peacebuilding, restorative justice processes, and effecting public policy are seen as critical skills for community work, as are grant-writing, asset-mapping, program evaluation, and social network analysis. We strive to ground any research efforts in the questions community groups have and to research collaboratively within participatory action and Indigenous research frameworks. Students are counseled to engage in continuous lifelong learning both from community members and in response to the needs that arise. This continued learning may be within one's chosen discipline or far from it, depending on the circumstances of a particular group. This approach addresses the needed reformulation of education in psychology, arguing for transdisciplinary and field-based approaches, grounded in liberatory theory and dialogical and participatory practices.

Mutual Accompaniment as a Pathway to Solidarity

Solidarity is an uneasy, reserved, and unsettled matter that neither reconciles present grievances nor forecloses future conflict.

—Eve Tuck and K. Wayne Yang[72]

I don't believe in charity; I believe in solidarity. Charity is vertical, so it's humiliating. It goes from top to bottom. Solidarity is horizontal. It respects the other and learns from the other. I have a lot to learn from other people. Each day I'm learning. Soy un curioso. I'm a curious man.

—Eduardo Galeano[73]

It is not possible for a Western-trained white psychologist—such as myself—to actively imagine and enact psychological practices that do not carry overtones and traces of coloniality. This reality requires accompanists like myself to engage in and be open to a state of continuing self-critique, as well as openness to the critical feedback of others who live and embody different standpoints. The accompaniment of those with fewer privileges by those with more—while an important step—is a step on a longer path: a path that moves away from the kinds of academic professionalization that have been common in European and American graduate programs, to forms of walking, as Fanon said, in "the company" of one another, "night and day, for all times."[74] It is, however, a necessary step in societies such as the United States that are so perniciously divided along class, racial, and ethnic lines. Will we one day be able to forego the professionalization of accompanying one another that social sciences promote? One day, will the kinds of useful knowledge that psychologists and social workers develop be sufficiently democratized so that they are both widely available outside of specialized training and more widely susceptible to cross-cultural analysis and critique? Will the tragic divides of privilege and scarcity be so erased that we can show up alongside one another less in the form of one person with more privileges accompanying another with fewer, and more as fellow musicians creatively exploring and playing music with one another? For even in a more just world, each of us would continue to be subject to life struggles where being accompanied is welcomed, where the deep hospitality of one to another can help to lift the burdens that weigh down one's spirit.

Sadly, all this seems a long way off. In the meantime, I propose accompaniment as a humble yet potent antidote to forms of psychological professionalism that misread symptoms of distress, that fail to see deeply enough, that insulate against the acute and chronic sufferings around us, and that unwittingly participate in sustaining the disastrous divides from which we suffer. Accompaniment may be able to grow up within more traditional roles for the psychologically minded, until it overflows the container of the discipline itself. There are signs of this happening already.

Due to its defection from hierarchical professionalism, accompaniment runs against the grain of human services regulated by a capitalist market. As those who accompany learn from others and share their own practices, they do indeed undermine bourgeois institutions and embody the kinds of negative work Basaglia spoke of.[75]

Solidarity emerges from a felt sense that our fates are interdependent and that our own well-being cannot be separated from that of others. As Martin Luther King, Jr., put it:

> As long as there is poverty in the world I can never be rich, even if I have a billion dollars. As long as diseases are rampant and millions of people in this world cannot expect to live more than twenty-eight or thirty years, I can never be totally healthy even if I just got a good checkup at Mayo clinic. I can never be what I ought to be until you are what you ought to be. This is the way our world is made. No individual or nation can stand out boasting of being independent. We are interdependent.[76]

Solidarity does not depend on a homogeneity of identity or shared origins. It depends on shared purpose, desire, vision, and action. It entails sharing equitably the work and risk of actions, often disproportionately borne by those with less privilege and power.

Collaborative solidarity as discussed by trans-activists Elle Hearns, Aaryn Lang, J. Mase, and Kei Williams assists the most marginalized to lead the work. It asks people to reflect on how they show up and centers communities to speak for themselves. It resists the language of inclusion.[77] Eve Tuck and K. Wayne Yang underscore that solidarity is not an endpoint; it is never finally achieved. It is not a resting place but a process where conflicts and challenges rightly emerge. They assert that from an Indigenous perspective, solidarity requires "the abolition of land as property and the uphold[ing of] the sovereignty of Native land and people."[78] In the absence of adequate national reparations, individual groups are beginning to try to live into this demand. For instance, the Possibility Alliance in Missouri, a land-based intentional community, actively sought the history of the land they were living on from Indigenous historians. When they discovered its roots, they decided to return most of it to local Native groups and to seek resettlement in Maine with the permission of the Wabanaki Nation. They have asked for permission to live on Wabanaki land and to ask how they can be of service.[79] Here "service" is understood correctly as reparation. Solidarity requires rightful returning of what we have taken or what has come to us through the unjust suffering of others.

When long-term efforts of accompaniment flower into the work of reparations and solidarity, the energies of co-creation are unleashed. The creation of commons becomes possible.

EIGHT

Nonhuman Animal Accompaniment

G. A. Bradshaw

Beginnings

How are we to become native to this land?

—Paul Shepherd

MY STORY OF ACCOMPANIMENT began in April 1996 with a first visit to the amazing land that had come to be known as South Africa. On top of the country's natural vibrancy, the air buzzed with a new, anxious exuberance. South Africans were disabling five decades of brutal machinery and mindsets put into motion by apartheid. The Truth and Reconciliation Commission commenced that very year. My attention was focused elsewhere, on nonhuman casualties of colonialism. I was there to investigate a series of baffling Lion deaths.[1]

The thrill of stepping on such primordial soil, however, immediately took on a minor key. This was not the Africa that I had expected. Having grown up privileged and white, immersed in dazzling images from *West with the Night, Born Free, The White Nile*, and other tales of landscapes bejeweled with huge and charismatic wildlife, I was unprepared to find the continent denuded. Centuries of escalating violence by European occupation had nearly bled dry the country's wildlife. Romantic stories of khaki-clad adventurers in rickety planes and dust-covered trucks hid the consequences of white colonialism. Almost all of South Africa's "big five"—Elephants, Leopards, Rhinoceroses, Cape Buffalos, and African Lions—had been extinguished.[2]

Now that post-apartheid South Africa was open to international eco-tourism, public and private landholders jumped at the opportunity to fill the empty spaces by implementing a mass wildlife extraction and transport program. Infant Elephant survivors of slaughter were grabbed, roped, and trucked to South African reserves. Lions and Leopards were hunted, darted, and netted to stock the same destinations.

Many imported immigrants failed to thrive. Lions were dying of an unexplained wasting disease, and young male Elephants had inexplicably and uncharacteristically killed over one hundred White and Black Rhinoceroses. These were just a few symptoms of trauma imploding Africa. The relational threads that sustained human and nonhuman indigenes for millions of years had been shred by colonial occupation, leaving a trail of raw, bleeding psyches. I saw the fallout up close the day after my arrival.

On the evening of our first stop, Pilanesberg National Park, we bundled up in jackets and jerseys and piled into a jeep. During the bumpy ride, our guide told us about young male Elephants who were at the time suspects in the deaths of Rhinoceroses. Their guilt had yet to be fully determined. The ranger also described a pair of fully mature male Lions living in the park. Originally, he explained, there had been three. The trio was formidable. They defeated even the boldest young males seeking to usurp territory. Failing time after time, ousted young males jumped the park fence to find ground elsewhere. The park simply did not afford Lions enough room. This, however, created a problem for humans.

African Lions had been vanquished from their ancestral lands for such a long time that only a handful of village elders remembered seeing one. Traditional ways of coexistence were lost. Once threaded in the minds and lives of villagers, Lions were now regarded as threatening strangers. Park personnel worried that the situation might spark already tenuous relationships between black and white South Africans. Parks and reserves were a flash point. Tribal lands had been appropriated and made exclusively white territory. The parks might be called African, but they were white African.

In light of current tensions, park administrators decided to topple the leonine hegemony by shooting one of the males. Their plan worked. The remaining pair was unable to stave off younger Lions. But an unexpected cost followed. "Losing their mate broke them," the ranger explained dolefully. "They howled and roared for days after he was killed. Then, they just retreated. They seemed to have lost the will to live." While he spoke, we sat under a sky white with stars. The two remaining males lay only a few feet away. They stared back, eyes dull, their tawny royalty draped over boney frames. I was witnessing Africa die in the first person.

There are moments, always unexpected, when everything changes. This was one such time. The Lions' eyes pierced the cocoon that social conditioning had wrapped around my senses, jerking me back to the transspecies existence of my youth. At the time, I did not recognize this ethical turning as a step along the path of "accompaniment." Indeed, an honest practice of accompaniment was not to follow until much later. But the Lions were the shockwave that brought me face to face with a staggering realization: I was living two contradictory realities.

Life was not always divided. Prior to formal schooling, I lived in a kind of eco-soup where species lines were virtually nonexistent. My world, my reality, *my people*, were populated with human and nonhuman family including our Dog, Cat, Rat, Tortoise, Iguana, Goose, and Parrot, and diverse inhabitants of the creeks—Planaria, Tadpoles, and Water Skimmers—and Red-Winged Blackbirds, Red-Tailed Hawks, and Mourning Doves of the fields and skies. Every morning, I woke, heart racing, anticipating the welcoming mysteries of Nature's greens and golds.

Kindergarten, that first transition from home to collective, interrupted this seamless pattern. Between eight in the morning and three in the afternoon, my friends were human. Owls, Sharks, Cats, and other Animals faded into the recesses of literary landscapes, reduced to objectified means to human ends. After school, I shed my skirts and penny loafers for peddle-pushers and sneakers and dove back into Nature.

A second separation occurred after leaving my ecodevelopmental context for university. Time "in Nature" was replaced by a life defined by humans to the point where being in the "Animal world" telescoped to sporadic forays to the beach and mountains. Mental preoccupation changed with physical context. I decided to major in what might be considered the most anthropocentric subject of all disciplines, linguistics. This interest was not new. I loved learning different human languages. My grandmother spoke five fluently and read to me variously in French, German, Danish, Swedish, and English. The characters and stories of *Les Misérables* and *Der Ring des Nibelungen* became part of my ancestral narrative; family facts and fantastic fiction blurred. Language was the medium that gave coherence to this relational matrix. Language, however, was rarely concerned with nonhuman Nature.

After graduating from university and a sojourn in Taiwan, I returned to the United States unmoored and uncertain as to how I might make a living. Then, one evening, I attended a lecture by a Harvard professor who studied slime mold communication. I sat in the audience, glued, as he described the amazingly complex and intense social life of these eukaryotes. At certain times, individuals gather together, each tasked with a specific role in the aggregate. Among other activities, they form exquisite flowering structures that spawn future slime mold generations. All this complicated organization, the lecturer told us, is coordinated via chemical telegraph. The slime mold members speak to each other! I was on fire. The next day I enrolled in science courses to learn about Animal languages.

As often happens, or at least in my case, one thing led to another, and my passion for slime molds gradually morphed into a love affair with the graceful arcs and glyphs of mathematics. Eventually a love of language and Nature came together in a doctoral dissertation on mathematical ecology and subsequent employment as a research mathematician. It was during this tenure with the government that the fateful journey to Africa came about and put my inner and outer worlds on a collision course. Unable to avert my gaze from the Lions' stare, that moment forced me to choose between three possibilities: stay inside the anthropocentric world of science, retreat into personal experience with Animals, or reconcile these two worlds. I chose the third. I would find a way to make the voices of Lions and other Animals heard by humans.

Once again seemingly by chance, I made another discovery—the work of C. G. Jung. I devoured one essay after another, amazed at the ease and elegance with which the Swiss psychologist traveled in the comfortable union of science, psyche, and Nature. Depth psychology provided a lexicon that, I believed, could faithfully serve and connect both human collective (science) and personal epistemes (Animal and my own experiences). In fits and starts, inner and outer worlds began to anneal under the umbrella of this reconceptualization. This process was midwifed by a second doctorate in depth psychology under the tutelage of Dr. Mary Watkins.[3]

I was driven to find a way to render an ontological turning into a language that could be used to communicate with fellow humans. A collectively valid means of communicating Animal experience was vital. Without such, nonhumans would remain silenced and disenfranchised. Unless their voices were recognized by humans, Animals would continue to be vulnerable to humanity's whims.

Ascribing qualities that are coveted as uniquely human, such as language, however, is regarded as sentimental anthropomorphic projection with little to no real scientific basis. Even the subjective experiences of great naturalists such as George Adamson and Daphne Sheldrick, who perceive and interact with Animals as sentient, linguistically competent beings, are not received with the same value and validity as scientists and other lettered scholars. Within the modern epistemic framing, personal experiences are denied the authority naturally bestowed to collectively sanctioned views.

So, with science in one hand and Animal psyches in the other, I set out to create a bridge that could faithfully grasp and communicate the meaning of the strange situation of the Rhinoceros-killing Elephants whom I had encountered during my visit with the Lions. Ironically, the science that proved so key in this process was neuroscience. I say "ironically" because it is neuroscientists who subject nonhumans to the most heinous experiments. These procedures are performed to extract information from Animal minds and bodies to understand those of our own.

On paper and in practice, researchers claim that Rats, Cats, Monkeys, Horseshoe Crabs, Rabbits, and other experimental victims are "less than" humans, lacking the higher-order faculties that supposedly make our species unique. Science demonstrates, however, that Animals do, in fact, possess the selfsame capacities that grant (at least in theory) humans immunity from exploitation and torture.[4] The evidence is plain: billions upon billions of dollars spent on biomedical and pharmaceutical research and testing that use nonhuman Animals as surrogates for humans (i.e., Animal models). Science learns about nonhumans to learn about humans using methods prohibited for our species. Although psychologically and physically comparable to humans, nonhumans are denied comparable ethical and legal protections. Scientific parity is ignored for the purpose of justifying ethical disparity.

This paradoxical paradigm is maintained by deliberate misrepresentation of species-similar science using species-dissimilar reportage. For example, in academic articles, while using a species common model to investigate both Monkey and human brain structures, researchers employ different language to describe the same phenomena. Researchers describe Monkey responses to experimentation as "abnormal behavior," but when observed in humans, the same symptoms are considered "neuropsychiatric disorders."[5] This linguistic parsing implies that Monkeys do not possess the brain structures, processes, and associated capacities (e.g., emotions, psychological suffering) that lead to psychological symptoms of distress in humans. Former vivisectionist in the pharmaceutical industry Michael Slusher describes how "the whole industry of animal research is built upon a foundation of willful ignorance, barbaric insistence on antiquated assumptions, and a perpetual need to maintain the status quo, 'because that's how it's always been done.' This illusion of necessity is funded quite well, of course, by the corporations and institutions interested in maintaining the profit stream earned at the expense of millions of lives."[6] The purpose of such distortion is used to control and oppress nonhumans and humans who eschew adapting to Western civilization and resist colonialism.[7] It has been an incredibly successful ruse. The accomplishments of human progress are directly proportional to the number of Animals and other nonhumans destroyed.

Science's internal contradiction became plain with the diagnosis of post-traumatic stress disorder (PTSD) of the South African Elephants—the first open recognition and assessment, using methods developed to probe and assess the human mind, of nonhuman psyches.[8] Elephant psychic pain described in the language of science demonstrates that what we know about Animals can be applied to humans and vice versa with equal rigor (bidirectional inference).[9] The only difference between the new field of transspecies psychology, the unified study of sentience of humans and all other

Animals, and standing science is that it *openly* recognizes cross-species comparability in brain and mind. Indeed, the purpose of naming trans-species psychology was to bring attention to the deliberate misrepresentation and selective use of science.

Elephant PTSD was the first drop of nail polish remover that, along with many other efforts, began peeling off the veneer of the reigning cultural agenda which has obscured scientific facts. Organic to Western culture, trans-species psychology is a cross-species liberation psychology (in the sense of Ignacio Martín-Baró[10]). It provides us with an accessible portal through which we may travel from the collective paradigm of anthropocentric domination to a nonhierarchical, species-inclusive ontology. Trans-species psychology joins traditions from both Western civilization (e.g., Gaia hypothesis, deep ecology, ecosemiotics) and Indigenous traditions of Nature-based consciousness (e.g., Sioux, Buddhists, Quechua).[11] Animal accompaniers are its pioneers.

Living at the "I Love Animals But . . ." Interface

When the suffering of another creature causes you to feel pain, do not submit to the initial desire to flee from the suffering one, but on the contrary, come closer, as close as you can to him who suffers, and try to help him.

—Leo Tolstoy

Today animal accompaniers largely live in a kind of no-man's land, embedded in the interface of two disparate paradigms with nonintersecting values (e.g., anthropocentrism/ecocentrism), means of living (e.g., urban industrial-technological/subsistence), and perceptions (e.g., human elite/trans-species equality). At one extreme, there is the dominant, modern human culture with its generative process of reductionism and agenda of systemic predation based on the idea that the world is made up of distinct parts. Carolus Linnaeus's classification system of plants and Animals, rendered in greater detail two hundred years later, reflects this view. For example, Western science envisions a Grizzly Bear this way:

Animalia (Kingdom)
Chordata (Phylum)
Carnivora (Order)
Ursidae (Family)
Ursus (Genus)
Ursus arctos (Species)
Ursus arctos horribilis (Subspecies)

Organism associations and divisions are arranged hierarchically from what is considered the most complex (humans) to the simplest (protozoa). This ordered string of relatedness, differences, and value, what the early Greeks referred to as *scala naturae* (great chain of being), undergirds European culture: an explicit political divide that appoints humans, and until recently only certain humans (i.e., Judeo-Christian white males), as superior to all other life forms. Perception, thought, law, economics, consumption, indeed all aspects of Western civilization, are shaped by anthropocentric stratification, control, and difference. Nature's flora and fauna are reduced to resource objects in service to human harvesting and exploitation. Lucy Hastings, nineteenth-century settler of Wisconsin, expressed this attitude in a letter to her family:

> Smead has now traded away our farm & done well. . . . We find it very good for poor folks out here to go on Government land make improvements, then sell, & and after a while get it to farming in good shape. . . . Timber there is plenty & Cheap, there. . . . I would like to send you some of the big fish we catch out of the Chippewa river. and the Huckleberries . . . I never saw them so thick, nor as large as they are here. I went out a little while one afternoon and picked 10 qts. Every bluff is covered with them. Cranberries are in great abundance.[12]

At the other extreme, similar to most Indigenous, nomadic humans, wildlife cultures are subsistence-based. Humans are not separate from the rest of Nature, neither are nonhumans "othered" or subjected to control and domination via domestication and other methods for pruning agency.

Settlers such as Hastings were beneficiaries of these harmonious trans-species relationships. North America was rimmed by oceans brimming with Fish and Insects; forests were rich with Deer, Puma, Bear, and Wolves; skies filled with a startling diversity of avian fauna who coexisted for millions of years with Indigenous humans. Precolonial humans killed Animals, but killing was spare relative to the wanton excesses of settlers and most of our ancestors were gatherers first and hunters occasionally.[13] Alberta Thompson, Makah elder, who with other tribal elders protested a Gray Whale hunt demanded by Makah men in the 1990s, reflects how the pulse of this philosophy is still alive: "Yes, my people once killed whales and yes the whale is important to us. . . . But now it's time to repay the whales for what they gave to us in the past, now is the time to protect them, not to kill them. The whale was once the salvation of the Makah. We now need to be the salvation of the whale."[14]

Inter-species relationships generally maintained an understanding of interdependence and even shared language. Sioux scholar Vine Deloria, Jr., described how his grandfather was known for his relationships with Plains Bison. He would confer with herd leaders to exchange information. There was an agreement that the Plains Indians would hunt Buffalo, but only for the necessary few and only at certain times. Outside the hunting season, Natives were able to walk among Bison without disturbing the herd.[15] The discordant clash between indigene and pioneer mentalities is vividly illustrated in the testimony of an Omaha elder. He not only speaks of the loss of land and traditional livelihoods caused by European occupation but of deep, imposed relational poverty:

> When I was a youth, the country was very beautiful. Along the rivers were belts of timberland, where grew cottonwood, maple, elm, ash, hickory, and walnut trees, and many other kinds. Also there were many kinds of vines and shrubs. And under these grew many good herbs and beautiful flowering plants. In both the woodland and the prairie I could see the trails of many kinds of animals and could hear the cheerful songs of many birds. When I walked abroad, I could see many forms of life,

beautiful living creatures which Wakanda (the Great Spirit) had placed here; and these were, after their manner, walking, flying, leaping, running, playing all about. But now the face of the land is changed and sad. The living creatures are gone. I see the land desolate and I suffer an unspeakable sadness. Sometimes, I wake in the night, and I feel as though I should suffocate from the pressure of this awful loneliness.[16]

Conqueror and conquered share time and space but have had radically different experiences.

Animal accompaniers inhabit the interface of these conflicting realities. It is not peaceful terrain. Human violence penetrates the lives of nonhuman species. Whether alive or as products, domesticated and wild Animal bodies and minds are used in nearly every aspect of human culture: consumption (e.g., meat industry), clothing (e.g., down jackets), entertainment (e.g., Orcas at SeaWorld), emotional support (e.g., Cats), labor (e.g., hunting Dogs), education (e.g., vivisected Frogs and Worms), decoration (e.g., feathers), sport (e.g., hunting), or extinction (e.g., Termites). Prosocial association with wildlife opens Animal accompaniers to similar violence. Trespassing species lines is akin to treason.

In most U.S. states, providing wildlife with food is illegal. Feeding is defined by law as "placing food materials out that attract wildlife for any reason other than baiting." However, baiting wildlife is not illegal. Baiting entails putting out food to attract wildlife but with the intent to "lure, or entice them as an aid in hunting." Eighty-one-year-old Mary Musselman fell victim of this contradictory law. A retired gym teacher in Sebring, Florida, Musselman was sent to jail for giving food to Black Bears and again incarcerated for putting out bread crumbs for Crows. Musselman was ordered to an assisted living facility where she died a few months later. In British Columbia, despite two Bear conflict-free decades, Allen Piche was charged with violating "the Wildlife Act, which maintains fines for feeding dangerous wildlife of up to $100,000 for a first offence, and/or a jail term." He was found guilty as were the Bears. Conservation officers shot seventeen Bears that spring because they were "too habituated to humans." According to a former fish and game law enforcement officer, the image of an angry dangerous bear is essential to sell the public that killing is necessary. If people find out that Smokey [the Bear] is really a nice guy, then there goes hunting fees, there goes your job. . . . Plus, most agency folks have a lot of personal and ego investment in being macho. It makes them look pretty silly if people realized that bears don't go out of their way to hurt you. That's why they go after individuals who don't pay attention to the myth and show the public that, yes, bears, pumas, and coyotes are nice! In the eyes of the agency, a human crosses that line and he or she is no different than the bear.[17]

While strong or sustained, positive attachments by humans to nonhumans can develop within the utilitarian paradigm of speciesism, statistically speaking, most relationships embody an internal contradiction, what psychiatrist Robert Jay Lifton referred to as "doubling," a psychological mechanism identified in his extensive interviews with German Nazi doctors. Doubling is a kind of mental compartmentalization that allows an individual to comfortably toggle between two distinct ethical contexts. Similar to dissociation, doubling is nonetheless distinct because it involves the creation of two autonomous, yet connected, wholes, not parts, within a single self. In the case of the Nazi doctors, an "Auschwitz self" existed free of the moral standards to which the "humane self" was held outside the camp.[18] A parallel situation is found in the utilitarian paradigm concerning attitudes about Animals.

Describing his childhood on an Oregon farm, the *New York Times* op-ed columnist Nicholas Kristof talks about how he learned to admire Geese:

Once a month or so, we would slaughter the geese. When I was 10 years old, my job was to lock the geese in the barn and then rush and grab one. Then I would take it out and hold it by its wings on the chopping block while my Dad or someone else swung the ax. The 150 geese knew that something dreadful was happening and would cower in a far corner of the barn, and run

away in terror as I approached. Then I would grab one
and carry it away as it screeched and struggled in my arms. Very
often, one goose would bravely step away from the panicked
flock and walk tremulously toward me. It would be the mate of
the one I had caught, male or female, and it would step right up
to me, protesting pitifully. It would be frightened out of its wits,
but still determined to stand with and comfort its lover. We
eventually grew so impressed with our geese.

While he now "draws the line at animals being raised in cruel conditions,"
Kristof goes on to say that, nonetheless, he "eat[s] meat (even, hesitantly,
goose)," and asserts that he will "enjoy the barbecues this summer" knowing "that every hamburger patty has a back story, and that every tin of goose
liver pâté could tell its own rich tale of love and loyalty."[19]

Individual psychological care/kill doubling is entrained in higher
levels of social organization. For example, with the public's increased concern for Animal welfare, many are calling for "humane farming":

Billions of animals [are] raised for food annually. . . . Factory
farming forces cows to stand in milking tie stalls 24/7, pigs to
live in gestation crates, and chickens to share small battery cages
with up to a half a dozen birds. These animals don't have places
to walk, root around, flap wings or live natural lives. At factory
farms, animals are not treated like animals, but like objects that
can be used and abused.

However, while Humane Farm Animal Care seeks to "improve the lives of
farm animals," it is with the understanding that Animals are intended for
food production. Consideration for their welfare begins with birth but ends
in slaughter: "The bottom line is this; just because an animal is raised for
food doesn't mean it shouldn't also be raised humanely."[20] Justifiable killing
is part and parcel of the dominant cultural narrative.

Iconic films such as *Babe, War Horse,* and *Old Yeller* feature farmers,
soldiers, and children in relationship with the Animals in their charge, yet

the exigencies of anthropocentric privilege inevitably overrule emotional bonds. While trauma and "grief imposed by the separation of the mother cow and her offspring is well discussed in the dairy industry," the unnatural practice is routinized into anthropo-crafted "facts of life" to maximize milk production.[21] In one town, the cries of mothers and calves were so loud and distressing that neighbors called local police to investigate these "strange noises." After confirming that the noise "was only farm animals," the officers stated, "We've been informed that the cows are not in distress and that the noises are a normal part of farming practices."[22] Similarly, farmers maintain that they have a "good and trusting relationship" with their herd. One dairy farmer cites as evidence the ease with which visiting veterinarians can insert an arm into Cow vaginas to perform artificial insemination.[23]

Martin, a veteran farmed Animal activist refers to these utilitarian relationships as the "I love Animals, but . . ." syndrome. He describes how a "love/kill" mindset is inculcated early in childhood:

> Everyone thinks that 4-H is such a wonderful way to get children to appreciate nature and learn an ethic of care. But when you look at it realistically, it is nothing more than setting up a child to be an emotionally dissociated abuser. What do you expect? A young boy or girl raises a chicken, sheep, or pig from infancy, gives the baby a name, spends time after school and weekends feeding, washing, and caring for the animal, then goes to the fair to win a prize and sell their former best friend for slaughter. It's the same attitude with the so called "humane and backyard farming."

Commenting on a video showing the brutality that free range Chickens suffer, Martin adds, "So Chickens get to be out of cages for a while. I guess it's better than being at a battery farm. But, Chickens are still living a conditional life when at any minute they can get lassoed and stuffed into a tiny crate with other live chickens or slaughtered on the spot. It is heartbreaking to hear their screams of fear and betrayal—they sound just like human babies."[24]

Similar to scientific reportage on Monkeys used in biomedical research, language is manipulated to retain the compartmentalization barrier to mask other Animal abuse. A biomedical researcher and vivisectionist for decades, Michael Slusher writes in his autobiography, "We may love the chickens in our yard, or the big friendly cow next door, but the plastic-wrapped chunks of meat at the grocery store aren't those animals. In fact, they aren't animals at all anymore. They are now called by names that disguise what they really are. They are now 'veal,' 'roast,' or 'sirloin.'"[25]

Doubling is destructive to humans as well as nonhumans. Reflecting on his career in the pharmaceutical industry, Slusher concludes,

> I was a monster. . . . I am very ashamed of my history and what I did to so many animals. . . . One would think that after so many years of my torturing and killing animals, the light bulb of compassion would have blinked on much sooner. The clues were all there, but I was still under the illusion that animals were nothing more than unfortunate, but essential commodities. However much I thought I loved animals, at least as wildlife and as pets, it's clear now that I was just like every other typical person when it came to exploiting them for utilitarian purposes or for my own pleasure.[26]

Virgil Butler was raised in a small town in rural Arkansas, home state of the world's largest poultry processor and where he worked in a factory killing Chickens. He describes how the experience changed him psychologically:

> I started catching chickens when I was 14 to help support my family, as I was the oldest, and we lived in extreme poverty. . . . When I first started killing, it really bothered me. It bothered me because the chickens were hanging there in those shackles, helpless, and couldn't run away. To me, it was extremely unfair simply because they were so innocent. And it really bothered me when I missed one and heard the poor bird go through the

scalder alive, thrashing and bumping against the sides of it as it
slowly died. I worked to become really good at killing so that I
wouldn't miss so many. I did become really good, but at a steep
price. The more I did it, the less it bothered me. I became de-
sensitized. . . . Most people that work in a chicken plant don't
eat chicken, even though they are meat-eaters.[27]

Later, with his partner, Laura Alexander, Butler became vegan and an Animal rights activist.

Andrew Sharo, a member of Direct Action Everywhere (DxE) and
committed farmed Animal rights activist, regularly takes part in open
rescue—a method inspired by Mahatma Gandhi's philosophy of nonviolence, *satyagraha*, used to save farmed Animals in industrial settings who
will not live without immediate veterinary care. Sharo attributes his path of
accompaniment to the way he was raised:

I grew up on the East Coast with a single mom who became
pregnant by choice with a sperm donor. She is [an] incredible
loving person when I was growing up and the way she saw the
world had an enormous impact on me. She would bring home
injured animals and try to nurse them back to health or get them
to a place where they needed to be. There was always a high
valuation of animals. I grew up with dogs and cats who were
part of the family. They were always in our photos and with us
as much as possible. This was my foundation. A lot of people in
Animal rights come from a background like this.[28]

Sharo's attachment experience resonates with precolonial ecocentric human
and nonhuman cultures. Animal societies and, on the whole, Indigenous societies, including 99 percent of our ancestors, reflect collective, prosocial
values—empathy and an ethic of care for others—that extended across
species.[29] I have noticed that individuals who are drawn to trans-species psychology, and in particular Elephants, retain close connection with
their human natal families. This has led me to reflect on the relationship be-

tween secure developmental contexts and trans-species identities, a sense of self that is not limited to one's biological species of origin or attached to any form.

Accompaniment and Identity

"I am protecting the rainforest" develops to "I am part of the rainforest protecting myself. I am that part of the rainforest recently emerged into thinking." What a relief then! The thousands of years of imagined separation are over and we begin to recall our true nature.

—John Seed

These personal narratives illustrate how individuals engaged in Animal issues do not necessarily share identities and values. Animal advocates and activists have widely varied philosophies that express in diverse ways such as personal habits (e.g., plant-based/Animal eaters), political philosophies (e.g., contrasting philosophies of People for Ethical Treatment of Animals and the Humane Society of the United States), and lifestyles (e.g., urban/rural). As sanctuary worker Beverly points out, not all who "love Animals" are accompaniers:

> We Animal people live in a kind of species No Man's Land, similar to the WWII Morocco portrayed in the film *Casablanca*, where rules and interpersonal expectations are uncertain. We may think of ourselves as being and feeling the same because we work with animals, but underneath there are so many different opinions, values, and ways of seeing other species. Accompaniment involves more than living close and spending time with animals. It really comes down to actions: what you do and don't do. Saying does not equate to doing.[30]

Commenting on Nicholas Kristof's articles on care/kill reflections, United Poultry Concerns founder Karen Davis underscores the difference between expressing and acting: "It's great that they care, but what next?

What are caring people going to do with their care? That, for the animals, is the question, the only one that counts."[31] Wayne Hsiung, cofounder of DxE, discusses the concept of direct action and how a demand for structural change is intrinsic to accompaniment practices such as slaughterhouse vigils and open rescue:

> The classic distinction between direct action and other forms of activism was, are you confronting the system? Are you working outside of the system to try and reshape it fundamentally or are you working within it? And my own view is that there's value in both of those approaches but any successful movement needs both of them. And so what we're trying to do is go back to this original conception of direct action which focuses on confronting the system.[32]

Another distinguishing feature of Animal accompaniers is an eco- and trans-species identity. Shifting from anthropocentric to ecocentric identity is considered core among eco-workers.[33] Most Animal accompaniers whom I have encountered believe that a commitment to plant-based eating (or veganism) is essential, indeed defines Animal accompaniment, because it represents a concrete and open expression of human deprivileging and nonhuman valuation. Harold Brown, longtime cattle rancher and dairy farmer, is now an Animal rights activist and staunch plant-based eater:

> Being vegan is not just a way of eating. . . . It is a practice of selfless service, unconditional love, and a holistic understanding of the biota. It is non-cooperation and non-participation with anything that does not allow another being to live on their own terms. There was now a conscious connection between my heart and my head and I now had a moral and ethical foundation upon which to live my life. . . . When we truly care, our intentions, words and deeds are acted out with integrity and are consistent with our core desires of compassion, empathy and love.[34]

Other human cultures have not traveled down the path of separation. For instance, the sense of self in many Indigenous cultures whose minds and lives are embedded and interlaced in the rest of Nature is ecocentric, similarly decentered from conspecifics and inclusive of nonhumans. Calvin Luther Martin writes about the Alaskan Natives, "A Yup'ik Eskimo handed me a scrap of paper whereon was penciled, 'I am a Puffin!' . . . Here was a man who effortlessly negotiated the porous, wafer-thin membrane separating Homo from the Other. . . . Still alive . . . standing before me . . . symmetrical, convergent consciousness: the world before."[35] Justo Oxa, a Quechuan schoolteacher in Peru, describes his trans-species culture in this manner:

> The community, the ayllu, is not only a territory where a group of people live; it is more than that. It is a dynamic space where the whole community of beings that exist in the world lives; this includes humans, plants, animals, the mountains, the rivers, the rain, etc. All are related like a family. It is important to remember that this place [the community] is not where we are from, it is who we are. For example, I am not from Huantura, I am Huantura.[36]

Cross-species and multicultural fluidity are also vividly documented among cross-fostered nonhumans, those who, similar to human feral children, have been raised by someone other than their own species and show a distinct affinity for relationships, identity, and cultural values reflective of their adoptive families.[37] Identification with their nonbiological species may be so dominant that conspecifics are eschewed. Psychological content does not always equate with external form.

Billy Jo was a wild-caught Chimpanzee who was raised as a human boy. His "owners" used Billy Jo in their entertainment business where he performed at private parties. At home, however, he dressed like a young man in t-shirts and pants, watched television and ate popcorn, and went fishing with his "dad." In his late teens, Billy Jo was sold to a biomedical lab where, for two decades, he underwent invasive procedures and lived alone in a six-by-six-by-four-foot cage suspended from a track. Eventually, he was rescued and brought to the Fauna Foundation, a Montreal-based sanctuary.

Unlike other Chimpanzees, Billy Jo was not able to integrate with conspecifics; in fact, he was almost killed by fellow residents. Sanctuary director Gloria Grow created for Billy Jo his own habitat, which included a night nest (similar to those that wild Chimpanzees build in trees) and access to "human" food. He loved to eat spaghetti twirled around a fork, drink coffee after carefully opening a packet of sugar and stirring it in with a spoon, wear different shirts and clothing, and watch women's exercise programs on television. Clearly, his sense of self and identity were predominantly human embodied in Chimpanzee form.[38] "Tim," another Chimpanzee at a second sanctuary who had also been in a circus, similarly illustrates the psychological importance of identity.

The sanctuary director called asking if I could explain why Tim had suddenly turned violent and destructive. When he arrived, Tim had been quite amiable and seemed to fit in well with his new home. After some discussion, I learned that the onset of his outbursts coincided with the removal of the baseball cap and plastic Hawaiian lei that he wore when he arrived. In an effort to help "put Tim's traumatic circus past behind him," the sanctuary had confiscated what they considered harmful symbols of Tim's slavery and brutal past. I suggested that they return the clothing because it was obviously of great importance to Tim, his sense of self, and security. If and when he was ready, and began to engage more fully with the "natural" setting of the sanctuary, the complex landscape, earth, and fruits, as well as other Chimpanzees, he might feel comfortable and secure enough to let go of his clothing. The sanctuary director had his clothing returned; Tim's angry, fearful outbursts subsided; and two months later, he dropped his cap and lei. Eventually, he ignored the articles of clothing entirely, and they were subsequently removed.

Empathy for another species may derive less from a shared developmental model than philosophy. Barney, a shelter volunteer, put it this way: "I am not an 'Animal person,' but I was drawn to help Animals in sanctuary as a social justice issue. Anyone who is treated cruelly and discriminated against should be protected." In other cases, a human may be drawn to nonhumans because of negative experiences with other humans such as trauma or, as in Barney's case, a rejection of society's treatment of nonhuman Animals. In these cases, affinity to nonhumans is less through a prosocial identity than disidentification with humans. A wildlife rescue volunteer recounts, "It's hard to feel very good about the species that has caused the problem I am trying to fix day-in day-out in sanctuary and rescue. Some days I am ashamed to be a human. And frankly, compared to Animals, most humans offer so little in terms of love, support, and honesty."[39]

A number of Animal workers express frustration with people who come to rescue and sanctuary primarily as a means to their own ends rather than a commitment to service: "When we work in rescue, we rescue many humans as well. . . . [However] I believe that when we put our self between Animals and our mission, we can lose sight of our goals. It's not about us!" While human trauma does not preclude ethical interactions with Animals, the accompanier needs to be keenly aware of his or her psychological state so as not to project damage on an Animal held captive and in recovery. This criticism has been levied at Animal-assisted therapy where Horses, Dogs, Parrots, and other species are used as recovery media for human adults and children with physical or psychological issues.[40]

A relationship grounded in wounding begins an interspecies relationship in very different ways than via trans-species identity, with the result that the Animal, who is psychologically vulnerable and in many cases traumatized, is at risk. A sanctuary professional asserts, "Very often these are people seeking self-fulfillment, needing to heal something within themselves by helping to heal the Animals, needing to belong to something and to be important somewhere." Animal care, then, may serve as a kind of psychological and emotional bandage or refuge where the human individual can avoid the challenges of intraspecies tension. These situations contrast with those of accompaniment where there is a sense of deep, empathetic, trans-species connection and shared or intersecting identity.

A trans-species sense of self and accompaniment do not require disidentification with one's biological origins, rather they entail cultivating an attitude that is not defined by external form. Kinship with, affinity to, and group identification with nonhuman Animals (if the latter are also open and positive toward such a relationship) fosters mutual psychological comfort and assurance. Natural historian and author of *Grizzly Heart*, Charlie Russell, describes his relationship with bears and sense of self this way:

> I consider bears, elk, and other animals like equals. We have different jobs as it were, but we live in the same community and what they are up to is at least as important as what I am doing or likely more so. There are some with whom I am particularly close and others I am not—much the same way I feel about humans. I know I am a human—there's a lot about me that is clearly human and not bear or elk, but there's also a lot that I relate to and share with the wildlife. I don't really think about who I am and who "they" are, just assume we are generally on the same wavelength and that any benign interaction with each other is completely normal. I guess I am not that hung up on what people look like on the outside. It's what's inside that counts.

Some accompaniers expressed a distinct preference for the values and culture of nonhuman species. Russell continues,

> For me, it's about the individual as we have both individual personalities and a group personality—for example, a shy bear may become very outgoing when in a group . . . and return to his/her shyness if/when not a group situation. . . . I am definitely a person who prefers to be with bears than people and definitely have a strong relationship and empathy with them compared with people.[41]

Not only do animal workers have diverse points of philosophical departure but of arrival too. Russell's fluidity of self and lack of preoccupation with human identity contrasts with the view of workers who, while actively campaigning for Animal rights, retain vestiges of *scala naturae* anatomy. Nonhuman Rights Project founder and attorney Steve Wise, who is litigating for Chimpanzee, Orca, and Elephant personhood, sees the necessity of drawing "lines," tailoring universal rights and self-determination based on an anthropocentric system of valuation: "Once we have broken through we intend to litigate which nonhuman animals should have what legal rights, based on what science tells us about each species."[42]

Social and self-identity may also vary with the situation. Daphne Sheldrick, founder of the David Sheldrick Wildlife Trust, and her carers play multiple roles in the lives of their Elephant charges: parent, therapist, advocate, friend, and teacher. Each relationship engages a different persona and part of one's self. Accompaniment requires an understanding of individual psyches and biographies in addition to natural history; a cross-species, bicultural perspective; and, if not an identification, then at least a deep connection to other-than-human sensibilities.[43]

Trans-species accompaniers often act as "culture brokers" helping Animals bridge personal experiences and cultures with those of other residents and humans in sanctuary. Carol Buckley, founder and director of Elephant Aid International, rescues Elephants from circuses and zoos. Historically, before widespread killing, social breakdown, homeland loss, and persistent human harassment, Elephants lived in a coherent, multitiered society whose nuclei were the natal family, a group of related individuals, a constellation of allomothers (female "aunties") and young Elephants ranging in age and led by a senior female. Captured and captive Elephants have been torn from or never experienced this (as in the case of captive-born individuals). Although they can and do form deep relationships with other Elephants in sanctuary, a reconstituted "family/herd" does not replicate what they would have experienced naturally in the wild. Similar to Gloria Grow, Buckley's accompaniment work in Elephant care is tasked with introducing unfamiliar, unrelated, and severely traumatized individual Elephants who come from disparate communities. Elephants in sanctuary learn to live at the intersection of Elephant cultures and those of humans.

Life outside the "Animal world" can be daunting. Jungian analyst and clinician psychologist Jerome S. Bernstein describes these individuals as "borderlanders." Their landscape is species-porous. Bernstein lists ten attributes characteristic of trans-species borderlanders:

1. Borderland personalities have a deep and primary connection to Nature. Most are more comfortable in relationship with animals than with people.

2. All have transrational experiences such as communicating with plants and animals and somatic identification with earth's suffering.

3. Many have experienced trauma as children or adults. Many have not.

4. Unlike the Borderline personality, the Borderland personality has a stable identity.

5. Most hide their Borderland Nature—often including from their therapist—for fear of being branded "crazy" or weird. This leads to living parallel and camouflaged lives—their hidden life in the Borderland (which is their primary identification), and their life in the mundane world.

6. Most feel isolated and lack a sense of community and belonging because they are unaware that there are many others like them.

7. All experience their Borderland reality as sacred.

8. Most tend to be hypersensitive on the somatic level. Many experience Environmental Illness. But, many do not.

9. 100% of all Borderland personalities with whom [Bernstein] has had contact say they would not give up that connection [with Nature] if they could—even if it were to diminish their suffering.

10. Although many would identify with being Nature's "canaries," most are at a loss as to the imperative for transformation that they have been given.[44]

Borderlanders often experience negative effects in the broader context of society, such as disparate wages, invalidation of cultural values, hostility, and isolation. Consequences for species trespass can weigh heavily. A physicist, Joe, shares a home with a Parrot (Tiki) and aquaria Fish whom he has rescued. The home in which they live is literally filled with Cockatoo habitat—large structures and piles of wood and indoor plants over which heavy ropes have been placed to emulate the flora of Cockatoo forests. Joe gently stewards the aquatic living quarters of Fish, carefully providing them with food that best suits their palates and heritages. He saves the barest of minimum for himself, his resources devoted to the nonhumans he has rescued. His deep appreciation for nonhumans is attended by excruciating pain caused by witnessing human indifference and cruelty:

> i try and take Tiki with me wherever i go (within reason). There are certain places that he is forbidden from being because of health code. i take issue with this of course mainly because there seems to be so much more to this banning. i think people just want nonhumans out and away. The bulk of people seem to at best regard Tiki as a fancy "object" of some value and entertainment. Or like zombies by comparison and i feel threatened for Tiki's sake as they can completely disregard him as being a viable Life. I am as alien as he is in those people's world. Every now and again, though, someone "connects" with Tiki with at least their whole heart if not their soul. These people appear as "alive" or, like me, half and half 'ers, half alive and half dead. For ten years now, I have watched my nonhuman family become a decimated memory. It is not lost on me how this is a "silhouette" of what is happening in the rest of the natural world around us. This does not offer or bring any relief from the constant grief that has engulfed me. The only way i have been able to survive, is through extreme focus on whatever i am endeavoring to accomplish for beings whose environment i can provide some semblance of freedom and even harmony. i get up between 2 and 4 every morning and walk for one hour around (through) the path between the trees and aquariums and kitchen + kitchen perches. Then i do yesterday's dishes (with a blue night light); feed the Elephant Nose (nocturnal Fish) and wait for Tiki to come down from the dormer window perch. He comes down and calls me and so i walk over and sing "daddy Loves Baby" and turn around

for him to hop over to my shoulder. Then we go crawl under the covers and snuggle for as long as he will stay. I fall asleep and actually rest (the only time in a 24 hour period) with his face and beak pressed against my face. This is the only thing i am certain of in life. This is what i am most grateful for and at the same time the most resentful for having lost time after time with each passing. How do i forgive Heaven for letting all of this happen?[45]

Social marginalization of Animals leads many Animal protection caregivers to feel "silenced" by denials concerning widespread suffering. Lauren Bailey, who is completing her degree in ethology at the University of Exeter, finds that

sometimes it is really difficult [to] speak up for what's right—difficult because I get angry that humans are in such denial of what they are doing. There is this overwhelming feeling of helplessness. At times I burst into tears because I can't do enough. Animal suffering is everywhere, I mean everywhere. I want to save everyone. I get exhausted. In Thailand, I witnessed such horrible cruelty to Elephants. How could people do that—steal a baby Elephant from her mother then beat and torture a *baby*?[46]

Annie, who has worked in a farmed Animal sanctuary for six years, observes,

Aside from a couple of co-caregivers, most people, including my family, don't really get why I do what I do. If I try and tell them about animals' plight and the terrible things that happens to them, I get "I don't want to hear about it" or "That's just the way life is" Or "What about human children? Don't they need our help first?" So, I have learned to steer away from the subject, keep the conversation "safe," and keep closed up.[47]

Individuals not infrequently express a sense of "no exit," nowhere to "escape," and no source of validation and camaraderie except fellow

Animal protection associates who are also struggling psychologically. These individuals feel that they have neither adequate at-work or in-home emotional and social support, an issue that has potentially adverse impacts on Animals outside sanctuary as well. Accompaniers express a pervasive sense of isolation, rejection, and empathetic strain, what Claire Mann refers to as "vystopia," an existential dystopia that, she maintains, many vegans experience. Even former refuges that provided temporary respite from the pain are gone.[48] Lena, a longtime shelter worker, describes her breakdown after witnessing the euthanasia of a Rooster at the shelter:

> I had witnessed countless situations almost identical to this. But something unexpected happened. Something inside me disintegrated, crumbled. As that gentle spirit was put to rest, I fled and before I could reach the bathroom, retched in the hall corner. After a few minutes, the center director came out. She waited silently while I washed up then said: "If you can't handle it, you shouldn't be here." She turned and left. The next day, I resigned. The following months found me gripped by a multitude of emotions—shame, anger, betrayal, grief, outrage, numbness, exhaustion, and confusion. Those feelings have muted, but remain. I still wonder what "handling it" really means.[49]

Yet almost all insist that the pain and difficulties of Animal accompaniment are attended by profound transformation. Similar to human-human accompaniment, partnered journeys of humans and Animals are twinned processes where accompanier and accompanied participate as co-transformative agents. Molly Flanagan teaches at a university in the California Bay Area. She describes her experience at a Chicken slaughter vigil:

> We stand at the entryway where the trucks unload the Chickens in crates to be slaughtered inside. It was so incredible to be so close and connecting. I really tried hard to connect with individuals. I tried to hold them in my gaze. I kept saying to them silently, "Don't look over there—stay with me." They remained

in eye contact until they were pulled out. I have never experienced such an honor to be able to be with them at that moment even though knowing that I/we could not prevent their terrible pain, fear, and deaths. It is a transformative experience. At the same time, I don't want to be there, I don't want to experience this, and yet the more connected that I feel with them, the stronger I become. I used to fear speaking up and causing social discomfort. Two days after the vigil, I was standing on BART when I overheard a man on his phone ordering burritos for dinner. I heard him request a veggie burrito and thought "oh, good, I don't have to say anything." But then he asked for a Chicken burrito. So I was compelled to say to him, "Hi, do you mind if I ask you a question?" He was open and said yes, and so I shared my experience at the slaughterhouse. He stayed very open. Vigil experiences have given me courage.[50]

Reflecting on his experiences of slaughterhouse vigils, Corey Rowland, a member of DxE and accompanier at slaughterhouse vigils, also speaks to deep internal shifts: "Even though, there they are, in cages with no chance. But somehow, being there, bearing witness, looking in each other's eyes, no matter how briefly, before they are slaughtered, there's a feeling of being paired allies. I think they can feel us standing there for them. It changes you, it changed me, so, in a way, those Chickens are part of me and I am part of them."[51]

Anita Krajnc holds a doctorate in political science and was an anti-nuclear activist before becoming involved in Animal rights. Her Animal accompaniment was catalyzed after watching daily truckloads of Pigs being taken to the slaughterhouse. In response, Krajnc cofounded the nonprofit Toronto Pig SAVE in 2010, which has expanded to over two hundred SAVE groups located around the world "who bear witness to pigs, cows, chickens and other farmed animals en route to slaughter." The vigils in which Flanagan, Rowland, and Sharo participate are part of the SAVE movement, organized by Bay Area Animal SAVE. SAVE's goal is to "raise awareness about the plight of farmed animals, to help people become vegan, and to build a mass-based, grassroots animal justice movement." Their primary strategy is "bearing witness to animals in their final moment as they approach slaughterhouses. We use a love-based community-organizing approach and develop team leadership in order to build a grassroots animal justice movement based on the principles of animal equality and freedom."[52]

Krajnc and others describe the reflexive nature of accompaniment:

> When I was about to be arrested, I remember starting to shake almost convulsively, I was so afraid of challenging authority. Since then, my fear has left me. . . . Toronto Pig Save (TPS) has vastly improved my life. Before TPS, I often was depressed about the state of the world. Paradoxically, I know more now about the unspeakable suffering of animals, and witness it personally each week, but I also see more changes.[53]

Krajnc became headline news when in 2015 she was arrested and charged with criminal mischief after she and other members of Toronto Pig SAVE tried to give water to the more than 190 Pigs through the metal vents in a truck outside Frearman Slaughterhouse, in Burlington, Ontario. A video taken by a SAVE member shows the Pigs dehydrated, stressed, and fearful, mouths dripping frothy saliva.[54] Anita was acquitted in 2017 but the judge included in his decision an insistence that Pigs—and Dog and Cats—are property, not persons. Further, he took umbrage with the defense counsel comparison of mass slaughter of Pigs and other farmed Animals to genocide and the Holocaust, finding "the comparison to be offensive and I will be attaching no weight to it in my decision."[55]

The issue of Animal personhood is pivotal. In Western cultures, "being a person" is generally defined as possessing consciousness over time, having agency and a sense of self, qualities synonymous with humans. Although U.S. corporations have been granted personhood, any attempt to demonstrate nonhuman personhood has failed. While some Westernized countries have extended personhood to Bears, rivers, and Great Apes, legal efforts on behalf of Elephants and Chimpanzees in the United States have been turned down by the courts.[56]

Steven Wise is founder and president of the Nonhuman Rights Project, whose mission is to "change the legal status of appropriate nonhuman animals from mere 'things,' which lack the capacity to possess any legal right, to 'persons,' who possess such fundamental rights as bodily integrity and bodily liberty." Wise has chosen litigation because of the recognition that

> there was a powerful structural bias in the law against protecting even the most fundamental interests of nonhuman animals. . . . The goal of the Nonhuman Rights Project is to break through the legal wall that has prevented all nonhuman animals from attaining legal rights for centuries. . . . From the outset we encountered numerous legal obstacles that we have been determined to surmount, one by one. We are slowly succeeding. We are also working with legal groups in ten countries on three continents to assist them in gaining legal rights for nonhuman animals in their jurisdictions. In November a court in Argentina found a chimpanzee named Cecilia to be a "nonhuman animal person" and ordered her transferred to a sanctuary in Brazil pursuant to a writ of habeas corpus.[57]

By bearing witness to Chickens, Pigs, and other Animals, accompaniers seek to dispel the imposed construct of species differences. Putting their bodies "on the line" is used as proof of a shared personhood with those who appear different on the outside but who have a common consciousness and soul.

Sea Change: Trans-Species Accompaniment as Emergent Culture

Love, by its very nature, is unworldly, and it is for this reason rather than its rarity that it is not only apolitical but antipolitical, perhaps the most powerful of all antipolitical forces.

—Hannah Arendt

Given the human-dominated context and language in which Animal accompaniment is set, it is easy to overlook the active participation of nonhumans.

Accompaniers are quick to point out that bearing witness recognizes engagement by the Animals for whom they are advocating. When Krajnc
stands next to trucks filled with Pigs, "I stand between [the Pigs] and the
managers and act as their voice and they know. . . . The pigs definitely know
who their friends are."[58] Andrew Sharo agrees:

> Some people say that Animals are voiceless, not able to advo-
> cate, but that is not true. Yes—at, say, an LGBT activist meeting,
> it is led by LGBT folks. Animal rights is led by human (Ani-
> mals). But is it being led by nonhuman or human Animals?
> This has to be an ongoing question. We have to remember that
> Animals are always the leaders. They may not use social media,
> they may be caged, but that is what we know how to use and we
> do so on their behalf to further their cause. Every direct action
> we report always tells their story, always.[59]

Corey Rowland recounts his experience at a Chicken slaughterhouse
vigil:

> It is difficult to explain to someone who has not been part
> of or witnessed a slaughterhouse vigil. But in my heart and my
> experience, we humans do play an important part not only in
> terms of making known what is hidden—the brutality to which
> Chickens and other farmed Animals are subjected—and waking
> up the humans who are involved in all that, but the Animals
> themselves. I can be their voice to humans who can't or won't
> listen to the Animals. Being there, being present physically, is
> very powerful. As best we can, we are putting our bodies on
> the line—not of course the way that the Chickens and Pigs
> are who we are witnessing and will die very soon—but being
> there with them is really different than writing a letter or giving
> a talk. I think it is because *we are with them at the terrible mo-
> ment before their death.* We are participating in their lives and
> deaths.[60]

Lauren Bailey has volunteered at farmed Animal sanctuaries and plans to craft a career dedicated to Animal rights and a life of accompaniment. She also disagrees that nonhumans are "voiceless" and makes the point that part of accompaniment entails not forcing Animals to "talk" on human terms:

> You just have to listen. We don't do that a lot in our culture. So rather than being in control of helping someone, like Matilda the Turkey in sanctuary, accompaniment means being there for them when they need you even if they don't say they need your help. Being a companion rather than someone in control or fixing something and letting them go at their own pace without forcing them to meet your expectation. With nonhumans, if you are quiet and listen, they will cue you. Once they know you are there with them and can be trusted, then gradually they tell you everything they need. At the sanctuary, so many of the other volunteers would talk right in front of the Animals as if they weren't there. You have to communicate the process to the Animal. Like "Matilda, I'm going to clean out your habitat because . . ." etc. The Animals pick up on this ethic of inclusivity because that is how they are. They don't assume that humans don't speak Turkey or whatever language. That's not important. What is important is how you feel about each other. After cleaning the enclosures, I would just sit on the floor and Matilda would come at her own time.[61]

Teri Walters founded the nonprofit Safe Haven Small Breed Rescue over twenty-five years ago and has rescued hundreds of mill Dogs, canines who are mass-produced in factory-like conditions.[62] On average, twenty to thirty Dogs live in her home that is the rescue-sanctuary. Walters is responsible for guiding physical and relational space that is shared by two score different personalities and experiences as well as preparing the Dogs to live in their adopted homes. Recognizing the exigencies that living within a human-dominated framework has created, she nonetheless emphasizes the need to create a trans-species way of living within those parameters that supports Animal agency, culture, values, and rhythms:

> Each and every one of the Dogs needs a psychological, social, moral, and physical sense of security—everything that was denied them when they were mill Dogs. It's up to me to craft that for all of the twenty-seven. First and foremost is I give them space, I watch them being with the others. I respond to their needs without forcing myself on them. Of course, at times I have to—for meds and things. But I try to let them take their own time and figure things out on their own. You provide the basics—good food, nice safe place to sleep, play, and live—when I say basic it really is more than that for them because they have never had this before, and we humans forget what it's like when you *don't* "have the basics." These traumatized Dogs need to have what they need on Dog time. For most, they don't even know what they want because they have never been asked. They have never been given a choice or opportunity. Dottie has always been timid and a bit standoffish. Then one day, and she had been here a while, I took a break from making Dog cookies and sat down on the couch. She came over. Then the timer rang, and I got up to turn the cookies. Dottie grabbed my pant leg trying to pull me back—her way of saying, "Hey! I'm not done with you yet!" It broke my heart. It was huge for her to initiate— she's never done that. It's times like that you know, you know they are starting to pull out of their past. It's also a time when they stop seeing things as "she and me" and start seeing "us."[63]

These nonhuman-human bonds do not stop at the level of individuals. They are embedded in a complex, multidimensional relational matrix of community and culture. Because nonhumans in these instances are included as equal partners, even privileged for the purpose of achieving parity, accompaniment acts as a culturally transformative reagent by dissolving the millennia-old barrier separating humans from Nature. Similar to trans-species psychology, methods employed by accompaniers are organic to the dominant paradigm but, when yielded in alignment with Animal rights, are deconstructive. Rowland describes his experience with nonviolence teachings:

> I recently got my first training in methods of nonviolence. It sounds odd but when you look at it, nonviolence is closely related to violence. It is not about avoiding conflict; it's about using conflict to solve a problem through reconciliation. We are faced with this profound disorder and tasked with bringing order, returning us to where [we] are supposed to be, converting negative peace into positive peace. Negative peace is when things appear to be going like they should and everything is quiet, but beneath all this is violence and injustice. Positive peace may not appear peaceful but everything is working well and in its natural order. It's the difference between modern human life and Nature. Just compare what modern humans have created with that of Nature—the first is neat, roads, building things, seems to be working, but it's ugly and so much violence has been done to create it and to maintain it. In Nature, things are happening all the time, it can be chaotic, but it all looks harmonious—the colors, the shapes, and the feeling.[64]

Both Molly Flanagan and Corey Rowland cite the "liberation pledge" as another powerful tool. "It really says to a fellow human, 'I won't sacrifice an animal to maintain our relationship' and *that* is radical."[65] The pledge is composed of three parts: to "publicly refuse to eat animals—live vegan, publicly refuse to sit where animals are being eaten, and encourage others to take the pledge." Names of pledgers and city and country of residence are displayed on the liberation pledge website, which, with its companion Facebook page, provide information and social support.[66]

Assessing the pledge as a radical move is accurate. By extending veganism to include human social interactions and rituals, the pledger refutes the hegemonic status of the human-human contract. But the pledge is far from being asocial. Rather, it resituates the human-human bond by grounding it in nonhuman Nature. Human relationships are valued but they are redefined by a trans-species ethic. This is consistent with one of the primary goals of Animal accompaniment: the deconstruction of human privilege and restoration of Animal and other Nature self-determination that simultaneously repairs human psyches damaged by the utilitarian paradigm.

Animal accompaniers openly discuss the importance of building community with conspecifics. Krajnc calls cultivating solidarity and collective activism with those sharing a common ethic "the best antidote on a personal and social level." She describes how

> what we see is hard, but what's positive is the suffering animals want us there to see them and to be their voice. If I were in that truck, I would want the same. It's made easier because we bear witness as a collective. The great artist Sue Coe said if you bear witness in a slaughterhouse by yourself, you will go insane. But collectively bearing witness is empowering and it builds community.[67]

Similarly, Andrew Sharo talks about how, after graduating from Princeton in physics and moving to Berkeley to enroll in a biophysics doctoral program, meeting other Animal activists and vegans made such a huge difference psychologically:

> Something changes when you meet other people who feel the same way you do. Suddenly, you stop feeling bizarre and so vulnerable. It was important for me to see other vegans who had vegan friends. I began to feel a part of a community. We all have different backgrounds but are united, together, because we are committed to the same cause. Having a diversity of like-hearted friends is really different from either being the only vegan or having one or two people you know who are vegan. Vigils are similar. They are community-building. It is really a positive experience

and has changed my perception about myself—it's a shared sense of self. I practice meditation daily to help me keep me sane.[68]

Social connection is not limited to within-movement members. SAVE workers even make a point of reaching out to foster human connection with those who are agents of Animal suffering. At vigils, they pass out educational DVDs and vegan BLTs to truckers hauling the Pigs: "We approach workers with respect as equals—but we don't always meet this standard, especially if we view a worker who is violent with the electric prod. . . . It is difficult remaining calm and talking in a respectful way, but it's an ideal we strive for."[69] Some meat workers have joined Pig SAVE groups.

Little by little the effects of this effort across sociopolitical lines make a mark:

> We also see the ripple effects of us standing there . . . it posi-
> tively affects the public and workers in the animal exploitation
> industry to see us there. It sends out the message "we're here,
> we care, we're sorry and we're trying." We plant some seeds and
> put the issue on the public agenda. Suddenly people start see-
> ing the transport trucks and looking and talking about it at
> home, at school and at work. We also get media attention which
> takes our message far and wide and we always take pictures at
> every vigil and post these on Facebook and occasionally create
> videos of the suffering animals and us activists bearing witness.
> Our vigils are 98% love-based and positive but occasionally
> there's a slip as in this video called Confrontation![70]

There is also increased attention to internal edges within the human accompanier community that, without tending, can undermine the spirit and intentions of accompaniment. Animal Liberationists of Color is an affiliate of DxE with common goals of increasing human ethnic diversity within Animal rights and addressing racism within the movement. Wayne Hsiung of both groups notes,

Roughly 95 to 97% of the public faces of [the animal rights] movement are still white. . . . The angriest and most hostile and aggressive campaigns have been focused on practices in foreign communities among people of color. . . . People were talking about murdering Michael Vick, which I thought was just shocking, the amount of angry and violent rhetoric, notwithstanding the fact that I agree that what Michael Vick did to these dogs was a terrible thing. And routinely whenever someone posts something about dogs being killed in China or cats being eaten or fur farms in China or Asia, you see people coming out of the woodwork saying things like, "The Chinese are a subspecies" or "I wish the entire Chinese population could be wiped out." And one of the most astonishing things I saw recently was a number of people responding to one of these pictures on Facebook saying that the Chinese are animals. Our movement talks about how much we love animals, how much we support animals, how much we want to protect animals. And yet we are seeing racial dynamics come out that reinforce the objectification of animals and violence against animals.[71]

lauren Ornelas, founder and director of Food Empowerment Project, discussed the link between racism and Animal rights, which powerfully intersect at food—what and who we eat. More specifically, she makes the point that the poor and marginalized frequently do not have ready access to healthy, plant-based foods to substitute for Animal products:

You have a lot of communities of color and low-income communities who do not have access to fresh fruits and vegetables. In our work at F.E.P., we know that some are immigrants who, after moving here, are being forced to eat unhealthier foods. Many are working several jobs to make ends meet and happen to live closer to a liquor store or fast food outlets with unhealthy foods. . . . The word vegan should not just be used when referring to people who choose not to eat animal products because being vegan includes doing our best to abstain from participating in the other ways animals are exploited, including animal testing.[72]

While considerable accompaniment work involves farmed Animals, there are many efforts to stand with the wild. Wolf Patrol, founded by Rod Coronado, is a response to the delisting of the North American Gray Wolf in the United States. It involves "citizen monitoring of public wildlife policies as a means towards exposing bad wolf policies, and using such documentation to empower citizens to become active in the reform of state wildlife agency policies. Wolf Patrol engages in community outreach and education to share strategy ideas and tactics, and information about the ecological importance of wolves and other predators."[73]

Coronado is a Pasqua Yaqui born in 1966 and former member of Earth Liberation Front and Sea Shepherds. In 1995, he was sentenced to five years in prison and charged $2 million for restitution for committing arson at Michigan State University, which caused $125,000 in damages to animal laboratory facilities. Prior to his founding of Wolf Patrol, he was accused of and jailed on successive occasions for alleged "terrorist" acts. In 2008, he wrote an open letter stating that he only participates in nonviolent protests exemplified by his founding of Wolf Patrol, which, he clarifies, is a "tactic," not an organization. Their approach is based on "principles of biocentricity, and indigenous cultural preservation. We believe in supporting the recovery of gray wolves in the lower 48 states and encouraging a greater understanding and tolerance for cultural world views that promote a harmonious co-existence with wolves and other predators."[74]

Wolves were effectively eliminated from the coterminous United States by the 1930s. In 1967, Gray Wolves were pulled from the precipice of extinction when they were listed under the Endangered Species Preservation Act, the precursor of the Endangered Species Act (ESA). By 1978, the Gray Wolf, including all its subspecies, were listed under the protective wing of the ESA. However, the new grace enjoyed by Wolves was short-lived. Twenty-five years later, in less than three Wolf generations, the U.S. Fish and Wildlife Service (USFWS) ruled that Gray Wolves should be down-listed from their endangered status to threatened. This meant that Wolves would become fair game for hunters. Federal courts countered by overruling the USFWS, claiming that the agency's proposal was "arbitrary and capricious." Nonetheless, the USFWS continued to campaign for delisting until 2011, when for the first time ever Congress delisted a species from the ESA. Individual states now have authority to decide to permit legal Wolf hunting.

Activists in Wolf Patrol travel to where Wolf or Bear hunts will be taking place and film the hunt. More often than not they are met with intense hostility. Hunters in trucks try to block and push Wolf Patrol vehicles off public roads. Their cameras have been confiscated by local police and they have received threats of being run down. Although Coronado and colleagues do not back down from gaining access to witness and film hunts, they are committed to nonviolence and dialogue.

In September 2017, a Bear and Wolf hunter with six Bear hounds in the back of his truck called Coronado over to sit down with him on the ground for an "Injun council." He then challenged Coronado to an "Indian style fight to the death." Coronado sat down but told the man that he was there to stop killing—the killing of Wolves, Bears, and humans. The man insisted that his hunting was legal. Coronado agreed and added that Wolf Patrol filming on public lands, too, was legal. Finally, after a tense discussion, including a second hunter attempting to block the meeting's filming, Coronado and the first hunter parted. As they stood up, Coronado wished the hunter, "Good day, Sir," and the hunter, replied, "Take care." Violence was averted, and some semblance of détente seemed to be achieved.[75]

These transactional flashpoints are symptoms of deeper currents. Many see Nature's recovery in need of a much more radical transformation, a "de-domestication" or re-wilding of domesticated humans and nonhumans alike. Others, such as Darcia Narvaez, a moral neuropsychologist at the University of Notre Dame, and Kevin Tucker, an anarcho-primitivist scholar of anthropology, beckon our species to return to its nomadic origins when humans lived in concert with the rhythms of Nature. Humanity's cultural chronosequence from horticulture to agriculture, and urbanization via industrialization and technology, Tucker maintains, has taken our species farther and farther away from the ability to adapt to Nature's vagaries. Civilization's proliferation does not reflect an evolution of advancement but rather an exponentially increasing hunger to substitute Nature's organization with our own:

> Domestication is, at its root, about the creation and maintenance of a synthetic order. It is about control. It reduces the fullness of the world into categories and systems of needs and resources. It turns wild communities into a sum of all parts rather than a single interconnected community. . . . As we rapidly approach the inevitable collapse of our own civilization . . . the implications of this critique become all the more important. We need to ask what does it mean in terms of our own future and how does that influence our decisions and directions now. . . . There is still some time to react to what we know about civilization and about wildness. There is time to work to apply some of these implications in our own lives and on the large scale.[76]

There is no question that the Animal rights movement and Animal accompaniment are demanding the most extreme changes in human psyche and society. With the cold realization of the damage that the project of progress has caused, our species is beginning to understand that nonhuman liberation is required for the survival of all species. By breaking down anthropocentrism, the mandate that has sought to outcompete Nature, a trans-species culture of accompaniment and the commons has returned as a human necessity and an existential reality.

NINE

Earth Accompaniment

Standing with Trees, Waters, Mountains, Earth, and Air

PRACTICES OF ECOLOGICAL accompaniment, the accompani-
ment of natural and built environments by humans, are a necessary foundation for sustainable and just life on Earth. Many culturally traditional forms
of eco-accompaniment have been radically disrupted by densely interrelated forces. The seizure of commons for the development of excess profit,
discussed in chapter 10, displaced people from the countryside to the cities
where rapid industrialization with the use and abuse of cheap labor took
root. Colonialism, with its racist constructs, waged genocidal assaults on
many Indigenous societies that embodied ecological mutual accompaniment as a cultural practice. These attacks go on as neoliberal capitalist
methods continue to treat the natural world solely as a source of short-term
economic profit. The West's radical individualism fundamentally recon-
ceived human beings as distinct from and superior to nature. The natural
world began to be seen as something separate from humans and to be used
for their sake—to be owned, mastered, and exploited. Instead of honoring
the natural world as a sacred web of reciprocal relationships of which we are
but a part, some humans came to see it as property to be managed and used.

Now humans' standing with trees, water, mountains, soil, seeds, and air
must provide not only witness to the ecocide that has been suffered but engagement in strategic struggles to stop the destruction and repair and restore
whole bioregions. Such accompaniment must prefigure truly sustainable and
equitable ways of living. Ecological accompaniment, like human-to-human
accompaniment, is marked by deep listening and responsiveness to the

Earth. Earth accompanists labor to stop humans' exploitative manner of relating to Earth.[1] This response-ability propels them into political struggles to secure and protect the rights of nature.

The psychological and community health of humans cannot be adequately addressed without sustained attention to environmental well-being. Psychosocial accompaniment must be indissolubly linked to ecological accompaniment. This chapter addresses a series of questions: What does ecological accompaniment look like? What are some of the grassroots models we should be aware of? How do we live into a deepened solidarity with the natural world at this perilous moment in Earth history and with those communities most affected by neoliberalism's destruction of their homeplaces? How can the classist and racist othering of poor communities and communities of color be understood as inseparable from the othering of natural entities, making psychosocial accompaniment and eco-accompaniment one?

Earth Democracy

The degree of democracy we can achieve is limited by our vision of who belongs, who counts among us, who and what has or does not have rights. In the United States, democracy was originally conceived to include white men who owned land. Only in time—and with great struggle—did propertyless men and men who were former slaves come to be included. Still later, women were also included. In the present, deep ideological battles continue over who can participate, who can register to vote, and to what extent people's votes count. Can prisoners and the formerly incarcerated vote? Can immigrant-neighbors without documents participate in local elections? Will precinct and district lines and the configuration of the Electoral College continue to be used to give more weight to some votes than to others, to favor a particular set of ideologies and interests over others?

Environmental legal scholar Christopher Stone proclaimed in his 1972 essay "Should Trees Have Standing? Toward Legal Rights for Natural Objects" that "the world of the lawyer is peopled with inanimate right-holders: trusts, corporations, joint ventures, municipalities, Subchapter R partnerships, and nation-states, to name a few." Yet we find other-than-human

sentient beings—rivers, mountains, forests, air—largely excluded from having legal rights.[2] Earth democracy, as described by environmental activist
and physicist Vandana Shiva, challenges this exclusion and proposes a
democracy founded on an awareness of the interconnectedness among
all living beings and on the rights and responsibilities that flow from these
connections.[3]

    Earth democracy is a radical corrective to the present reality of busi-
nesses and governments that accord no sentience and legal rights to the
other-than-human beings of nature. When nature is viewed as having
no rights, it is prey to commodification and the mindless extraction of non-
renewable "resources" for the profit of a small number of humans. The
hyper-extraction and excess consumption of these resources too often
leaves behind sickened and destroyed ecosystems, byproducts of normalized destructive business practices. This is done without recognition of the
harm perpetrated not only on nature but on adjacent human communities
as well. In part, this is due to a lack of deep comprehension of our interdependence and a resulting failure to value *all* communities. Poor communities and communities marginalized due to race and/or ethnicity experience
a double devaluing—of themselves and the land on which they live, including the larger landscapes that surround them. These cruel diminishments
set the stage for environmental exploitation that leaves behind bioregions
and human communities as devastated sacrifice zones.

    Shiva articulates key principles of Earth democracy: that all species,
peoples, and cultures have intrinsic worth; that diversity in nature and culture be defended; and that all beings have a natural right to sustenance.
Earth democracies, for Shiva, are created through a synergy between living
economies, living democracies, and living cultures. Living economies, built
on local economies, work to create and ensure sustainability and share
prosperity across people. Living democracies work to uphold our freedom
and human rights through our own active participation "to protect life on
earth, defend peace, and promote justice." They honor all species. Living
cultures are life-nourishing. They are marked by their "nonviolence and
compassion, diversity and pluralism, equality and justice, and respect for
life in all its diversity."[4]

Movements for Earth democracy seek to protect the local commons that exist and to create new commons where water, forest, and Earth are not exploited and destroyed. Instead, these are understood as having their own right to exist and thrive. Shiva describes living economies as those that protect life on Earth and contrasts these to suicidal economies, based in violence, that lead to the destruction of human and other-than-human life. Living economies do not eschew globalization but found it on "ecological processes and bonds of compassion and solidarity, not [on] the movement of capital and finance or the unnecessary movement of goods and services."[5]

Shiva describes Earth democracy as connecting "people in circles of care, cooperation, and compassion."[6] Thus, Earth democracy requires practices of mutual ecopsychosocial accompaniment. Qualifying accompaniment with the adjective "ecopsychosocial" points us in two interrelated directions. First, it requires that we accompany with awareness of the sociocultural, historical, and ecological contexts in which a particular accompaniment unfolds. Second, it refers to the interrelated realms across which accompaniment is needed: psychological, social, and ecological. At a local level, in an embodied Earth democracy, humans would accompany other-than-human nature to try to meet the needs and create the conditions for flourishing of all community members, human and nonhuman.

Accompaniment to Secure and Protect the Rights of Nature

While many Indigenous communities throughout the world have long histories of listening to the voices and attending to the well-being of mountains, rivers, oceans, forests, fields, seeds, and air, these voices are not listened for and attended to in neoliberal offices and boardrooms. Ecological accompaniment is necessary to bring these "voices" into the center of human attention and create legal structures where their rights can be recognized and protected. In the last fifty years, we have witnessed progress along these lines at global, national, and local levels. We have also witnessed the brutal repression of movements to protect nature, including the assassination of hundreds of environmental activists.

In 1972, Christopher Stone prefaced his case for the rights of nature by noting that every time a new group without rights sought to gain rights, its demands appeared ridiculous to many at the time—be they men without land, slaves, women, or children. "There is something of a seamless web involved: there will be resistance to giving the thing 'rights' until it can be seen and valued for itself; yet, it is hard to see it and value it for itself until we can bring ourselves to give it 'rights'—which is almost inevitably going to sound inconceivable to a large group of people."[7]

Stone clearly demonstrated that U.S. law was not concerned with the loss and harm suffered by natural entities. A homocentric perspective could only see natural entities in their use and monetary value for humans. Natural entities cannot institute legal actions, have their injury taken into account, or have relief assigned for their benefit. Stone proposed a guardianship approach, where a friend or friends of a forest or river, for instance, could represent the situation, arguing that it is not difficult to assess the state of well-being of a natural entity. He was aware that the movement to give legal standing to trees and other natural entities ultimately rests on humans' capacity to see the Earth as one organism of which they are a part. Is accompaniment of natural entities done for the sake of the entities themselves or for the humans that rely on their well-being? Stone answers, "Because the health and well-being of mankind depend upon the health of the environment, these goals will often be so mutually supportive that one can avoid deciding whether our rationale is to advance 'us' or a new 'us' that includes the environment."[8]

In 1968, the United Nations World Commission on Environment and Development called for a new charter to help guide sustainable development. In 1982, the UN General Assembly offered the global community a resolution entitled the World Charter for Nature. It articulated five important general principles:

1. Nature shall be respected and its essential processes shall not be impaired.
2. The genetic viability on the earth shall not be compromised; the population levels of all life forms, wild and domesticated,

      must be at least sufficient for their survival, and to this end necessary habitats shall be safeguarded.

3. All areas of the earth, both land and sea, shall be subject to these principles of conservation; special protection shall be given to unique areas, to representative samples of all the different types of ecosystems and to the habitats of rare or endangered species.

4. Ecosystems and organisms, as well as the land, marine and atmospheric resources that are utilized by man, shall be managed to achieve and maintain optimum sustainable productivity, but not in such a way as to endanger the integrity of those other ecosystems or species with which they coexist.

5. Nature shall be secured against degradation caused by warfare or other hostile activities.[9]

While UN resolutions are not binding, they do direct and encourage nations to craft their laws in the light of articulated principles.

In 2010, 35,000 people meeting in Cochabamba, Bolivia, at the World People's Conference on Climate Change affirmed the Universal Declaration of the Rights of Mother Earth. Mother Earth and all the "beings of which she is composed" were declared to have the

      right to life and to exist; the right to be respected; the right to regenerate its bio-capacity and to continue its vital cycles and processes free from human disruptions; the right to maintain its identity and integrity as a distinct, self-regulating and interrelated being; the right to water as a source of life; the right to clean air; the right to integral health; the right to be free from contamination, pollution and toxic or radioactive waste; the right to not have its genetic structure modified or disrupted in a manner that threatens its integrity or vital and healthy functioning; the right to full and prompt restoration for violation of the rights recognized in this Declaration caused by human activities.

Box 9.1 The Earth Charter

Mikhail Gorbachev, last leader of the Soviet Union, and Maurice Strong, controversial oil businessman and former secretary general of the United Nations Conference on the Human Environment, took to heart the United Nations' 1968 call for a new charter. The Earth Charter Commission was initiated as a follow-up to the 1992 Rio de Janeiro Earth Summit. The commission's goal was to create a global consensus of values and principles that could help construct a sustainable future. Over a six-year period (1994–2000), five thousand people contributed to the writing of the Earth Charter, and since then thousands of individuals and groups have signed on to the charter, using it to guide their actions.[a]

Unlike the Universal Declaration of Human Rights, which focuses entirely on human rights, the Earth Charter includes "life in all its diversity" and focuses on human responsibilities. It articulates sixteen principles on four interdependent pillars: respect and care for the Earth community; ecological integrity; social and economic justice; and democracy, nonviolence, and peace. The four principles of ecological integrity are

> 1) Protect and restore the integrity of Earth's ecological systems, with special concern for biological diversity and the natural processes that sustain life. 2) Prevent harm as the best method of environmental protection and, when knowledge is limited, apply a precautionary approach. 3) Adopt patterns of production, consumption and reproduction that safeguard Earth's regenerative capacities, human rights and community well-being. 4) Advance the study of ecological sustainability and promote the open exchange and wide application of the knowledge acquired.[b]

Despite the fact that many hoped this charter would include the rights of nature, it does not. Nevertheless, these four principles, taken together, aptly lay out the work of ecological accompanists.

---

a. Steven Rockefeller, "Universal Rights and Responsibilities: The Universal Declaration of Human Rights and the Earth Charter," April 2009, http://earthcharter.org/virtual-library2/universal-rights-and-responsibilities-the-universal-declaration-of-human-rights-and-the-earth-charter/.
b. The Earth Charter (text), http://earthcharter.org/virtual-library2/the-earth-charter-text/.

Further, the statement declared that "each being has the right to a place and to play its role in Mother Earth for her harmonious functioning," and the "right to well-being and to live free from torture or cruel treatment by human beings." For the rights of nature to be respected, human beings must shoulder their obligations to respect and live in harmony with Mother Earth. These obligations include defending her rights, establishing laws for this defense and protection, and learning how to live in harmony with Mother Earth.[10]

The Universal Declaration of the Rights of Mother Earth seeks to help ensure that the pursuit of human well-being contributes to the restoration and well-being of Mother Earth. Economic systems should support human harmony with Mother Earth and not harm the integrity of species and biosystems.

Navdanya is a multilevel initiative in Dehradun and New Delhi, India, that supports the Universal Declaration of the Rights of Mother Earth and development of Earth democracy (See Box 9.2).

These global initiatives now rest alongside several national initiatives. The inclusion of the rights of nature in the Ecuadorean Constitution in 2008 is a stunning example of the respect of and care for other-than-human nature. It proclaims that nature has rights to exist that can be legally enforced: "Nature or Pachamama, where life is reproduced and exists, has the right to exist, persist, maintain and regenerate its vital cycles, structure, functions and its processes in evolution."[11] Further, the constitution opens the door for every person, community, or nationality to "be able to demand the recognitions of rights for nature before the public organisms," welcoming "natural and juridical persons as well as collectives to protect nature."[12] Here accompaniment is called for—by individuals, communities, and collectives. The state itself assumes the responsibility for restoring and protecting ecosystems. Unfortunately, as the country's financial difficulties have deepened, the state has not upheld the law. Instead of decreasing oil production, in 2017 it was increased to gain revenue.

Across the globe, many Indigenous groups are leading local and regional struggles for governments to include the rights of nature among their central priorities and responsibilities, and to resist neoliberal globalization's

Box 9.2 Navdanya's Earth University/Bija Vidyapeeth
Dehradun, India

India's best ideas have come where a man was in communion with trees
and rivers and lakes, away from the crowds. The peace of the forest has
helped the intellectual evolution of man. The culture of the forest has
fueled the culture of Indian society. The culture that has arisen from the
forest has been influenced by the diverse processes of renewal of life,
which are always at play in the forest, varying from species to species,
from season to season, in sight and sound and smell. The unifying
principle of life in diversity, of democratic pluralism, thus became the
principle of Indian civilization.

—Rabindranath Tagore

In 1917, the "Bard of Bengal," Rabindranath Tagore, on a visit to
Santa Barbara and the orange groves of Los Angeles, began to dream about
a new kind of university where people could learn in and from nature. He
used his father's ashram to begin Visva-Bharati University. Its motto:
"Where the whole world meets in one nest."[a] Both Navdanya's Earth
University/Bija Vidyapeeth in India and Schumacher College in England
take their inspiration from Tagore's dream of "an essential education that
takes account of the organic wholeness of human individuality, needing a
general stimulation of all faculties, bodily and mental."[b] Bija Vidyapeeth
has grown out of a program founded by Vandana Shiva in 1984, the Research Foundation for Science, Technology, and Ecology. Bija Vidyapeeth
is a nature sanctuary and learning center for Earth citizenship and sustainability.

Navdanya, the umbrella NGO for Earth University, began the Earth
Democracy movement. This alternative worldview sees humans as embedded in the Earth, not lords over it. Greed, consumerism, and competition
are replaced by ecological responsibility and economic justice. Through
multiple initiatives and campaigns, Navdanya mobilizes grassroots struggles for seed, food, water, land, and knowledge sovereignty, resisting biopi-
racy and the corporate privatization of the commons.

The word *navdanya* means nine seeds, and it is used to symbolize
the protection of precious biological and cultural diversity. While holisti-
cally learning—using hands, hearts, and heads—students give the gift of
their labor (*shramadana*) to assist with needed activities such as seed sav-

ing, food harvesting, and food preparation. At Earth University, nature and farmers are the teachers as students live into the potential of Earth citizenship and more consciously engage their membership in the Earth family (*Vasudhaiva kutumkam*).[c] In such an intentional setting, accompaniment between humans and the natural world can be experienced as bidirectional, reciprocal, and mutual.

---

a. Krishna Dutta and Andrew Robinson, *Rabindranath Tagore: The Myriad-Minded Man* (New York: Tauris Parke, 2009), 220.

b. Rabindranath Tagore, *Rabindranath Tagore: An Anthology,* ed. Krishna Dutta and Andrew Robinson (New York: St. Martin's Press), 258.

c. This description of Navdanya and the Earth University is drawn from http://www.navdanya.org/.

injurious incursions that sicken, denude, and destroy nature. The Inuits' Petition to the Inter-American Commission on Human Rights Seeking Relief from Violations Resulting from Global Warming Caused by Acts and Omissions of the United States in 2005 is an exemplary effort that links the well-being of human communities with the well-being of the atmosphere and other-than-human animal communities. Average global temperature increases due to climate change doubled in the Arctic, creating rapid and severe effects. The increased temperatures cause thinning and melting of ice, necessary for Inuit transportation between villages and for subsistence marine and agricultural harvesting. Their sustainable harvesting practices are a traditional pathway for spiritual and cultural affirmation, allowing intergenerational transmission of skills, knowledge, and values.[13]

Maoris in New Zealand live with a sense of interdependence with the natural world, using the saying, "I am the river and the river is me." They feel at one with and equal to mountains and rivers, not superior to them. Indeed, they experience living entities like rivers as their ancestors, part of their family, not as property to be owned. For 140 years, the Maori have been negotiating with the New Zealand government to have the third largest river in New Zealand, the Whanganui River, and all its tributaries granted the same legal rights as a human being. In 2017, they finally achieved this goal. Two guardians were appointed, and money was set aside for redress.[14]

The Maoris' living philosophy has also been guiding a transition from the government's ownership of a large national Park, Te Urewera, to the land being recognized as a legal entity with "all the rights, powers, duties and liabilities of a legal person." The Te Urewera Act of 2014 enables lawsuits to be brought on behalf of the land.[15]

The Ganges River, considered to have the attributes of a deity, is India's holiest and dirtiest river. After decades of eco-accompaniment by river activists and inspired by the success of the Maoris, the north Indian state of Uttarakhand has now granted the Ganges and Yamuna Rivers the rights of living entities, with the right to sue. This means that polluting the river is deemed equivalent to harming a person.[16] These are examples of what Cormac Cullinan calls "wild laws," ones that seek to protect "the freedom of communities of life to self-regulate."[17]

In the United States, efforts are under way to seek the rights of nature for several rivers, including the mighty Colorado River. In a recent court action, the Colorado River was named as the plaintiff in a case arguing that its rights of the river "to exist, flourish, regenerate, be restored, and naturally evolve" had been violated. The accompanist or friend of the river is the environmental group Deep Green Resistance. The river supplies water to 36 million people. It has been adversely impacted by pollution and massive draining.[18] In 2010, the Pittsburgh City Council banned natural gas extraction, maintaining that nature has "inalienable and fundamental rights to exist and flourish." Instead of being subject to deals made between corporations and government, residents claimed both their own rights to determine what happens in their area and legally binding rights for nature.[19]

The UN-backed International Criminal Court at The Hague widened its mandate in 2016 to include environmental crimes that result in the destruction of the environment (e.g., destroying rainforests and polluting water sources), "exploitation of natural resources," and the "illegal dispossession" of land.[20]

Global and national frameworks are helpful as ethical blueprints as we engage particular struggles. Ultimately, however, when the curtains of the idealistic and lofty rhetoric of global, interregional, and national initiatives open, we see into regional and local conflicts, where the rights to mindlessly extract and pollute and to maximize use of fossil fuels imperil all living communities. In too many such places, corporations use paramilitary, military, and police force to fight off and even criminalize Earth accompanists, protectors, and activists. Nevertheless, struggles over time can yield success, opening paths to redress and restoration. We can examine this through the Ogoni people's campaign in Nigeria against Shell and Chevron.

Ecological Accompaniment and the Struggle for Environmental Self-Determination: The Ogoni People Versus Shell and Chevron

To the Ogoni, the land and the people are one and are expressed as such in our local languages. It emphasizes, to my mind, the close relationship between the Ogoni people and their environment.

—Ken Saro-Wiwa[21]

The work of witnessing is compounded when it is one's own community or people being undermined by ecological devastation caused by powerful elites. This is the situation in which Nigerian playwright Ken Saro-Wiwa and other Ogoni found themselves. Nigeria's independence from British colonial rule in 1960 did not mean greater representation and self-determination for the Ogoni, a micro-minority of 500,000 living in the Niger River Delta. The national borders drawn by Britain comprise three hundred ethnic groups of vastly different size. British colonialism seamlessly morphed into domestic colonialism in the service of neoliberalism. A death-dealing collusion among Shell, Chevron, the Nigerian National Petroleum Corporation, and successive military regimes permitted the oil giants to extract oil without care for the environment and without fair compensation to the Ogoni. Despite $600 billion in oil revenues, 69 percent of Nigerians live on less than a dollar a day. Once the Ogonis' land and water were polluted, they could not supplement this with their own subsistence farming and fishing.

Nigeria's Indigenous colonialism carried forward the racism that was an essential ingredient in how European colonialism functioned. In Indigenous colonialism, small ethnic communities are not granted rights for self-determination; larger ethnic groups claim the political and economic power, suppressing the will and desire of less-populous minorities. The oil companies failed to hold themselves to any of the regulatory standards they observed in Europe or the United States, fully aware of the destructive consequences that would ensue. Clearly, the welfare of the non-European, non-white, human inhabitants was of little concern to these corporations, as they satisfied their lust for oil and gas profit at the Ogonis' expense. Those in the government shared this lack of concern, reflecting the ethnocentrism that pitted larger ethnic groups against smaller ones.

Neither the military government nor the oil companies could succeed in fulfilling their greed without the other. A leaked Nigerian government memo in 1994 put it plainly—and chillingly: "Shell operations still impossible unless ruthless military operations are undertaken for smooth economic activities to commence."[22]

While the Nigerian Constitution of 1960 promised that such communities would receive 50 percent of revenues from oil production on their territory, the Ogoni have received approximately 1.5 percent. One report notes, "Shell, Chevron, and successive Nigerian regimes have siphoned $30 billion worth of oil from beneath Ogoni earth. Yet the locals find themselves lacking a hospital, electricity, piped water, basic roads, housing, and schools. The community has found itself, in the fullest sense of the word, utterly undermined."[23] The Ogoni had no representation in Nigerian institutions and no job opportunities in federal or state agencies or in public- or private-sector companies.[24]

"Environmental pollution" is too vague and detached a term to allow us to begin to grasp what the Ogoni and countless other groups are suffering. It is painful to describe. The constant gas flares for thirty-three years eliminated the night darkness. The flares made it impossible to breathe clean air, filling it with hydrocarbons, carbon monoxide, and carbon dioxide. Oil spills and blowouts of oil coated agricultural fields, streams, rivers, and houses. There is no water untainted by oil, and thus no fish left in the rivers. Groundwater is tainted with benzene and hydrocarbons, both carcinogens. When the spills were burnt, they left four meters of crust on the earth, making the growing of food impossible. Rain was no longer sweet but acid. Saro-Wiwa wrote, "What used to be the bread basket of the delta has now become totally infertile. All one sees and feels around is death. Environmental degradation has been a lethal weapon in the war against the indigenous Ogoni people."[25]

Protests and organized campaigns were met by police and military "suppression." Here too the word "suppression" is too vague. People were killed and intentionally maimed. Their houses and what was left of their fields were burned. In short, they were violently displaced, removed. In 1993, several hundred Ogonis peacefully protested the injustice of their situation. Their demands were answered with the destruction of twenty-seven villages; two thousand were killed and eighty thousand displaced.[26] While Shell moved on to new fields in 1993, Ogoniland was left without adequate resources to do any meaningful cleanup and restoration.

Like Victoria Earle Matthews, whom we visited in chapter 1, Ken Saro-Wiwa was deeply affected by the death of one of his sons in 1992. In the face of this loss, he turned from being a prolific writer, playwright, and creator of a hit TV series to using his words—spoken and written—in the service of his Ogoni brothers and sisters and the land they call home. Environmental scholar Rob Nixon describes him as "the first African writer to articulate the literature of commitment in expressly environmental terms."[27] While Saro-Wiwa's initial efforts to gain the accompaniment of international groups failed, he continued to travel and study other environmental and Indigenous rights movements. He became increasingly able to name and describe what he was seeing in Ogoniland and to link it with other catastrophes and movements. "In virtually every nation-state," he observed, "there are several 'Ogonis'—despairing and disappearing people suffering the yoke of political marginalization, economic strangulation and environmental degradation, or a combination of these."[28]

Sociologist Kai Erikson, in studying the social consequences of environmental disasters in the United States, warned us of "a different species of trouble."[29] In natural disasters, victims often reach out to help one another, strengthening community bonds in the face of shared losses. In large-scale toxic events, however, it is clear that the disaster is a consequence of *human* decisions and actions, and that the possible ill-effects on individuals and communities were known beforehand. People intentionally made a decision to pursue a profitable project, placing the community in harm's way, clearly failing to adequately value the health and lives of its members and the eco-system of which they are a part. Erikson describes such human-wrought environmental trauma as "a blow to the basic tissues of human life."[30]

Erikson has been invited to accompany communities in the wake of environmental assault for over three decades. Through interviewing those who are suffering the effects of a catastrophe, he is able to write a revealing research report on the psychological and community repercussions of this "new species of trouble," and to appear on the community's behalf in court to help argue for deserved recompense. Environmental disasters caused by fellow humans, he says, are "one of the social and psychological signatures of our time." They carry with them distinctive assaults on individual and com-munity trust, undermining a sense that one can rely on fellow humans: "Hu-man beings are surrounded by layers of trust, radiating out in concentric circles like ripples in a pond. The experience of trauma at its worst, can mean not only a loss of confidence in the self but a loss of confidence in the scaf-folding of family and community, in the structures of human government, in the larger logics by which humankind lives, and in the ways of nature itself."[31] Accompaniment is an antidote to tears in this delicate fabric of trust. It will in most instances prove insufficient to restore full confidence in human beings, but without it such assaults cannot be metabolized so that life can continue in any way resembling the time previous to the insult. Such accompaniment may, of course, come from many corners—family members, neighbors, healthcare providers, lawyers, emergency workers, or psychologists.

Erikson describes how difficult it can be for community members to understand what is happening: "A chronic disaster is one that gathers force slowly and insidiously, creeping around one's defenses rather than smashing through them. People are unable to mobilize their normal defenses against the threat, sometimes because they have elected consciously or unconsciously to ignore it, sometimes because they have been misinformed about it, and some-times because they cannot do anything to avoid it in any case."[32] In such situ-ations of environmental disaster, accompaniment of other-than-human nature and accompaniment of affected community members must be linked. The latter often need spaces for dialogue not only to voice their losses but to understand the societal dynamics of the situation to which they fell prey.

Once Saro-Wiwa understood the species of trouble he was witnessing in Ogoniland, he was able to link the nonviolent Movement for the Survival of the Ogoni People (MOSOP) to both international Indigenous rights movements and environmental justice movements in order to gain traction. What the Ogoni needed to confront was the interlinked damage to both cultural and ecological survival. Their demands to the Nigerian government needed to reflect the indivisibility of these two areas of critical concern. The Ogoni Bill of Rights, signed by Ogoni elders in 1990, laid out their tragic situation and their demands for environmental and political self-determinism, reparations for the harms perpetrated, and financial recompense for the revenues diverted from the Ogoni to the government and corporations who had colluded against them. The Ogoni wanted adequate and direct representation in all Nigerian national institutions, the use and development of Ogoni languages in their own territory, the right to religious freedom, and the full development of Ogoni culture.[33] The right to protect the Ogoni environment from further assault was indissolubly linked to the right to protect their languages and culture. Saro-Wiwa advocated for a federalism under which cultural and ecological survival would be in the hands of those who live in a particular region.

As Saro-Wiwa along with other Ogoni leaders successfully mobilized an international audience concerned about Indigenous rights and environmental protection and justice, both the Nigerian government and the oil executives understood how much the leaders were a threat to their profitable but exploitive and destructive pursuits. The Nigerian government pursued its strategy of further militarizing commerce. It banned public gatherings in Ogoniland and made any disturbance of oil production an act of treason. Nine Ogoni environmental activists, including Saro-Wiwa, were falsely accused of murder, imprisoned, subjected to a masquerade of a trial, and then hanged in 1995. In speaking of environmental martyrs, Rob Nixon called it "witnessing through the body."[34] Saro-Wiwa's son, Ken Saro-Wiwa, Jr., pursued Shell for its role in his father's death and for their payments to soldiers who carried out human rights abuses against the Ogoni.[35] Shell settled out of court for $15.5 million, which largely went into a trust for the Ogoni people.

To gain recognition in the eyes of the government and oil companies, Saro-Wiwa called out for accompaniment by the international community, turning to human and environmental rights groups. Sister Majella McCarron, an Irish nun, was teaching science in Nigeria when she met Saro-Wiwa. She responded to his need for help in getting MOSOP's message beyond Nigeria by bringing it to the Africa Europe Faith and Justice Network. Their relationship blossomed into one of accompaniment. McCarron shared with Saro-Wiwa the pedagogical method of Brazilian Paulo Freire, as he sought ways to raise Ogonis' critical consciousness about their plight. One time when he was imprisoned, she visited his family in London and was able to send him news of their well-being, including that of his newborn son whom he had not yet met. She spent her sabbatical creating Ogoni Solidarity Ireland, which provided a platform for her to educate the Irish about his imprisonment and the trials of the Ogoni 9 activists. Some in Ireland were receptive to the Ogonis' struggle because the Irish too were battling with Shell in Rossport, County Mayo, where the oil giant failed to provide a sufficient environmental impact assessment. Saro-Wiwa was grateful for McCarron's "presence among us," for her witnessing of the Ogoni struggle for environmental self-determination. On a personal level, her careful recounting of news of his family in her letters raised his spirits. She said in a telling phrase that she had the "good fortune of accompanying the campaign" in Nigeria and in Ireland.[36]

The Nigerian government requested that the UN Environmental Programme assess the environmental pollution in Ogoniland. In 2011, the program deemed the area one of the most polluted inhabited areas in the world and recommended a twenty-five-to-thirty-year cleanup, to begin with a $1 billion investment. UN engineers, Shell, and the government co-crafted a plan that was to begin in 2016.[37] As of 2018, no cleanup had yet been initiated.

The concerted and persevering nonviolent activism of MOSOP resulted in Shell's removal from Ogoniland but has not succeeded in winning the estimated $6 billion that is believed necessary for a true cleanup. Meanwhile, there are ongoing spills from old oil infrastructure that have not been decommissioned, as well as from pipelines that cross Ogoni lands. There are also outstanding calls for reparations. Shell moved to other communities, repeating their destructive practices elsewhere.

For the Ogoni people, accompanying the land and the water in their travail and accompanying the Ogoni themselves are one and the same. The well-being of humans and the well-being of earth, air, and water are interdependent. In the face of the destruction of the ecosystems and suppression of their culture, the Ogoni requested accompaniment from various sectors of the international community. The widening rings of accompaniment, from McCarron to citizens of Rossport, Ireland, to Greenpeace, Amnesty International, and the UN were a fitting and necessary antidote to the destruction of trust created by the Nigerian military government's corrupt militarization of commerce with Shell and Chevron.

After Saro-Wiwa's death the Nigerian-based Environmental Rights Action joined forces with Acción Ecológica in Ecuador to launch a global movement to "leave the oil in the soil": Oilwatch International. Journalist Naomi Klein traces the current scale and mutual accompaniment of anti-extraction activists to the earlier struggles in the Niger Delta.[38] Nevertheless, the full restoration of the water, earth, and air the Ogoni so deeply desire is yet to come. The accompaniment of nature that leads to its regeneration is also regenerative of human community and individual well-being, underlining our interdependence.

Ecological Accompaniment: The Labor and Joy of Restoration

Brazilian photographer Sebastião Salgado has provided an unusual kind of accompaniment in his decades-long dedication to photography. In his autobiography, he writes of his love for Rwanda. As a young economist, he had traveled to the most fertile parts of Rwanda to help farmers establish tea plantations. Decades later, he photographed the Rwandan genocide, the forced migration of 2 million Rwandans, and walked the scorched, formerly verdant earth of the tea farms, scattered with human bones of people he had known for years. He shares, "And at that horrific time, I photographed it with all my heart. I thought the whole world needed to know. No one has the right to protect himself from the tragedies of his time, because we are all responsible, in a certain way, for what happens in the society in which we have chosen to live. This is our world, we have to assume responsibility for it."[39]

Yet as he offered his eyes and photographic art to documenting the violence, he says he began to feel as though he was dying: "The nine months I spent in Rwanda were so shocking that at a certain point my mind and body started to give way.... Until then, I had never imagined that man could be part of a species capable of such cruelty to its own members and I couldn't accept it. I was depressed and sinking into a deeply pessimistic state of mind. I was equally despairing about how economic, social and political upheavals had altered the planet. The felled trees, the ruined landscapes, the destruction of entire ecosystems."[40] He put down his camera and returned home, believing he was leaving photography forever.

Salgado had grown up on a cattle ranch in Minais Gerais, Brazil, in a verdant landscape, graced by the Atlantic Forest. He and his wife, Lélia Deluiz Wanick Salgado, had to go into exile at a young age due to the military dictatorship in Brazil (1964–1985). When they returned to the area where he had grown up, there were no longer families living there, the trees were gone, the springs had run dry, and the extraordinary biodiversity had vanished. Land erosion and drought prevailed and were worsening.

Seeing how shaken her husband was, Lélia proposed a project of restoration and reforestation for the land that was at the same time a potential project of restoration for Sebastião's spent and despairing spirit. Instituto Terra was to become a way for the Salgados to accompany the landscape and to assist in its regeneration. The process was mutual, however, as the restoration of the forest and its biodiversity were balm to the Salgados' disheartened souls. After witnessing brutal, senseless killing and destruction, the project Sebastião and Lélia Salgado undertook would allow them to witness the re-creation of a forest and a flourishing lifecycle.

Before colonization, the Atlantic Forest covered 3,500 kilometers of Brazil's coastline and stretched inland for 350 kilometers. Humans' uncontrolled exploitation of natural resources slowly devastated much of the region and reduced it to 8 percent of its original size. This grand forest was decimated by the overcutting of trees for housing and for the production of wood coal to fuel the steel industry, by mining projects, by the clearing of land for agriculture and cattle grazing, and by the vast sprawl of urbanization. The springs dried up. Without trees, rain water flowed away, beginning the process of desertification.

The Salgados carefully assembled financial backers. They procured an expert in the recovery of ecosystems, Renato de Jesus. They engaged a legal process to create a community nonprofit NGO and a "Private Natural Heritage Reserve." The Instituto Terra was born in 1998 in the valley of the River Doce between Minais Gerais and Espiritu Santos. They called this 1,754-acre tract Bulcão Farm.

When their first crop of seedlings was ready to be planted, the couple enlisted local schoolchildren to help, knowing the children would share the experience with their parents. Twenty years later, over 2 million trees have been planted, and the land has been returned to a subtropical rainforest. The farm has the capacity to grow another 1 million seedlings each year, which will be planted at Bulcão Farm and shared with others replicating this restoration. Now a single uninterrupted stretch of Atlantic Forest has been restored, and with this 8 springs have come alive again; 172 species of birds, 15 kinds of reptiles, 15 sorts of amphibians, and 33 types of mammals are living in the forest. Even jaguars have returned.[41]

Instituto Terra is committed to education about forest recovery. One hundred public schools are involved, as are hundreds of small farmers who want to plant trees on their dry and eroding land. There have been over 700 educational projects engaging 65,000 people in 170 municipalities of the region.

Sebastião shares that "initially, my father was skeptical about our project. He was convinced that our city-dweller's utopia would ruin us. But when he died at the age of ninety-five, he had time to see the trees reclaim their rights."[42] In effect, the Salgados have been acting as accompanists, as ombudspeople or friends, enabling the rights of the forest, the springs, and the animals to be restored.

The devastation unfolding on Earth today calls for eco-accompaniment. Throughout the world, groups have mobilized to protect nature and ways of life that depend on their relationships with nature. The intertribal groups that work in solidarity at Standing Rock in North Dakota name themselves not protestors but "protectors," water protectors. Tribes' members are protected *by* water, and they offer their protection *to* water in a deeply reciprocal relationship and commitment that acknowledges the sacred nature of water. Protecting water and themselves is one and the same effort.

The Civic Council of Indigenous and Popular Organizations of Honduras (COPINH), formerly led by Berta Cáceres, is an exemplar of such reciprocal protection.

Ecological Accompaniment: Protection, Defense, and Care

The Lenca people of Honduras and El Salvador have been able to maintain a number of their pre-Columbian traditions as well as their cosmovision, their way of seeing the world and existence, despite the impositions of colonialism, Catholicism, and unbridled capitalism. They understand the world as an interrelated order that deserves respect and gratitude. The Lenca understand each being as sacred, having a life, image, heart, and spirit that all beings share. Each has a mother and a father and needs to be fed. Each is a part of every other that exists, and each has a language.[43] They value relations among themselves and their neighbors, celebrating each year Guanasco, a ceremony to promote peace and friendship with neighboring communities. They also value their relations to the natural world, which is understood as sacred. Mountains and hills are viewed as holy places. Water is the essence of life, and rivers are life in movement that nourish the whole. When rivers are strangled by dams, the placental circulation of Mother Earth's sacred waters is stopped, bringing harm to the whole. When waters are contaminated, a needed harmonious balance is disrupted, affecting each part of the whole, including the forests and biodiversity.

In this comprehensive eco-vision, efforts to defend rivers and the earth are expressions of love for Mother Earth. Each individual has a role to play within the totality of relationships.[44] It is in this cultural context that Berta Cáceres as a young woman decided to found COPINH in 1993. She created it to support Indigenous rights, which are seen as inextricable from land rights and the defense and care of nature. The group addressed illegal logging and the presence of U.S. military bases on Lenca territory. Lenca from the town of Rio Blanco approached Cáceres and COPINH to investigate why construction machinery had suddenly appeared near their community. The investigation discovered that there were four hydroelectric dams slated for development on the Gualcarque River. International law that requires consultation with the affected community or communities had been disregarded. The dams threatened to disrupt the Lencan way of life, limiting their access to water, food, and traditional medicines.[45]

Cáceres organized a year-long protest in 2013, involving community meetings and legal actions to fight the construction of the dams. Like Ken Saro-Wiwa, she understood that COPINH needed to mobilize the international community. She took the case to the Inter-American Commission on Human Rights and later to Amnesty International. The protestors prevented construction at the dam sites by their continued presence at these places. Security guards and employees of the three companies who had planned to create the dams and the Honduran military threatened and harassed the protestors, even firing on them on July 15, 2013. One person died, three were injured, and intimidation of COPINH continued. In 2014, members of COPINH were again attacked, resulting in two deaths and three serious injuries. Two of the companies withdrew from the project, leaving one, DESA (Desarrollos Energéticos).

Cáceres had bogus charges filed against her for "usurpation, coercion, and continued damages" to DESA, in addition to multiple attempts to smear her name and discredit her. In 2016, more than one hundred protestors were detained and intimidated by security forces. On March 3, 2016, Berta Cáceres was murdered in her own home, after years of death threats and placement on a military hit list. As of 2018, it is clear that company employees of DESA, private security forces, and agents of the state were complicit in her assassination.[46]

At her acceptance speech for the Goldman Environmental Prize in 2015, Cáceres appealed to all of us, as she shared the cosmovision that inspired her accompaniment of the Gualcarque River:

In our world-views, we are beings who come from the Earth, from the water and from corn. The Lenca people are ancestral guardians of the rivers, in turn protected by the spirits of young girls, who teach us that giving our lives in various ways for the protection of the river is giving our lives for the well-being of humanity and of this planet.

COPINH, walking alongside people struggling for their emancipation, validates this commitment to continue protecting our waters, the rivers, our shared resources and nature in general, as well as our rights as people.

Let us wake up! Let us wake up, humankind! We're out of time. We must shake our conscience free of the rapacious capitalism, racism, and patriarchy that will only assure our own destruction. The Gualcarque River has called upon us, as have other gravely threatened Rivers. We must answer their call. Our Mother Earth—militarized, fenced-in, poisoned, a place where basic rights are systematically violated—demands that we take action. Let us build societies that are able to co-exist in a dignified way, in a way that protects life. Let us come together and remain hopeful as we defend and care for the blood of this Earth and of its spirits.[47]

From Ecopsychology to Environmental Justice

Western psychology has been slow to explicitly understand and grapple with humans' interdependence with other-than-human nature and with both the natural and built environments in which we all live. In the 1980s in the United States, an effort to correct Western psychology's neglect of natural and built environments began to gain traction through the emergence of ecopsychology as a new discipline. Ecopsychology initially sought to understand the human-nature relationship and to heal individuals' separation from nature, offering various forms of ecotherapy, deep ecology workshops, and wilderness experiences, as well as conducting research on the benefits of exposure to nature.

Unfortunately, the idea of the separate self, born out of the radical individualism of the West—which had caused the neglect of human- and other-than-human-nature relationships—also limited the initial focus of ecopsychology: the healing of *humans'* dissociation from the natural world. The ill effects of this disassociation on psychological well-being were increasingly noted, as efforts to have people spend time in the natural world proved conducive to their well-being. This early articulation of ecopsychology can be faulted, however, for its often one-sided focus, turning to other-than-human nature to increase the well-being of humans and neglecting the study of how to alter humans' own deleterious effects on nature. Following Aldo Leopold, the father of wildlife ecology, ecopsychologists hoped that those who developed connections to the natural world would be better able to defend it, operating out of a love of the natural world. In 1949, Leopold wrote that "we can only be ethical in relation to something we can see, understand, feel, love, or otherwise have faith in."[48]

The early iterations of ecopsychology suffered from another blindspot, pointed out in 1995 by architect, urban planner, and visionary Carl Anthony. Eurocentrism, he said, led ecopsychology to an aesthetic approach, concerned with the preservation of the beauty of wilderness. The predominantly white movement of ecopsychology had left out environmental racism. Anthony pointed out that in the United States, the exploitation of the land and the brutal abuse of Africans forced into slavery co-arose with white small farmers discovering the fortunes that could be made by monocrops of tobacco and cotton, if free labor was available. While both nature and African Americans were "othered," early ecopsychology largely attended to only the othering of nature, failing to see the interlinkage between racism and environmental destruction. "An ecopsychology," Anthony wrote, "that doesn't deliberately set out to correct the distortion of racism is an oxymoron."[49]

Three decades later—amid planet-altering climate change, unprecedented raging wildfires, hurricanes, earthquakes, tsunamis, droughts, and poisoned waters—it is clear that humans need to focus on the destructive effects of *human* action and inaction on forests, waters, mountains, earth, and air. But it is not just many humans' dissociation from the natural world that has opened the door to these disastrous effects on the environment; it is also some humans' dissociation from other humans by dint of racism and ethnocentrism that has compromised both natural and built environments.

The burdens of environmental degradation are not suffered equally. Many marginalized communities and regions disproportionately suffer what Rob Nixon calls "slow violence," "a violence that occurs gradually and out of sight, a violence of delayed destruction that is dispersed across time and space . . . a violence that is neither spectacular nor instantaneous, but rather incremental and accretive, its calamitous repercussions playing out across a range of temporal scales." It is this slow violence that has led to the "environmentalism of the poor." Many insults to the environment—for example, toxic spills, poisoning in war as in Agent Orange, and radiation—play themselves out, says Nixon, in the "cellular drama of mutations . . . particularly in the bodies of the poor," where they "remain largely unobserved, undiagnosed, and untreated."[50] In attending to the effects of violence on individuals and communities, accompaniment in the face of this slow and ongoing environmental violence is urgently needed. This work is also "psychosocial," not only because of the psychological and social damage that is suffered but because many environmental assaults are caused or exacerbated by racial, ethnic, and class inequities.

This means that ecological accompaniment is needed not just by wild places threatened with fracking and pipelines and by mighty rivers strangled by dams, but in cities and urban regions where communities of color are burdened with toxic waste, poisoned water, polluted air, and seized public gardens. Carl Anthony and Paloma Pavel, president of Earth House Center, accompany regional and urban organizations to help them create urban planning that addresses both economic and environmental sustainability and justice. Rather than moving pollution from wealthy areas to poorer ones—which often means moving it from white communities to communities of color—regional thinking is deployed to address the root causes of environmental degradation and to clarify the resources available and needed to improve the well-being of the whole bioregion and all that lives within it.[51]

Andy Fisher defines "critical" ecopsychology as "an effort to under-stand the social links between two areas of violence: between the violation we recognize as the ecological crisis and the violation we recognize in hu-man suffering." A society that is organized primarily to serve the expansion of capital—rather than to serve life—must increasingly exploit both humans and the natural world, and so generate a state of psychospiritual ruin and continual ecological crisis. For these reasons, Fisher sets the tasks of a radi-cal and critical ecopsychology to be both resistance to the necrophilic ten-dencies within modern society and assistance in building an ecological society. These tasks require that ecopsychology "act more like a social movement than an academic discipline."[52]

In understanding well-being through the lens of radical interdepen-dence, ecopsychosocial accompaniment is—of necessity—also a political and economic undertaking. It necessarily involves a search for biophilic forms of organization that redress destructive Earth practices contributing to the hyper-accumulation of capital by one group at the expense of all oth-ers. Fisher proposes the alignment of ecopsychology with ecosocialism. Ecosocialism integrates psyche and nature with society, having as its telos societies of life that meet genuine human needs while maintaining the integ-rity of ecosystems. The needs of life are the central concern, not the accu-mulation of capital. Ecosocialism offers a postcapitalist vision of societies where alienation among humans, between humans and non-human nature, and between humans and their own labor have been healed. In such societ-ies, relational, spiritual, and creative sustenance replace hyper-materialism. Eco-accompaniment that begins with conservation and protection, that grapples with restitution and reparation, and that lives into Earth democ-racy is part of what Buddhist eco-philosopher Joanna Macy calls the Great Turning, the turn from an industrial growth society that requires ever-increasing consumption to a life-sustaining society that satisfies its needs while protecting the prospects of coming generations.[53]

Increasingly, I witness my psychology graduate students turning their attention to ecopsychology and environmental justice: notably, wilderness vision questing with formerly incarcerated youth, liberatory education about permaculture with formerly incarcerated men, joining into and learning from permaculture projects in Palestine and on Navajo reservations, working to legally establish rights for the polluted Gowanus Canal in Brooklyn, being an accomplice during Standing Rock.[54] Such work is slowly weaving a path between deepening one's own connection to nature and critically addressing humans' destructive effects on both nature and poor communities; indeed, it is a weaving made possible by the mutuality of accompaniment. These ecopsychosocial approaches deepen or sustain humans' connections to the natural world while also engaging in environmental struggles and projects of restitution and restoration.

In reflecting on the uncertain start of ecopsychology, Robert Greenway, a father of ecopsychology, argues that it would have been better to announce a focus—understanding human-nature relations—rather than to announce a form of psychology. When one appends "eco-" to "psychology," the latter term is neither clear nor singular in its reference. *Which* kind of psychology—behavioral, humanistic, liberation, cognitive?[55] Fisher argues that ecopsychology is not a subdiscipline of psychology but a "radical ecological transformation of the entire psychological enterprise. This means," he says, "that it is still psychology, but of a very different sort—one that makes its arena of practice the whole terrain of ecological and social relations or interdependencies."[56] The telos of a radical ecopsychology, for Fisher, is to build ecological societies. Ecological societies are founded on both social and environmental justice and on a dynamic understanding of these as indissolubly linked. I offer ecopsychosocial accompaniment as a set of practices that share this goal, and that, in company with Fisher and Anthony, refuse the divorce of the ecological from the social and both from history. Such accompaniment surely has a psychological dimension, but it is not necessarily housed within or only within psychology as a professional discipline.

Integral Ecology

At first, I thought I was fighting to save rubber trees, then I thought I was fighting to save the Amazon rainforest. Now I realize I am fighting for humanity.

—Francisco Chico Mendes[57]

For many who are part of cultures that have managed to preserve practices of Earth accompaniment, neoliberal assaults to literally take the earth from under their feet and to engage in actions that compromise their air, soil, and water have intensified. For others who come from cultures that have subjugated and exploited natural entities for profit, there needs to be what Pope Francis has called in his encyclical *Laudato Si'* "an ecological conversion" to become a protector of the ecologies of which we are a part.[58] Significantly, "conversion" is the same term used by some of the psychosocial accompanists explored in chapters 3, 4, and 6. Throughout the globe, we are witnessing the growing solidarity between members of Indigenous groups and those who have undergone ecological conversion.

Anthropologist Philippe Descola nests human societies within and alongside of other-than-human societies, offering the holistic term "societies of nature."[59] In societies of nature, where there is an integrated focus on the well-being of all human and non-human beings, human societies are members, not dominators. Members do have a special ethical responsibility in helping to ensure that they themselves do not radically disrupt the equilibriums within nature. Instead of separating nature from culture, Descola departs from anthropocentric dualism and urges us to understand the complex relationships between the human and nonhuman. He cites the variety of kinds of affinity and consanguinity that many Amazonian groups, among other Indigenous peoples, experience with nonhuman others. Plants and animals are ascribed a spiritual principle of their own, and maintaining personal relationships with them is customary. Descola recounts that these may be in the form of friendships or matrimony; they may be hostile, seductive, or reciprocal. For instance, Achuar women treat the plants in their gardens as their children. The men behave toward hunted animals through the relational norms of marriage. Plants and animals are experienced as imbued with "intentionality, subjectivity, affects, even speech in certain circumstances."[60]

As we can see from our own relational experiences with other-than-human nature and from those of photographer Sebastião Salgado, even when a given culture does not honor this degree of intense, familial intimacy with nature, when we draw close in our relationships, surprisingly similar feelings arise. Salgado describes as babies the small bushes that emerged from tree saplings at Bulcão Farm:

> A bush is like a baby; when it is born it is, in effect, a human being. A baby needs love, protection, it has to learn to walk, but it already possesses all the emotions of a human being. It is the same for a bush: at six months, when it measures only 70 centi-meters, it already has the structure of a fully-grown tree. Insects come to feed off its tiny flowers and when its tiny leaves fall to the ground, the ants grab them. It is already a whole world. Lé-lia always used to say "We have a baby forest," but it was a forest already.[61]

The work at Instituto Terra enabled Salgado to pick up his camera again in order to document places throughout the globe that are relatively untouched. During the time of photographing for his work *Genesis,* his "love letter to nature," he found himself building relationships with animals in much the same way he had done with the people he had photographed over the years, getting to know them, establishing trust, empathically trying to place himself in their situations.[62] One day in the Galapagos Islands, he was looking closely at the front feet of an iguana, a reptile, that seemed to bear little resemblance to humans. He describes this encounter:

> But, looking closely at one of his front feet, suddenly I saw the hand of a Medieval knight. Its scales made me think of a suit of chain mail, under which I saw fingers similar to my own! I said to myself, this iguana is my cousin. I had before my eyes the proof that we all come from the same cell, each species having evolved in the course of time in its own way and in conformity with its own ecosystem. . . . I wanted to recount the dignity and beauty of life in all its forms and show how we share the same origins.[63]

Critical ecopsychologist Andy Fisher reflects that when "more-than-human beings are granted personhood, agency, power, or interior depth of their own, then the natural world may be regarded as a psychological and social field."[64] Experience in this field that we share suggests the need to extend our understandings of relationship and of subjectivity beyond the human, as well as the wisdom we gain from doing so.

Descola calls for a holistic ethical system where the emphasis is not on particular shared properties but "on the need to preserve the common good and not inconsiderately upset the relations of interdependence that unite all the organic and biotic components of an environment." He describes this as a "truly moral approach to the duties of humans toward the whole collectivity of living entities and the rights that this collectivity might intrinsically possess."[65] Eco-accompaniment is an expression not only of this moral stance but of the forms of intimacy humans can experience with nonhuman nature.

Pope Francis in *Laudato Si'* underlines the inseparability of psychosocial and ecological accompaniment: "We are faced not with two separate crises, one environmental and the other social, but rather with one complex crisis which is both social and environmental." "Today," he continues, "we have to realize that a true ecological approach *always* becomes a social approach; it must integrate questions of justice [into] debates on the environment, so as to hear *both the cry of the earth and the cry of the poor.*"[66]

Mutual accompaniment between humans and other living entities is expressive of an integral ecology. It is part of the turn from what Thomas Berry called an "exploitative anthropocentrism to a participative biocentrism."[67] Instead of using and objectifying living entities, instead of trying to be the lord and master over them, eco-accompanists acknowledge their intimate interdependence with nature. They listen, observe, and learn. They offer what they can—witness, defense, energies for protection and restoration—while knowing all the while that their own lives unfold in and depend on the sacred web of creation to which they have apprenticed themselves.

Mutual Accompaniment and the Commons-to-Come

"The Long Shipwreck"

The life path that led me to the psychosocial accompaniment of asylum seekers and those facing deportation, described in chapter 1, has been a long one. However, the societal path that has led us to demean, cast out, and harm "strangers" is much longer and continues to breed inhospitable and often carceral holding spaces throughout the fabric of our communities. This path has developed over the last five hundred years of colonialism, and it remains embedded in the present entrenched state of coloniality. How and why is it that we have normalized such destructive ways of being with each other, with animals, and with Earth? In repudiating these ways, we can replace them with a mutual accompaniment in which we seek attunement to those around us, enabling our responsiveness, care, and love, and galvanizing our action in solidarity with others to resist and overturn systemic injustices and injuries.

Over the first decade of this century, my husband, Ed Casey, and I became witnesses to and students of the extension and fortification of the U.S. wall at the U.S.-Mexico border. We studied the humanitarian and ecological crises that erupted as the United States tried to divert economic migrants from crossing the border in urban areas like San Diego to the perilous deserts and mountains of Arizona and New Mexico. In the wake of the North American Free Trade Agreement (NAFTA) and 9/11, bulldozers were unleashed from environmental regulations and their operators were instructed to destroy nature preserves, fragile marshes, and other delicate ecosystems for the sake of building the wall. Because of fortifying the wall in urban areas, children and their parents were forced into the desert to cross the border. Their deaths were touted as an effective way to deter others contemplating migration.[1] Women were—and still are—forced to endure rape and extortion to arrive in a land where they harbor the hope of feeding and educating their children. When we began to study the border in 2002, I thought that U.S. society had reached the lowest possible point in how it was treating forced migrants, and I expected the situation to improve. Sadly, year after year, it has worsened. Now, for instance, Central American parents living in the United States are threatened with the charge of child trafficking for helping their own children escape drug gang induction, murder, and rape in their home countries. The United States, under the presidency of Donald J. Trump, has pulled out of the United Nations' global compact on migration. In 2018, three thousand migrant children—including infants and toddlers—were forcibly separated from their parents at the border and placed in detention, presumably to warn families to stop traveling to the United States to request asylum.

As I studied the U.S. wall at the border, it multiplied right before my eyes. In 2006, a border patrol public relations officer proudly boasted to me that representatives from other countries and regions were coming to our border to learn how to build their own walls. Indeed, our wall building has been a tragic inspiration, as well as providing a panoply of advanced technological tools to apprehend people pressed into migration by the daily circumstances of their lives at home. We now see walls and other barriers used to separate groups and stop the migratory flows of people displaced by violence, war, poverty, and environmental disruption in Cyprus, Egypt, India, Israel, Kuwait, Lebanon, Malaysia, Saudi Arabia, the United States, Syria, the West Bank, Brazil, Hungary, the Czech Republic, Romania, Slovakia, Northern Ireland, Slovenia, Macedonia, Morocco, and Greece.[2]

As I began to grasp the extent of the deepening migration crisis, I started to study and visit other walls. I went to Derry and Belfast to learn about the walls built in Northern Ireland. Derry, in the north of Ireland, has a rare intact city wall built by English and Scottish settlers between 1613 and 1619. It was built to keep the Irish out—that is, the people whose land had been seized from underneath them. The people who had lived on the land were removed, and the area was then surrounded by a wall to keep them out. The British called their first settlement in Ireland "the Pale." Those displaced were outside, "beyond the Pale."

Many, including the Martinican poet and founder of the Negritude movement Aimé Césaire, have argued that colonialism first involved the violent and forced extension of Western Europe into Latin America, then Africa and Asia, and that later these brutal practices bled back into Europe, creating Nazism and the Holocaust.[3] I learned in Derry that colonialism is much older. The Normans invaded Ireland in 1169. The British colonized the country from 1200 to 1250. In 1494, England claimed Ireland as its own. In Derry, English and Scottish settlers built a wall around their own settlement to keep Natives out. A plantation system was created, rewarding those loyal to the English crown with land that had belonged to the Irish. The colonial practices that would be malevolently perfected later in the southern hemisphere were first devised and practiced on the Irish. English invaders, who constructed the native population as uncivilized and in need of governance by others, displaced this population from the land desired by settlers, ceded lands to absentee landlords from the colonizing country or to English settlers, controlled the native population through terror and violence, created laws superseding those of the original people, and outlawed Indigenous languages and rituals. Resisting and rebellious populations were punished through violence, torture, and starvation. The native population was excluded from power, politics, and land ownership, becoming used as a cheap labor force, divested of their lands. For instance, Catholics who still owned land were unable to pass it to their heirs.[4]

Once those Indigenous to the land were locked into a subservient and disempowered position, the land was stripped of its resources. Following philosopher John Locke's proposition that land ownership issues from labor performed on the lands create "improvements," the British looked down on the Irish for leaving land idle. They quickly deforested it for building, including the construction of British naval ships. In step with all of these colonial so-called improvements, prisons were created for the poor and insurgent. Unlike the biblical verses of Isaiah, 65:21–22, that prophesize a time when people "shall plant vineyards and eat the fruit of them . . . [as well as a time they] shall not plant and another eat," in Ireland Catholics were forced into labor to grow food for Britain. In particular, they had to produce food for the British Army, even to the point of their own starvation.[5] In the 1700s, this wave of conquest and displacement that unfolded in Ireland was called the long *briseadh,* the long "breaking" or "shipwreck."[6] Those who suffered it were suffused with hopelessness.

Enclosing the Commons and Outlawing Hospitality: Removal and Imprisonment

And, it is clear, the loss of a local commons heralds the end of self-sufficiency and signals the doom of the vernacular culture of the region.

—Gary Snyder[7]

The practice of intentionally wrecking the "boats" of communities and cultures for the sake of accumulating capital and oligarchic power began with what is called "the enclosure of the commons." Commons refer to those lands that are used and sustained for the common good. It is land that is not owned by an individual. Early stewardship of commons in England involved not only appropriate use but also obligations and duties, ensuring sharing and sustainability. Commoning rights included being able to pasture one's animals, gather firewood and construction materials, and glean food and seeds that were left behind, often for the benefit of those who most needed them.[8]

According to poet and environmental activist Gary Snyder, the commons was an "ancient mode of both protecting and managing the wilds of self-governing regions."[9] The people belonged to the land and the land belonged to the local community members, not as property but through ongoing and interdependent relationship. "The commons is a level of organization of human society that includes the nonhuman. The level above the local is the bioregion."[10] When some land or water was considered part of the commons, it did not mean that everyone could take from this common resource as much as he or she wanted. Access was regulated to avoid the excess of exploitation. Commoners stinted, refraining from overuse. Being part of the commons involved mutual obligations among people, as well as between people and the local natural system. Indeed, "commons" comes from the Latin *communis*, which combines *com* (together) and *munis* (ready to be of service, to oblige): bonded together under obligation or, as Snyder suggests, "service performed for the community."[11]

The practice of the commons in England and Ireland was disrupted by the enclosure movement. Village-held land was stolen from communities, fenced off, and turned over to private interests, disrupting sustainable and communal agriculture. In 1847, the Bishop of Meath in Ireland, Thomas Nulty, described his personal recollection of the evictions in a pastoral letter to his clergy:

> Seven hundred human beings were driven from their homes in one day and set adrift on the world, to gratify the caprice of one who, before God and man, probably deserved less consideration than the last and least of them. . . . The horrid scenes I then witnessed, I must remember all my life long. The wailing of women—the screams, the terror, the consternation of children—the speechless agony of honest industrious men—wrung tears of grief from all who saw them. I saw officers and men of a large police force, who were obliged to attend on the occasion, cry like children at beholding the cruel sufferings of the very people whom they would be obliged to butcher had they offered the least resistance. The landed proprietors in a circle all around—and for many miles in every direction—warned their tenantry, with threats of their direct vengeance, against the humanity of extending to any of them the hospitality of a single night's shelter . . . and in little more than three years, nearly a fourth of them lay quietly in their graves.[12]

I want to underline the outlawing of hospitality and mutual aid by force: people's lives were threatened if they responded to the needs of a neighbor. The capacity and courage to respond—to the neighbor, the stranger, the animal, the Earth—so crucial to the building and sustaining of the commons were forcibly disrupted.

When wealthy lords began to seize these lands, often to provide grazing ground to vast cattle holdings or to market timber, those people who lived in and by the commons, who cared for and sustained the commons, were massively and violently displaced.[13] Some became the first industrial working class in the burgeoning cities.[14] During the enclosures in England and Ireland, those who could not find work in the cities fell into vagrancy and poverty. Many were imprisoned.

Poor laws began to legislate where the responsibility for helping these people lay. Legislation dictated that vagrants, beggars, the disabled, and the "deserving" poor should be returned to and taken care of by the community or parish from which they had come, where they might still have family and may have once contributed their labor. This minimized people being called on to pay taxes to support people from outside their own community. But for many, the community to which they were supposed to return no longer existed. Categories were created to divide those considered deserving from the undeserving poor, the latter being subject to torture and imprisonment. Indeed, the birth of the prison is directly related to the creation of the urban poor due to enclosures.[15]

In England and Ireland, both those who fell through the cracks and into unremitting poverty and those who rebelled against their evictions were imprisoned. Before 1776, more than 50,000 were sent into indentured servitude in the United States from Britain alone. After the American Revolution, between 1787 and 1868, 164,000 prisoners were transported to Australia. In both the United States and Australia, European settlers enclosed and destroyed the commons—called by other names—of those living there before them, committing genocide to seize the land.

The rise of capitalism and indenturement, slavery, and the invention of prison systems went hand in hand in the Western world. Peter Linebaugh, a renowned historian of the commons, says incisively,

> The commons is destroyed in two ways, by imprisonment and privatization. Each process produces its requisite emotional

environment, wrath and fear. Those in prison are angry, those with property are fearful. Restorative justice therefore must include both the restoration of the commons and the restoration of liberty to the prisoner. This cannot be done as long as commoners are locked up. Since the commons and liberation are inseparable, the abolition of privatized, capitalist property and the abolition of prison must go together.[16]

Erasing commons requires two kinds of walls and fences: those to keep people out and those to keep people in, a walling-out and a walling-in.[17]

"A Clash of Commons"

When the Puritans came from England to New England in the 1600s, they brought both practices of the commons and practices of exclusion and enclosure. The new settlers did not understand the complex relationships with nature and one another that the Indigenous peoples in New England had been practicing for centuries. They too practiced forms of commoning, but in modes that differed in significant respects from the settlers'. This "clash of commons" resulted in appropriation of lands from native communities and an undermining of subsistence practices that led to continual displacement and community fragmentation.[18]

Historian Allan Greer describes how settlers had been used to both an "inner" commons and an "outer" commons.

In Europe, where agriculture typically involved the raising of livestock and the growing of crops in close proximity, "open-field" practices developed in many (by no means all) regions, whereby land was held individually but managed collectively, and where the cattle and other animals of a given community grazed either in a special pasture or on portions of the arable land that were not currently bearing crops. The commons might be thought of both as a place—the village pasture—and as a set of access rights, such as gleaning and stubble grazing. This portion of the commons located in the tillage zone of a given community might be designated the "inner commons." "Outer commons" can then be used to refer to collectively owned resources in the surrounding area beyond local croplands. This was called "the waste" in England: the zone of moor, mountain, marsh, or forest that rural folk used as rough pasture for their livestock as well as for cutting wood or peat for fuel, gathering herbs, taking rushes for basketry or thatching, felling timber for construction, and so on.[19]

When the settlers arrived in the "new world," they misunderstood Native commons. What they perceived as waste and open land was filled with particular places serving designated functions (fishing, hunting, foraging, grazing, wood-cutting) to support subsistence, as well as cultural and spiritual life. The settlers did not perceive that the Natives were busily managing the "forests and waterways, burning underbrush, diverting streams, and generally altering the environment." Indeed, as Greer says, "America was a quilt of native commons each governed by the land-use rules of a specific human society."[20] While settlers interpreted land agreements to be conferring them exclusive ownership of the land, Natives thought they were offering to share with settlers "a right of ownership identical to their own: not to possess the land as a tradeable commodity, but to use it as an ecological cornucopia. Save for cornfields, no Indian usufruct rights were inherently exclusive."[21]

Settlers felt free to cut trees for firewood and buildings and to let their cattle, hogs, and horses roam in what they considered the "outer" commons. Native dispossession was accelerated by the large number of domesticated animals that settlers brought. Left to graze freely, these animals ate their way through Native commons and were used to expand the land claims of settlers. The activities of deforestation and free grazing destroyed areas the Natives depended on for their sustenance—their hunting, fishing, foraging, and cultivation—leading to their ongoing displacement. Greer describes how the settlers' sense of the "outer" commons as an area freely available to them for their own pursuits was a "significant agent of [Native] dispossession." To the settlers, nature was seen through the lens of commodities that could be extracted and sold. Whereas settlers understood property as clearly bounded, Natives understood land "in terms of central places, lines, and waterways."[22] Native villages were not fixed in place. Villagers moved in response to seasonal food opportunities, careful not to exhaust these supplies. In the eyes of the settlers, this mobility reduced Native claims to the land they moved through.

Settlers were initially invited to share in the "common pot" of Native commons, "a vast web of familial, political, and geographic relationships." Greer notes that "plantations could be integrated, at least in theory, into an existing Indigenous commons as part of an extensive network of places and resources governed by recognized rules of access." For the Wabanakis, a confederation of five Indigenous groups (the Mi'kmaq, Maliseet, Passamaquoddy, Abenaki, and Penobscot) living in the region of what is now Maine to southwestern Massachusetts, the common pot referred to "a way of seeing and being in the land." They clearly understood that the health of the common pot requires sharing, reciprocity, and equal distribution for balance. Taking more than one needs and hoarding are antithetical to the ethic of the common pot. Abenaki historian Lisa Brooks elaborates: "All inhabitants of the pot were fed from the pot and were part of the pot. Every part affected the whole. If one person went hungry, if certain individuals were excluded from the bounty of the dish, the whole would face physical and/or psychological repercussions from this rupture in the network of relations."[23]

In time, Natives discovered that the settlers did not share their ways of seeing and being. They acted individualistically and with greed, rather than seeing and acting through the eyes of interdependence. The Abenakis, for instance, realized that the sharing they had offered was not only unreciprocated by the settlers but that the settlers took actions to undermine the well-being of the Abenakis through land encroachment and excess resource depletion and extraction. At that juncture the Abenakis announced that they would no longer share their "pot" with those who seek only for themselves and warned settlers not to continue to take from areas that were not designated as their settlements.[24]

While Natives had struggled to negotiate how settlers and Natives could share in the common pot, settlers did not invite Natives to share in their commons. Natives gave settlers gifts but seldom were these customary gifts reciprocated. Brooks describes how Monhegan Mahomet I decried the settlers' threatening to hang three Monhegans for simply warming themselves in a cellar on a freezing night. Another Monhegan leader asked how could the settlers turn Monhegan women and children out of their houses and into the snow. Why after offering to share their space and to help defend the settlers were the latter acting in such bewildering and shameful ways, they wondered? Increasingly settlers' sharing of common fields for grazing and communal agriculture even among themselves gave way to strict land ownership of private parcels that were often fenced.[25]

Lisa Brooks and Cassandra Brooks describe the conflicts that arose between Puritans and the Wabanaki people. Brooks and Brooks argue that in order to grasp the significance of the Wabanaki's protest of settlers' damming of the Presumpscot River, "we must come to understand the matrix of social and ecological relationships that governed its participants, those human and non-human beings who 'belonged' to the river and to the principle of reciprocity that allowed life to thrive."[26] Initially, the Wabanaki asked for the payment of a tribute from those Puritans living in their region. The Puritans offered corn but then stopped paying it. The Wabanaki accepted those who had already moved into their region but requested they not bring more settlers, afraid that it would disrupt a sustainable equilibrium between humans and the other-than-human animals and places. The settlers did not comply. They moved into the Wabanaki's traditional hunting regions and constructed multiple dams on the Presumpscot River, disrupting the seasonal movement of fish on which the Wabanaki depended for their sustenance.

The Wabanaki had a sense of belonging to the rivers and watershed they lived in and advocated on their behalf. They had a feeling of responsibility to the river and related aspects of the natural world. In 1739, a leader of the Wabanaki, Polin, met with the governor of the Massachusetts Bay Colony, Jonathan Belcher, to ask that an area be made in the blockages along the river so that the fish could move through freely. While the settlers experienced the supply of fish as endless, the Wabanaki understood and respected the seasonal cycles of abundance and scarcity that they were familiar with across many generations. According to Brooks and Brooks, "In declaring their 'belonging' to the river, Polin and his counselors expressed an awareness of this intimate, interdependent relationship with a diverse environment. Wabanaki people had developed an embedded knowledge based on longstanding resource use and reciprocal relationships of exchange with their human and 'other-than-human' relations in this place."[27] Mindful of being part of an interdependent web, the Wabanaki were careful to redistribute their food so that not only all members of a given community had adequate supply but members of other interrelated communities did as well. Hoarding was culturally rejected. Some settlers were offered kinship, but they did not understand that this obligated them to also carry certain responsibilities in the reciprocal networks that included the redistribution of food and supplies.

What knowledge settlers gleaned of the Wabanaki's intricate system of relationships with the beings of their environment was used against them, as some settlers intentionally attempted to disrupt the seasonal practices that were necessary for Wabanaki survival. The deadly strategy of starvation waged against the Irish was now repeated on the Wabanaki. This assault was instigated in order to move settlers further into Wabanaki territory so that further capital could be accumulated from extensive logging.

The same brutal practices of taking the land out from under commoners in England and Ireland were now put into use against Native Americans across the New World. To seize control of the land, full assaults on the peoples and their cultures were justified under the self-serving slogans of "progress" and "civilization," supported by racist ideas of Native Americans as uncivilized and inferior. The Puritans greeted decimation of Native villages by European diseases as a sign from God that he was making room for them. With these self-serving and racist ideas, genocidal practices against Native Americans were unleashed and normalized.

For both settlers and Natives, commons were not places where anyone could come and take what he or she desired. Commons were particular places for particular communities with recognized rules of usage and responsibility. When two or more communities desire to equitably share particular places, the principles of mutual accompaniment are needed for understanding to develop. Different communities practice "the commons" differently. It is best to begin by not assuming that one knows how another community of humans relates to a given place, its human inhabitants, and other living beings, both plants and animals. Without efforts to not assume others hold the same or "lesser" values, projection and misunderstanding prevail.

In 1836, Pequot William Apess delivered the "Eulogy on King Philip" in Boston.[28] Although Apess did not use the word accompaniment—with its meaning of sharing bread together—he anticipated much of what we have come to understand about it as he focused on the lessons of the common pot. First, the kind of relationship that is desired is mutual and initiated by invitation or free consent. The accompaniment he requested is *not* that of the missionary, the overtaker, or the settler teacher. Too often, these figures have assisted the settler community in acts of cultural invasion and destruction, hastening the dispossession of Natives. Instead, he asked settlers to acknowledge and confront the violence of their ancestors and themselves, to act as brothers and kin, to think and act with the welfare of the whole in mind, rather than with the promotion of individual interests.[29]

The accompaniment needed begins with rigorous self-examination, a critique of how one is living from self-interest and holding on unjustly to power. From the acknowledgment of responsibility and shame comes the labor of reparation, of ceding back what has been stolen and treating "colored people they have around them like human beings." Apess appealed to the image of the common pot, urging his listeners to lay down greed and to take up the sharing of equal distribution. In this way, divisions can be healed. As Brooks points out, Apess alternated between a "we" that includes settlers and a Native "we." He did not ask to be included in the colonial space of the settlers but rather asked settlers to join an Algonquian-centric family and to walk side by side in peace, as brothers and sisters. He insisted that aggrieved communities that had been usurped be given the lead. He warned that violence against the Natives would breed violence within white settler communities.[30]

Today the work of such mutual accompaniment is still upon us. The creation of intercommons is essential, as forced migrations due to war, economic necessity, and climate change are affecting every corner of the Earth.

Such places where two or more communities dedicate themselves to equitably and sustainably living with one another require welcoming "the stranger" and slowly and committedly forming relationships where mutual understanding and a sense of belonging can be engendered, and where the other-than-human natural world can be cared for and equitably and sustainably shared.

The Assault on Relationships, On Belonging

Most settlers not only excluded Natives from their commons and communities but settler strangers as well. Families in colonial New England were not allowed to shelter strangers. Strangers in need would be asked to return from where they came. Indeed, there was a profession of "warners" who, like Robert Love in colonial Boston, made their daily rounds to determine if any strangers had come to town and where they were staying. Strangers were given fourteen days to leave, and were encouraged to go back where they came from. As in England, this practice was intended to protect local treasuries from caring for the poor who were not originally from their jurisdiction.[31]

In the United States, despite a dominant narrative of success in welcoming the "stranger," the vulnerable, and the immigrant, our history is laced with xenophobic and racist attacks and legislation that oppose those deemed "outsiders." These attacks have roots going back to the enclosure of the commons in England and the subsequent rise of Elizabethan poor laws in England and Ireland in the early seventeenth century. Few U.S. citizens are aware of how they and others carry forward this tradition of inhospitality in their thoughts and actions.

When the forced labor of Native people failed to satisfy settlers' rapacious hunger for cheap labor, the kidnapping of 12.5 million Africans for the slave trade in the "New World" was sanctioned through racist ideas, policies, and laws. Roughly 1.8 million died in the Middle Passage alone. Little thought was given to the human costs of the severing of Africans' relationships to their own land, families, and cultures left behind. Poet Aimé Césaire observed, "I am talking about millions of men torn from their gods, their land, their habits, their life—from life, from the dance, from wisdom."[32]

Once in the Americas, family members were mercilessly and continuously separated. An ideology of Eurocentric white supremacy took strong root in the United States and was used to rationalize the inhumane and exploitative treatment of both Africans and Native Americans.

For many of the Indigenous groups in what is now the United States, human disassociation from nature and the propelling human greed and gluttony that leads to such destruction and brutal treatment are seen as a form of disease. This disorder is regarded as a type of cannibalism called *Wétiko* in Cree, *windigo* in Ojibway, and *wintiko* in Powhatan.[33] Cree author Jack Forbes contrasts the preconquest "pollen path" of the Navajo and "the good red road" of the Lakota with the evil destruction wrought by colonialism. While these Native paths understand the interrelationship of all forms of life and promote living life in a sacred manner, the conquest introduced a completely foreign reality: the consumption of others' lives for the sake of one's own private profit.[34] Because most of those directly implicated in the terrorism of the conquest did not experience themselves as part of nature and as brothers and sisters to all beings, they were seen by Natives to act with an "icy heart," without empathy and compassion.[35] Many were seemingly unaware of the harm they were doing to others, as well as to their own spiritual paths and the welfare and integrity of their own communities.

Throughout the Americas, the exploitation of Native Americans and Africans forced into slavery went hand in hand with the denuding of forests, the mining of the Earth, the pollution of water, and the exhaustion of the soil through monocrops like sugar, coffee, and cotton. Colonialism and neocolonialism have disrupted Indigenous commons all over the world through the deadly twins of disregard for other people and for the other-than-human beings and places of the natural world.

Raj Patel and Jason Moore argue that for colonialism to propel itself, it sorted people and animals into the dualistic categories of nature and society, the uncivilized and the civilized. The idea of race was invented and deployed to powerfully assist with this deadly ranking. The patriarchal devaluing of women and their labors of care continued and contributed to the derogatory categorization necessary to a capitalist ecology. Moore argues that other-than-human animals, women, people of color, and white people in colonized regions were designated as nature, as outside what is civilized, while white colonizers and their cultures were deemed civilized. This division defined whose lives were valued and whose were susceptible to exploitation, forced displacement, and discarding, a deadly division still in practice today. This created access to the free and/or cheap human labor necessary to fuel capitalism's rapid excess accumulation of capital. It also justified, asserts Moore, the appropriation of the free work of forests, oceans, trees, plants, and animals.[36] Patel and Moore describe capitalism as having its own ecology, a set of relationships that integrate power, capital, and nature. Capitalist ecology requires cheap nature, cheap money, cheap work, cheap care, cheap food, cheap energy, and cheap lives.[37] Capitalism continuously reproduces this cheapening of life by finding new parts of nature that have not yet been commodified.

Through this analysis we can reperceive nature and society as one, a unity that has been falsely severed for too many. From this vantage point, the accompaniment of humans pushed to the margins and of other-than-human animals, rivers, mountains, and forests is crucial to restoring the commons. Capitalist exchange has wrought alienated and exploitative relationships, leading to the cheapening and expendability of some forms of life. Mutual accompaniment refuses this cheapening and seeks to replace these destructive dealings with relationships that are generative and just. By understanding accompaniment in historical context, we can reject framing it through the idea of charity and perceive, instead, that critical practices of accompaniment are part of needed reparative processes that directly address both historical and contemporary injustice and abuse and the psychospiritual poverty that fuel their perpetration.

Philosopher Nelson Maldonado-Torres describes the perversion of human relationships during the seizure and enclosure of the commons as a metaphysical catastrophe. This catastrophe turned "a potential world of human relations into one of permanent forms of conquest, colonization, and war":

> When it comes to conceptions of humanity and to ideals of inter-human contact, modernity/coloniality represents a veritable catastrophe (which means a "down-turn") whereby the world populations started to be divided according to, not merely specific

practices or beliefs, but degrees of being human. This catastrophe can be considered metaphysical because it transformed the meaning and relation of basic areas of thinking and being, particularly the self and the other, along with temporality and spatiality, among other key concepts in the basic infrastructure that constitutes our human world. This metaphysical catastrophe is informed by and helped to advance the demographic catastrophes of indigenous genocide in the Americas and the middle passage, as well as racial slavery, among other forms of massacre and systematic dehumanization in the early modern world. Both demographic and metaphysical catastrophe continued and continue in the colonization of Asia, Africa, Australia and all other colonized and peripheralized territories in the modern world-system.[38]

Philosopher Jacques Derrida describes the societal autoimmune response of one portion of a society turning on another similar to the perception of *wetiko*. One serious and destructive potential in our body is actualized when it incorrectly identifies a part of itself as something foreign, something to be eliminated. One's immune system, for instance, can attack the thyroid, destroying a biological basis for energy and well-being.[39] The displacement, impoverishment, and unjust maltreatment of individuals and communities falsely deemed as separate from one's own constitutes an autoimmune response within the society at large, a self-destructive and quasi-suicidal response. Turning against other-than-human animals and against the places of Earth as though their presence exists for some humans' profit also constitutes an autoimmune response that destroys the very habitats and creatures of which our lives are but a part in a shared ecological commons.

The Relational Reweaving of Commons

In 2006, when Nelson Mandela was asked to define the Nguni Bantu term *ubuntu*, he shared, "In the old days when we were young, a traveler through a country would stop at a village, and he didn't have to ask for food or water; once he stops, the people give him food, entertain him."[40] A villager was a neighbor to a stranger and welcomed the stranger as a friend. The spiritual ethic of *ubuntu*, which means humanity, understands that I am a person through other people. I am because of you. A person with *ubuntu* is a person who is generous, hospitable, friendly, caring, and compassionate. Archbishop Desmond Tutu describes a person with *ubuntu* as one who "is open and available to others, affirming of others, does not feel threatened that others are able and good, for he or she has a proper self-assurance that comes from knowing that he or she belongs in a greater whole and is diminished when others are humiliated or diminished, when others are tortured or oppressed, or treated as if they were less than who they are."[41]

Violence, lies, theft, deceit, corruption, and exploitation have destroyed such delicate interdependent ties among peoples, communities, and families. They have assaulted the most fragile membranes of exchange in the mind where we metabolize differences and recover psychic space for multiplicity, contradiction, ambiguity, and the not-yet-known. In the literature on the commons, insufficient attention is given to the quality of our relationships. And yet it is these relationships that are reflective of the autoimmune response and the metaphysical catastrophe Derrida and Maldonado-Torres describe. To create new intercommons or intercultural commons we must attend to our relationships to both other humans and other-than-human beings.

Because of the walling-in and walling-out that are essential ingredients to the enclosure of commons, accompaniment is often both a movement across constructed borders and an effort to create inclusive, intercultural counterspaces and contact zones where a different ethic of relationship, belonging, and mutuality can be tended. It also entails strategic efforts to dismantle divisive borders and create in their stead places for mutual thriving, that is, intercommons.

We can liken accompanists at these borders to what Chicana scholar-activist Gloria Anzaldúa describes as *nepantleras*, those who facilitate passage between worlds. Where others see borders, *nepantleras* see bridges. This bridging, she says, "is an act of will, an act of love, an attempt toward compassion and reconciliation, and a promise to be present to the pain of others without losing themselves to it." When we bridge, we loosen our borders, refusing to close off to others: "Bridging is the act of opening the gate to the stranger, within and without."[42] It is a threshold we step into that places us in unfamiliar territory. Many of the examples in this book display the generativity and love that are possible in these in-between spaces, these intercultural and interspecies commons.

The psychosocial and Earth accompaniment necessary for the creation of the commons requires the kinds of intra- and intersubjective work that have been discussed in these chapters. It is about slowly and steadily building relationships, relationships that are responsive and respectful, that open to solidarity and radical imagination. Regardless of our original social locations, the building of commons and beloved communities require our conversion to each other through an ethic of love. They also require addressing the destruction of Native commons by settlers.

Once we begin on a path of accompaniment and learn to respond, we enter a new orientation and our life may begin to unfold in deeper and more profound relationship to others. Brazilian liberatory pedagogist Paulo Freire says that conversion "requires a profound rebirth. Those who undergo it must take on a new form of existence; they can no longer remain as they were. Only through comradeship with the oppressed can the converts understand their characteristic ways of living and behaving, which in diverse moments reflect the structure of domination."[43] For some of us this will mean turning away from culturally normalized, individualistically oriented self-interest and hedonistic pursuit; it will entail, instead, a decided turn toward others. It will require grappling with the injustice born from our histories and developing the capacity to face into the storm of catastrophes unfolding in our midst. It will necessitate our responding to the needs for accompaniment in our own communities as well as listening for and responding to calls for accompaniment from outside of our own local groups and community.

Self-proclaimed deprofessionalized intellectual Gustavo Esteva names intercultural dialogue as the main challenge of the twenty-first century and enjoins us to create intercultural commons, where we learn how to engage with the radical otherness of the Other.[44] He urges us to promote commonism. Commonism or commoning goes beyond the nation-state,

beyond socialism and communism. He suggests that our unit of understanding be the commons, not the person. Unlike fundamentalist-minded
communities that close off their borders completely, the localism he is advocating develops interrelations with other collectives that are working on
similar issues. It is based on hospitality instead of development. Esteva
names three pillars for the recovery of the commons: friendship, hope, and
surprise. Instead of waiting for the utopia over there, he says, we can create
it in our own place.

Gary Snyder would agree, offering us advice about where to start in
the recovery of the commons: "The sum of a field's forces becomes what we
call very loosely the 'spirit of the place.' To know the spirit of a place is to
realize that you are a part of a part and that the whole is made of parts, each
of which is whole. You start with the part you are whole in."[45] When such
places are fragile or have become unavailable, the work is to restore or create
them. Thich Nhat Hanh and Daniel Berrigan call such creations "communities of resistance." By "resistance" they mean "opposition to being invaded, occupied, assaulted, and destroyed by the system." The purpose of
resistance, they write, is to seek the healing of oneself and one's community
in order to be able to see clearly. Such local efforts of mutual accompaniment
and renewal are crucial to the regeneration of solidarity. Communities of
resistance, Thich Nhat Hanh observes, "should be places where people can
return to themselves more easily, where the conditions are such that they can
heal themselves and recover their wholeness."[46] It is crucial to observe that
when such public homeplaces are established and nourished, art, music,
and joyful interactions thrive, expressing the spirit and feeding the soul.

Amid and in opposition to violence and injustice, it is necessary for
people to join together to create communities where justice and peace on a
small, local scale are possible. This allows those who visit such communities to experience that life is possible, that a future is possible. Through
their commoning, these communities resist the dehumanizing forces present in dominant cultures. This book has sought to nourish our vision of
what these places and spaces can look like, so that our imagination regarding a relationally responsive life can be quickened. Hull-House, the White
Rose Mission, L'Arche communities, Fountain House, MOSOP, Partners in

Health initiatives, and Catholic Worker Houses, among others, create or strengthen relationships in the face of division. These organizations open the way for accompaniers to be on paths of learning that deepen their critical and empathic understanding, and thereby refine their response-ability and actions.[47] Paths of accompaniment open us to a reverence for life, a re-sacralization of life, as they suture false divisions between self and other, self and animals, self and the natural world. "Reverence for life," says environmental scholar-activist Vandana Shiva, "is based on compassion and caring for the other, recognition of the autonomy and subjecthood of the other, and the awareness that we are mutually dependent on each other for sustenance, for peace, for joy." The Sanskrit word for culture, says Shiva, means activities that hold a society and community together.[48] Accompaniment is at the heart of culture.

Just as we try to reclaim the integrity of places that have been undermined, so we must also create spaces in which basic aspects of relational practice can be established and enjoyed. The recovery of the commons requires a corollary recovery and creation of dialogical practices that mend the fabric of community. To realize the possibility of the commons, we must create psychic and social spaces where we can unfurl our thoughts, images, and desires with one another, and listen to each other in order to find modes of thinking and acting in solidarity with one another. Paulo Freire wrote,

> Solidarity requires that one enter into the situation of those with whom one is solidary; it is a radical posture. The oppressor is solidary with the oppressed only when he stops regarding the oppressed as an abstract category and sees them as persons who have been unjustly dealt with, deprived of their voice, cheated in the sale of their labor—when he stops making pious, sentimental, and individualistic gestures and risks an act of love. True solidarity is found only in the plenitude of this act, in its existentiality, in its praxis.[49]

Freire adds that to cross over into the practice of accompaniment replaces seeing others abstractly, that is, with sentimentality or through distorting stereotypes. As we can see from the examples given here, the activity of accompaniment flows outward, creating homeplaces, alliances, and networks, inspiring others to join forces and craft places locally and responsively.

In speaking of commons, Gary Snyder writes, "A place on earth is a mosaic within larger mosaics—the land is all small places, all precise tiny realms replicating larger and smaller patterns."[50] Mutual accompaniment reverses the autoimmune response in our social bodies, building solidarity between these realms, rather than division and self-destruction. Recovering and creating commons through accompaniment proceeds small mosaic by small mosaic, and in many instances leads to wider transformation through a slow and steady process of diffusion and integration.[51]

In Chiapas, Mexico, the Zapatista communities have created such mosaic pieces in the form of autonomous communities, each a type of commons. Such communities are horizontally governed through shared leadership and methods of consensus, and connected into a network for mutual solidarity. Through communal processes, they are seeking the well-being of the land and of all members of the community, including women and children. The Zapatistas imagine that one day these autonomous zones will be so numerous on Earth that they may finally create a global shift.

In 1998, Checo Valdez and a group of community members helped to inaugurate a new Zapatista autonomous community named Ricardo Flores Magón by painting a mural, *Vida y Sueños de la Cañada Perla* (The Life and Dreams of the Perla Ravine).[52] A portion of this piece graces the cover of this book. It imagines a deeply desired time, a time after the ravages of colonialism and neoliberalism, when the community lives in peace and with justice. Women can safely circle together as children playfully refresh themselves in the clear and clean waters of the river. Birds, jaguars, and other animals live side by side with humans. A man tends the sacred maize.

This visionary mural of a beloved community was destroyed fourteen hours after its creation by paramilitary forces on April 11, 1998, and its artist along with others were imprisoned. Subcomandante Marcos, the spokesperson for the Zapatistas, in a call for survivance, of living to nourish Indigenous ways of knowing, asked for it to be repainted throughout the world. This has now happened, expressing solidarity from diverse places: San

Francisco, Toronto, Munich, Barcelona, Madrid, Bilbao, Ruest, Bortigiadis, Florence, Mexico City, Brussels, Paris, and Oakland. In 2005, Mexican artists Guadalupe Serrano and Alberto Morackis invited Valdez to oversee its replication on the U.S. border wall in Nogales, Mexico, where I first encountered it in 2006.[53] Here a monument to violent division, the United States' separation wall, was used as a canvas to express the commons-to-come.[54]

Some of the small mosaics of commons described in this book have also been assaulted and destroyed; some accompanists have been imprisoned, and others assassinated. Like the original mural, however, these attempts to defeat resistance and erase alternative visions for how we can live together are foredoomed. Each mosaic of a commons, when witnessed, inspires the creation of many others. The mutual accompaniment from which such mosaics are composed is a source of critical hope and offers "bread" for our daily sustenance.

Notes

Foreword

1. Toni Cade Bambara, "What It Is I Think I Am Doing Anyhow," in *The Writer on Her Work*, ed. Janet Sternberg (New York: Norton, 1992), 155.
2. Linda Janet Holmes, "Poised for the Light," in *Savoring the Salt: The Legacy of Toni Cade Bambara*, ed. Linda Janet Holmes and Cheryl A. Wall (Philadelphia: Temple University Press, 2008), 8.
3. Doris Sommer, *The Work of Art in the World: Civic Agency and Public Humanities* (Durham, NC: Duke University Press, 2014), 89.
4. Hannah Arendt, *The Origins of Totalitarianism* (New York: Harvest, 1973), 478.

Introduction

1. Paul Farmer and Gustavo Gutiérrez, "Re-Imagining Accompaniment: Global Health and Liberation Theology," Ford Family Series, Notre Dame University, South Bend, IN, October 24, 2011.
2. M. Brinton Lykes, Rachel M. Hershberg, and Kalina M. Brabeck, "Methodological Challenges in Participatory Action Research with Undocumented Central American Migrants," *Journal for Social Action in Counseling and Psychology* 3, no. 2 (2011), http://www.psysr.org/jsacp/Lykes-v3n2-11_22-35.pdf; Ravi Ragbir, New Sanctuary, www.newsanctuarynyc.org/accompaniment.html.
3. Oscar Romero, "Fourth Pastoral Letter: Misión de la iglesia en medio de la crisis del país," in *La Voz de los sin voz: La Palabra viva de Monseñor Romero*, ed. Jon Sobrino, Ignacio Martín-Baro, and R. Cardenal (San Salvador, El Salvador: UCA Editores, 2001), 123–172.
4. Patricia Mathes Cane, Kathryn L. Revtyak, and the Capacitar en la Frontera Team, *Refugee Accompaniment: Capacitar Practices of Self-Care and Trauma Healing* (Santa Cruz, CA: Capacitar, 2016); Jesuit Refugee Services, http://jrsusa.org/accompaniment.

5. World Council of Churches' Ecumenical Accompaniment Programme in Palestine, https://www.oikoumene.org/en/what-we-do/eappi.

6. Survivors of Torture International, https://notorture.org/.

7. Stella Sacipa-Rodríguez et al., "Psychosocial Accompaniment to Liberate the Suffering Associated with the Experience of Forced Displacement," *Universitas Psychológica Bogatá* 6, no. 3 (2007), http://www.scielo.org.co/scielo.php?script=sci_arttext&pid=S1657-92672007000300011.

8. Liam Mahoney and Luis Enrique Eguren, *Unarmed Bodyguards: International Accompaniment for the Protection of Human Rights* (Bloomfield, CT: Kumarian Press, 1997).

9. Chris Hedges and Joe Sacco, *Days of Destruction, Days of Revolt* (New York: Nation, 2012).

10. Hussein Bulhan, "Stages of Colonialism in Africa: From Occupation of Land to Occupation of Being," *Journal of Social and Political Psychology* 3, no. 2 (2015): https://jspp.psychopen.eu/article/view/143.

11. G. A. Bradshaw, *Elephants on the Edge: What Animals Teach Us About Humanity* (New Haven, CT: Yale University Press, 2010); G. A. Bradshaw, *Carnivore Minds: Who These Fearsome Animals Really Are* (New Haven, CT: Yale University Press, 2017).

12. Communality, says Regina Day Langhout, "goes inward, outward, and weaves between us. It is a practice of entanglement and resistance . . . a praxis of liberation." Langhout, "This Is Not a History Lesson; This Is Agitation: A Call for a Methodology of Diffraction in US-Based Community Psychology," *American Journal of Community Psychology* 58, nos. 3–4 (2016): 5.

13. Glen Coulthard, *Red Skin, White Masks: Rejecting the Politics of Recognition* (Minneapolis: University of Minnesota Press, 2014), 12.

14. William Cronon, *Changes in the Land: Indians, Colonists, and the Ecology of New* England (New York: Hill and Wang, 2003); Lisa Brooks, *The Common Pot: Recovery of Native Space in the Northeast* (Minneapolis: University of Minnesota Press, 2014).

15. Max Haiven, "Reimagining Our Collective Powers Against Austerity," *Roar Magazine,* June 5, 2015, https://roarmag.org/essays/max-haiven-common-austerity/.

Chapter 1. Accompaniment

1. I have drawn a composite portrait of a typical detainee, lacking in specific details, since all visitation is confidential.

2. Mary Field Belenky, Lynne Bond, and Jacqueline Weinstock, *A Tradition That Has No Name: Nurturing the Development of People, Families, and Communities* (New York: Basic, 1997).

3. bell hooks, *Yearning: Race, Gender, and Cultural Politics* (Boston: South End Press, 1999).

4. Bulhan, "Stages of Colonialism in Africa."

5. Roxanne Dunbar-Ortiz, foreword, in Jordan Flaherty, *No More Heroes: Grassroots Challenges to the Savior Mentality* (Chico, CA: AK Press, 2016), 5.

6. Paulo Freire, *The Pedagogy of the Oppressed* (New York: Bloomsbury, 2000), 45.

7. Gada Mahrouse, *Conflicted Commitments: Race, Privilege, and Power in Solidarity Activism* (Montreal: McGill-Queen's University Press, 2014).

8. Local efforts toward ecological sustainability must develop linkages with efforts elsewhere to ensure that practices that clean up and work to sustain one ecological region do not deleteriously affect others, as in transporting toxic waste from one place to less privileged ones or locating polluting companies in disadvantaged neighborhoods or regions. Without viewing local efforts in the context of other regions and the globe as a whole, the environmentalism of privileged communities too often fails to work effectively against creating what Rob Nixon calls "the environmentalism of the poor." Nixon, *Slow Violence and the Environmentalism of the Poor* (Cambridge, MA: Harvard University Press, 2013).

9. Paul Farmer, *To Repair the World: Paul Farmer Speaks to the Next Generation* (Berkeley: University of California Press, 2013), 234.

10. Staughton Lynd, *From Here to There: The Staughton Lynd Reader*, ed. Andrej Grubačić (Oakland, CA: PM Press, 2010), 295.

11. Staughton Lynd and Andrej Grubačić, *Wobblies and Zapatistas: Conversations on Anarchism, Marxism, and Radical History* (Oakland, CA: PM Press, 2008), 241.

12. See discussion of public homeplaces and sites of reconciliation in Mary Watkins and Helene Shulman, *Toward Psychologies of Liberation* (New York: Palgrave Macmillan, 2008).

13. Carter Heyward, *Saving Jesus from Those Who Are Right: Rethinking What It Means to Be Christian* (Minneapolis, MN: Fortress Press, 1999), 62.

Chapter 2. Creating Social Democracy Through Mutual Accompaniment

1. O. Hill and A. Mearns, *Homes of the London Poor and the Bitter Cry of the Outcast Poor* (1883; London: Routledge Revivals, 2015), 90.

2. Victoria Bissell Brown, "The Sermon of the Deed: Jane Addams's Spiritual Evolution," in *Jane Addams and the Practice of Democracy*, ed. Marilyn Fischer, Carol Nackenoff, and Wendy Chmielewski (Urbana: University of Illinois Press, 2009), 33.

3. University and Social Settlements and Social Action Centers, www.infed.org/mobi/university-and-social-settlements.

4. Jane Addams, *Twenty Years at Hull-House: With Autobiographical Notes* (Urbana: University of Illinois Press, 1990), 51.

5. Ibid., 52.

6. Ibid., 53.

7. Ibid., 5.

8. Ibid., 55, 57.

9. Belenky, Bond, and Weinstock, *A Tradition That Has No Name*, 175.

10. Addams, *Twenty Years*, 244.

11. Ibid., 61, 245, 249, 89.

12. Ibid., 88.

13. Ibid., 199.

14. Mary Jo Deegan, *Jane Addams and the Men of the Chicago School, 1892–1918* (New Brunswick, NJ: Transaction, 1988), 40.

15. Addams, *Twenty Years*, 178.

16. Louise W. Knight, "Jane Addams's Theory of Cooperation," in Fischer, Nackenoff, and Chmielewski, eds., *Jane Addams and the Practice of Democracy*, 65–86.

17. Deegan, *Jane Addams and the Men of the Chicago School*.

18. Jane Addams, "The Subtle Problems of Charity," *Atlantic Monthly*, February 1899, 163, https://socialwelfare.library.vcu.edu/settlement-houses/jane-addams-on-the-problems-of-charity-1899/.

19. Addams, *Twenty Years*, 175.

20. Keith Morton and John Saltmarsh, "Addams, Day, and Dewey: The Emergence of Community Service in American Culture," *Michigan Journal of Community Service Learning* 4, no. 1 (1997): 140.

21. Addams, "The Subtle Problems of Charity," 178.

22. Jane Addams, *The Second Twenty Years at Hull-House: With a Record of Growing World Consciousness* (New York: Macmillan, 1930), 421.

23. Fischer, Nackenoff, and Chmielewski, eds., *Jane Addams and the Practice of Democracy*.

24. Addams, *Twenty Years*, 69.

25. Ibid., 53, 168.

26. Ibid., 255.

27. Ibid., 159.

28. Belenky, Bond, and Weinstock, *A Tradition That Has No Name*.

29. Addams, *Twenty Years*, 309.

30. Ibid., 165, 162–163.

31. Ibid., 16–17, 315.

32. Emily Scarbrough, "'Fine Dignity, Picturesque Beauty, and Serious Purpose': The Reorientation of Suffrage Media in the Twentieth Century" (M.A. thesis, Eastern Illinois University, 2015), http://thekeep.eiu.edu/theses/2033.

33. Jane Addams, "The Modern City and the Municipal Franchise for Women," speech, National American Woman Suffrage Association Convention, 1906.

34. Addams, *The Second Twenty Years*, 174.

35. Fischer, Nackenoff, and Chmielewski, eds., *Jane Addams and the Practice of Democracy*.

36. Harriet Hyman Alonso, "Can Jane Addams Serve as a Role Model for Us Today?" in ibid., 203–218.

37. Wendy Sarvasy, "A Global 'Common' Table: Jane Addams's Theory of Democratic Cosmopolitanism and World Social Citizenship," in ibid., 183–202.

38. Ibid.

39. Deegan, *Jane Addams and the Men of the Chicago School*, 310.

40. Quoted in ibid., 319.

41. Ibid., 314.

42. Deegan, *Jane Addams and the Men of the Chicago School*, 320.

43. Deegan, *Jane Addams and the Men of the Chicago School*, 255, 39.

44. Morton and Saltmarsh, "Addams, Day, and Dewey," 142.

45. Mary Louise Pratt, "Arts of the Contact Zone," *Profession* 91 (1991): 33–40.

46. James Linn, *Jane Addams: A Biography* (Melbourne: Swinburne Press, 2007), 113.

47. Staughton Lynd, "Jane Addams and the Radical Impulse," *Commentary*, July 1, 1961, https://www.commentarymagazine.com/articles/jane-addams-the-radical-impulse/.

48. Jane Addams, "The Subjective Necessity for Social Settlements," 6, https://www.dunmoreschooldistrict.net/site/handlers/filedownload.ashx?moduleinstanceid=93&dataid=615&FileName=Jane%20Addams%20on%20Settlement%20Housing.pdf.

49. In 1949, it was renamed the National Federation of Settlements and Neighborhood Centers.

50. Carol DuBois and Lynn Dumenil, *Through Women's Eyes: An American History with Documents* (Boston: St. Martin's Press, 2012).

51. Jane Addams, *Second Twenty Years*, 401.

52. Elisabeth Lasch-Quinn, *Black Neighbors: Race and the Limits of Reform in the American Settlement House Movement, 1890–1945* (Chapel Hill: University of North Carolina Press, 1993).

53. Ibid., 111.

54. Ibid., 101.

55. Ibid.

56. M. K. Smith, "University and Social Settlements, and Social Action Centres," in *The Encyclopedia of Informal Education,* 1999, www.infed.org/mobi/university-and-social-settlements.

57. Stephen Kramer, "Uplifting Our 'Downtrodden Sisterhood': Victoria Earle Matthew and New York City's White Rose Mission, 1897–1907," *Journal of African American History* 91, no. 3 (2006): 245–246.

58. Victoria Earle Matthews, "The Awakening of the African-American Woman," lecture, Society for Christian Endeavor, San Francisco, 1897, 139.

59. Victoria Earle Matthews, *Aunt Lindy: A Story Founded on Real Life* (New York: J. J. Little, 1893).

60. Kramer, "Uplifting Our 'Downtrodden Sisterhood,'" 247.

61. Ibid., 247–248.

62. Victoria Earle Matthews, Hampton Negro Conference Proceedings, July 1898, 63.

63. White Rose Mission and Industrial Association Collection, Schomburg Center for Research in Black Culture, Manuscripts, Archives and Rare Books Division, New York Public Library.

64. Morton and Saltmarsh, "Addams, Day, and Dewey," 137–149.

65. Addams, "The Subtle Problems of Charity."

66. Deegan, *Jane Addams and the Men of the Chicago School,* 317.

67. Michael Ignatieff, *The Needs of Strangers* (New York: Chatto and Windus, 1984); Morton and Saltmarsh, "Addams, Day, and Dewey."

68. Morton and Saltmarsh, "Addams, Day, and Dewey," 146–147, 137.

69. David B. Schwartz, *Who Cares? Rediscovering Community* (Boulder, CO: Westview Press, 1997), 29, 36, 44, 49.

70. Robert A. Nisbet, *The Quest for Community: A Study in the Ethics of Order and Freedom* (New York: Oxford University Press, 1953).

71. Ibid.

72. Ivan Illich, "Hospitality and Pain," paper presented at the McCormick Theological Seminary, Chicago, 1987, http://brandon.multics.org/library/illich/hospitality.pdf.

73. Schwartz, *Who Cares?* 122, 69.

Chapter 3. Radical Hospitality and the Heart of Accompaniment

1. Jim Forest, *All Is Grace: A Biography of Dorothy Day* (Maryknoll, NY: Orbis, 2011), 100.

2. Robert Coles, *A Spectacle unto the World: The Catholic Worker* Movement (New York: Viking Compass Press, 1974), 11.

3. Forest, *All Is Grace*, 105.

4. Ibid., 102, 114.

5. Ibid., 121.

6. Coles, *A Spectacle unto the World*, 40.

7. Eric Anglada, "Growing Roots: Peter Maurin and the Agronomic University," *Houston Catholic Worker,* March–April 2011, http://cjd.org/2011/04/01/growing-roots-peter-maurin-and-the-agronomic-university/.

8. Forest, *All Is Grace*, 109.

9. Ibid., 124.

10. Ibid., 164.

11. Ibid., 164, 158.

12. Robert Coles, *Dorothy Day: A Radical Devotion* (Reading, MA: Addison-Wesley, 1989), 102–103.

13. Dorothy Day, *The Long Loneliness* (San Francisco: Harper Collins, 1951), 87.

14. Forest, *All Is Grace*, 192.

15. Robert Ellsberg, "Day by Day: The Letters and Journals of Dorothy Day," *U.S. Catholic,* November 2010, 34–36, http://www.uscatholic.org/church/2010/09/day-day-letters-and-journals-dorothy-day; Coles, *Dorothy Day: A Radical Devotion*, 111, 28.

16. Forest, *All Is Grace*, 207.

17. Coles, *Dorothy Day*, 140, 113.

18. Coles, *A Spectacle unto the World*, 57.

19. Coles, *Dorothy Day*, 111, 142.

20. Ibid., 18.

21. Dorothy Day, *All the Way to Heaven: The Selected Letters of Dorothy Day*. (Milwaukee, WI: Marquette University Press, 2010), 309.

22. Dorothy Day, *The Duty of Delight: The Diaries of Dorothy Day* (Milwaukee, WI: Marquette University Press, 2008).

23. Coles, *A Spectacle unto the World*, xxi.

24. Day, *The Duty of Delight*, 318.

25. Jean Vanier, *Becoming Human* (Mahwah, NJ: Paulist Press, 1998), 129.

26. Bernard Allon, "Jean Vanier and L'Arche," CatholicIreland.net, November 30, 1999, http://www.catholicireland.net/jean-vanier-and-larche/.

27. Ibid.

28. Ibid.

29. Jean Vanier, *Community and Growth* (Mahwah, NJ: Paulist Press, 1989), 249, 196.

30. Ibid., 26.

31. Ibid., 77.

32. Ibid., 249–250.

33. Ibid., 117.

34. Ibid., 308.

35. Schwartz, *Who Cares?* 122–129, 124 (Vanier quotation).

36. Ibid., 125.

37. "The History of Kingsley Hall," http://kingsley-hall.co.uk/kingsleyhall.htm.

38. Kelly Oliver, *Witnessing: Beyond Recognition* (Minneapolis: University of Minnesota Press, 2001), 7.

Chapter 4. Psychosocial Accompaniment

1. Frantz Fanon, *Toward the African Revolution* (New York: Grove Press, 1967), 53.

2. Frantz Fanon, *Black Skin, White Masks* (New York: Grove Press, 1967), 51.

3. Frantz Fanon, *The Wretched of the Earth* (New York: Grove Press, 2004), 236, 239, 238; Fanon, *Black Skin, White Masks*, 332, 42.

4. Marie Dennis et al., *St. Francis and the Foolishness of God* (Maryknoll, NY: Orbis, 2015), 11.

5. Gustavo Gutiérrez, quoted in Michael Griffin and Jennie W. Block, eds., *In the Company of the Poor: Conversations with Dr. Paul Farmer and Fr. Gustavo Gutiérrez* (Maryknoll, NY: Orbis, 2013), 75, 99, 104.

6. James Cone, *A Black Theology of Liberation* (Maryknoll, NY: Orbis, 2013), 103, 101.

7. Jon Sobrino, *No Salvation Outside the Poor: Prophetic Utopian Essays* (Maryknoll, NY: Orbis, 2015).

8. María López Virgil, *Oscar Romero: Memories in Mosaic* (London: Darton, Longman, and Todd, 2000), 248; Barbara Tomlinson and George Lipsitz, "American Studies as Accompaniment," *American Quarterly* 65, no. 1 (2013): 1–30.

9. Gustavo Gutiérrez, *The Power of the Poor in History: Selected Writings* (Maryknoll, NY: Orbis, 1983), 45.

10. Rubem Alves, quoted in Mev Puleo, *The Struggle Is One: Voices and Visions of Liberation* (Albany: SUNY Press, 1994), 194, 191.

11. Roberto S. Goizueta, *Liberation, Method, and Dialogue: Enrique Dussel and the North American Theological Discourse* (Atlanta, GA: Scholars Press, 1988).

12. Roberto S. Goizueta, *Christ Our Companion: Toward a Theological Aesthetics of Liberation* (Maryknoll, NY: Orbis, 2009), 192, 199.

13. In 2007, Jon Sobrino, a Jesuit priest who was away from his home in El Salvador when it was attacked in 1989 by a paramilitary squad trained in the United States, was sanctioned by the Vatican for errors in his teachings and writings. This was seen as a censoring of an important voice in liberation theology, an advocate for the poor and the dispossessed. Tracy Wilkinson, "Vatican to Punish Priest, Sources Say," *Los Angeles Times,* March 14, 2007, http://articles. latimes.com/2007/mar/14/world/fg-sobrino14.

14. Cone, *A Black Theology of Liberation*; Marc H. Ellis, *Toward a Jewish Theology of Liberation* (New York: Maryknoll, 1987); S. Akhtar, *The Final Imperative: An Islamic Theology of Liberation* (London: Bellew, 1991); H. Dabashi, *Islamic Liberation Theology: Resisting the Empire* (London: Routledge, 2008); F. Esack, *Qur'an, Liberation and Pluralism: An Islamic Perspective of Interreligious Solidarity Against Oppression* (Oxford: Oneworld, 1998); Sharon D. Welch, *Communities of Resistance and Solidarity: A Feminist Theology of Liberation* (Maryknoll, NY: Orbis, 1985); Elisabeth Schussler Fiorenza, *The Power of Naming: A Concilium Reader in Feminist Liberation Theology* (Maryknoll, NY: Orbis, 1996).

15. Paul Farmer, quoted in Griffin and Block, eds., *In the Company of the Poor*, 24.

16. Paul Farmer, http://www.pih.org/.

17. "Our Mission at PIH," http://www.pih.org/pages/our-mission.

18. Paul Farmer, quoted in Griffin and Block, eds., *In the Company of the Poor*, 19–22.

19. Jonathan Weigel, Matthew Basilico, and Paul Farmer, "Taking Stock of Foreign Aid," in *Reimagining Global Health,* ed. Paul Farmer et al. (Berkeley: University of California Press, 2013), 298.

20. D. R. Thomson et al., "Community-Based Accompaniment and Psychosocial Health Outcomes in HIV-Infected Adults in Rwanda: A Prospective Study," *AIDS Behavior* 18, no. 2 (2014): 368–380. doi: 10.1007/s10461-013-0431-2.

21. Farmer et al., eds., *Reimagining Global Health*, 295, 241.

22. Paul Farmer, "Accompaniment as Policy," Kennedy School of Government, Harvard University, May 25, 2011, https://www.lessonsfromhaiti.org/press-and-media/transcripts/accompaniment-as-policy/.

23. Weigel, Basilico, and Farmer, "Taking Stock," 301.

24. Ibid., 295–296.

25. Jonathan Weigel, introduction, in Farmer, *To Repair the World*, xxv, xxvi.

26. Ibid., xxvii.
27. Ignacio Martín-Baró, *Writings for a Liberation Psychology* (Cambridge, MA: Harvard University Press, 1994), 46.
28. Ibid., 26, 121, 183.
29. Ibid., 25, 24.
30. M. Brinton Lykes, "Liberation Psychology and Social Change: An Introduction to Ignacio Martín-Baró and Challenges for the 21st Century Practitioner," Center for Human Right and International Justice, Boston College, December 6, 2013, https://vimeo.com/81222221.
31. Martín-Baró, *Writings for a Liberation Psychology*, 37, 120.
32. Ibid., 27, 28.
33. Ibid., 29.
34. Ibid., 46.
35. Ignacio Martín-Baró, *Accion y ideologia: Psicologia social desde Centroamérica* (El Salvador: UCA Editores, 1990), http://www.uca.edu.sv/coleccion-digital-IMB/wp-content/uploads/2015/11/1983-@-Acci%C3%B3n-e-ideolog%C3%ADa-psicolog%C3%ADa-social-desde-centroamerica.pdf.
36. Martín-Baró, *Writings for a Liberation Psychology*, 43, 40–41.
37. Ibid., 125, 135.
38. Kleinman, *Re-Thinking Psychiatry*, 154.
39. Joao Biehl, *Vita: Life in a Zone of Social Abandonment* (Berkeley: University of California Press, 2005).
40. Ellen Danto, *Freud's Free Clinics: Psychoanalysis and Social Justice, 1918–1939* (New York: Columbia University Press, 2005).
41. Nancy Caro Hollander, *Uprooted Minds: Surviving the Politics of Terror in the Americas* (New York: Routledge, 2010).
42. Nancy Caro Hollander, *Love in a Time of Hate: Liberation Psychology in Latin America* (New Brunswick, NJ: Rutgers University Press, 1997).
43. Marie Langer, "Psicoanálisis y/o revolucion social," in *Cuestionamos,* ed. Marie Langer (Buenos Aires: Granica Editor, 1971), 262–263.
44. Nancy Caro Hollander, introduction, in Marie Langer, *From Vienna to Managua: Journey of a Psychoanalyst* (London: Free Association, 1989), 1–22.
45. Hollander, *Uprooted Minds.*
46. Hollander, "Introduction," 9.
47. Marie Langer and Ignacio Maldonado, "Nicaragua Libre," unpublished, 1983, cited in Langer, *From Vienna to Managua.*
48. Hollander, "Introduction," 9.
49. Sacipa-Rodríguez et al., "Psychosocial Accompaniment to Liberate the Suffering."

50. Stella Sacipa-Rodriguez and Maritza Montero, eds., *Psychosocial Approaches to Peacebuilding in Colombia* (New York: Springer, 2014).

51. Stella Sacipa-Rodriguez, "To Feel and to Re-Signify Forced Displacement in Colombia," in *Psychosocial Approaches to Peacebuilding in Colombia,* ed. Stella Sacipa-Rodriguez and Maritza Montero (New York: Springer, 2014), 67.

52. Stella Sacipa-Rodríguez et al., "Psychological Accompaniment: Construction of Cultures of Peace Among a Community Affected by War," in *Psychology of Liberation: Theory and Applications,* ed. Maritza Montero and Christopher Sonn (New York: Springer, 2009), 222.

53. Ibid.

54. Ibid., 223, 224.

55. Maritza Montero, "Una orientación para la psicología politica en América Latina," *Psicología Política* 3 (1991): 38.

56. M. Brinton Lykes, "Activist Participatory Research and the Arts with Rural Mayan Women: Interculturality and Situated Meaning Making," in *From Subjects to Subjectivities: A Handbook of Interpretive and Participatory Methods,* ed. Deborah L. Tolman and Mary Brydon-Miller (New York: New York University Press, 2001), 183–199.

57. M. Brinton Lykes and Marcie Mersky, "Reparations and Mental Health: Psychosocial Interventions Towards Healing, Human Agency, and Rethreading Social Realities," in *The Handbook of Reparations,* ed. P. De Grieff (New York: Oxford University Press, 2006), 589.

58. Lykes, Hershberg, and Brabeck, "Methodological Challenges in Participatory Action Research," 5.

59. Ibid.

60. Ibid.

61. M. Brinton Lykes, "'I Am Not Going to Stay with My Arms Crossed If I See Another Woman's Suffering': Accompanying Maya Protagonists Through Community-Based Activist Scholarship Post-Genocide," Seymour Sarason Award Talk, Society for Community Research and Action Conference, Ottawa, Canada, June 24, 2017.

62. Ibid.

63. Immigration Rights Committee, *In the Shadows of Paradise: The Experiences of the Undocumented Community in Santa Barbara* (Santa Barbara, CA: PUEBLO Education Fund, 2008).

64. M. Brinton Lykes and Geraldine Moane, eds., "Editors' Introduction: Whither Feminist Liberation Psychology? Critical Explorations of Feminist and Liberation Psychologies for a Globalizing World," *Feminism and Psychology* 19 (2009): 293. doi:10.1177/0959353509105620.

65. Linda Tuhiwai Smith, *Decolonizing Methodologies: Research and Indigenous Peoples* (New York: Zed, 2012); Shawn Wilson, *Research Is Ceremony: Indigenous Research Methods* (Black Point, NS: Fernwood, 2009).

66. Irene Edge, Carolyn Kagan, and Angela Stewart, "Living Poverty in the UK: Community Psychology as Accompaniment," 2003, www.compsy.org.uk/LivingPoverty5b.pdf.

Chapter 5. After the Asylum

1. The Treatment Advocacy Center (http://www.treatmentadvocacycenter.org/) reports that, in 2014 in the United States, there were 383,000 prison and jail inmates with severe mental illness, ten times the number of mentally ill patients in state psychiatric hospitals in the same year—about 35,000 people. In addition, according to the National Coalition of the Homeless (http://nationalhomeless.org/), 20–25 percent of the U.S. homeless population of 500,000 suffers from mental illness.

2. *Asylum*, dir. P. Robinson, 1972.

3. Ibid.

4. Philadelphia Association, https://www.philadelphia-association.com/.

5. Mary Barnes was the most famous resident of Kingsley Hall due to her autobiographical account, written in 1971 with her therapist, Joseph Berke—*Mary Barnes: Two Accounts of a Journey Through Madness* (New York: Other Press, 2002). She translated her psychotic experiences into artistic images and lived as an artist after her residence at Kingsley Hall.

6. Philadelphia Association.

7. "Houses," Philadelphia Association, https://www.philadelphia-association.com/houses.

8. Loren Mosher, "Alternatives to Psychiatric Hospitalization: Why Has Research Failed to Be Translated into Practice?" *New England Journal of Medicine* 309, no. 25 (1983): 1579–1580; Loren Mosher and Samuel Keith, "Research on the Psychosocial Treatment of Schizophrenia: A Summary Report," *American Journal of Psychiatry* 136, no. 5 (1979): 623–631.

9. John Weir Perry, *The Far Side of Madness* (Upper Saddle River, NJ: Prentice-Hall, 1974); Harry Stack Sullivan, *Schizophrenia as a Human Process* (New York: Norton, 1974); Thomas Scheff, *Being Mentally Ill* (Piscataway, NJ: Aldine Transaction, 1984); Frieda Fromm-Reichman, *Psychotherapy and Psychosis* (Madison, WI: International Universities Press, 1989); Harold Searles, *Collected Papers on Schizophrenia and Related Topics* (New York: Routledge, 1986).

10. Loren R. Mosher, "Soteria and Other Alternatives to Acute Psychiatric Hospitalization: A Personal and Professional Review," *Journal of Nervous and Mental Disease* 187 (1999), http://www.moshersoteria.com/articles/soteria-and-other-alternatives-to-acute-psychiatric-hospitalization/.

11. Loren R. Mosher, "Non-Hospital, Non-Drug Intervention with 1st Episode Psychosis," in *Models of Madness: Psychological, Social and Biological Approaches to Schizophrenia,* ed. John Read, Loren R. Mosher, and Richard P. Bentall (New York: Routledge, 2004), 351.

12. Ibid., 350.

13. Nancy Remsen, "Dream House: Soteria Vermont Welcomes Mental Health Patients," Seven Days, June 3, 2015, https://www.sevendaysvt.com/vermont/dream-house-soteria-vermont-welcomes-mental-health-patients/Content?oid=2643104.

14. Judy Siegel-Itzkovich, "Jerusalem Mental Health Home Modeled After the 'Prince and the Turkey,'" *Jerusalem Post*, September 3, 2017, http://www.jpost.com/HEALTH-SCIENCE/Jerusalem-mental-health-home-modeled-after-the-Prince-and-the-Turkey-504046.

15. Mosher, "Non-Hospital, Non-Drug Intervention," 115–130.

16. As I discovered, this mode of separating oneself from those one is working with was not practiced by many psychotherapists in the late 1800s. Some of the early phenomenologically and existentially oriented psychiatrists began their professional lives by living in the home of a patient and sharing daily life with him or her; see Rollo May, Ernst Angel, and Henri Ellenberger, eds., *Existence: A New Dimension in Psychiatry and Psychology* (New York: Basic, 1958). In the small European asylums of the late nineteenth and early twentieth centuries, chief psychiatrists often sought to create the asylum like a home. They and their families dined nightly with their patients. At times, they were the ones to open the front door to greet newcomers, carrying the patients' bags to their rooms, as a host would for an invited guest.

In the mid-1880s, Samuel Woodward was the superintendent of Worcester State Hospital in Massachusetts. When incoming patients arrived at the door, Woodward would personally greet them and remove them from any manacles or cages in which they arrived. Then he would escort them into the dining room where he and his family ate each night. He would seat the newcomer at the head of the table with his family. David Schwartz, in recounting this story in *Who Cares?* sees "a vestige of the medieval monastic traditions of hospitality in which guests, treated as the hidden Christ, were greeted by the abbot, who washed their hands and sometimes their feet as a ritual of reception" (92).

17. Courtenay Harding et al., "The Vermont Longitudinal Study of Persons with Severe Mental Illness, I: Methodology, Study Sample, and Overall Status," *American Journal of Psychiatry* 144, no. 6 (1987): 718–726.

18. Kleinman, *Re-Thinking Psychiatry*.

19. Angelo Barbato, *Schizophrenia and Public Health* (Geneva: World Health Organization, 1998), http://www.who.int/mental_health/media/en/55.pdf.

20. In his *Description of the Retreat for the Insane: An Institution near York for Insane Persons of the Society of Friends* (York, UK: W. Alexander, 1813), Samuel Tuke advised, "As experience demonstrates, that the recovery of insane patients, frequently depends on their being removed from their connexions, and put under proper care and treatment, in the early stages of the disorder, it is earnestly recommended to their friends, to remove them at an early period after the disorder appears to be fixed" (88).

21. Barbato, *Schizophrenia and Public Health*, 28.

22. Larry Davidson, Jaak Rakfeldt, and John Strauss, *The Roots of the Recovery Movement in Psychiatry: Lessons Learned* (Hoboken, NJ: Wiley Blackwell, 2010).

23. Ibid., 83.

24. Ibid., 176.

25. Ibid., 219, 221, 98.

26. Ibid., 235.

27. Patricia E. Deegan, "There's a Person in Here," lecture, Sixth Annual Mental Health Services Conference of Australia and New Zealand, Brisbane, Australia, September 16, 1997.

28. Patricia E. Deegan, "The Recovery of Hope," lecture, Sixth Annual Mental Health Services Conference of Australia and New Zealand, Brisbane, Australia, September 16, 1997.

29. In Algeria, Fanon observed that Tosquelles's model worked well for European patients but less well for native Algerians who were suffering under the multiple collective traumas imposed by colonialism. David Macey, *Frantz Fanon: A Biography* (New York: Picador USA, 2000), 231.

30. I am grateful to the following sources for this section on Geel, Belgium: James Broderick, "The Geel Model: Cultivating Love and Justice for the Mentally Ill," lecture, Pacifica Graduate Institute, 2013; Angus Chen, "For Centuries, a Small Town Has Embraced Strangers with Mental Illness," NPR, July 1, 2016, http://www.npr.org/sections/health-shots/2016/07/01/484083305/for-centuries-a-small-town-has-embraced-strangers-with-mental-illness; Eugeen Roosens, *Mental Patients in Town Life: Geel—Europe's 1st Therapeutic Community* (Beverly Hills, CA: Sage, 1979); Eugeen Roosens and Lleve Van De Walle, *Geel*

Revisited: After Centuries of Rehabilitation (Antwerp, Netherlands: Garrant, 2007); and Judy Molland, "Meet the Town Where the Mentally Ill Are Welcomed as Family," Care2, 2014, http://www.care2.com/causes/the-town-where-the-mentally-ill-are-welcomed-as-family.html.

31. In the past, there have been critical reports of insufficient hygiene and medical care, the shackling of out-of-control boarders, and the exploitation of boarders' farm labor. The residents of Geel, however, have developed an ethic of care that has now been incorporated into the larger system of mental health care in the town. For instance, it would be considered unethical for a family not to include a guest at their meal table or to give the guest a bedroom inside the family house. In addition, the development of psychiatric medications has made appeals for shackling no longer necessary. Families are supported by a case management team with a visiting nurse as the key bridge between family care and community supportive services.

32. Roosens and Van De Walle, *Geel Revisited*.

33. Broderick, "The Geel Model."

34. Roosens and Van de Walle, *Geel Revisited*, 59.

35. Ibid., 62.

36. A. Hauben, *Geel* (television documentary), OPZ Geel & Woestunvis, 2006.

37. Roosens and Van de Walle, *Geel Revisited*, 11, 12.

38. *Healing Homes: Recovery from Psychosis Without Medications*, dir. Daniel Mackler, 2014, https://www.youtube.com/watch?v=JV4NTEp8S2Q. The quotations in this section are from the film.

39. The quotations in this section are from the documentary film *Open Dialogues: An Alternative Finnish Approach to Healing*, dir. Daniel Mackler, 2014. See also Jaako Seikkula, Mary Olson, and Douglas Ziedonis, "The Key Elements of Dialogic Practice in Open Dialogue," The University of Massachusetts Medical School, Worcester, MA: 2014; Jaako Seikkula and T. E. Amkil, *Dialogical Meetings in Social Networks* (London: Karnac, 2006).

40. Seikkula, Olson, and Ziedonis, "The Key Elements of Dialogic Practice."

41. *Open Dialogues*.

42. Franca Ongaro, "Nota introductivo," in *L'Istituzione negata,* ed. Frano Basaglia (Turin: Einaudi, 1998), 3.

43. This is an excerpt from Basaglia's resignation letter from his work at the Gorizia asylum, quoted in John Foot, *The Man Who Closed the Asylums: Franco Basaglia and the Revolution in Mental Health Care* (New York: Verso, 2015), 228.

44. Ibid.

45. John Foot, "Franco Basaglia and the Radical Psychiatry Movement in Italy, 1961–78," *Critical Radical Social Work* 2, no. 2 (2014): 235–249.

46. Nancy Scheper-Hughes and Anne M. Lovell, "Breaking the Circuit of Social Control: Lessons in Public Psychiatry from Italy and Franco Basaglia," *Social Science and Medicine* 23, no. 2 (1986): 159–178; Nancy Scheper-Hughes and A. M. Lovell, eds., *Psychiatry Inside Out: Selected Writings of Franco Basaglia* (New York: Columbia University Press, 1986).

47. Foot, "Franco Basaglia."

48. John Foot, *The Man Who Closed the Asylums*, 267.

49. Ibid., 263.

50. Elena Portacalone et al., "A Tale of Two Cities: The Exploration of the Trieste Public Psychiatry Model in San Francisco," *Culture, Medicine, and Psychiatry* 39, no. 4 (2015): 3, https://www.researchgate.net/publication/277078425_A_Tale_of_Two_Cities_The_Exploration_of_the_Trieste_Public_Psychiatry_Model_in_San_Francisco.

51. A. J. Frances, "World's Best and Worst Places to Be Mentally Ill," *Psychology Today*, December 28, 2015, https://www.psychologytoday.com/us/blog/saving-normal/201512/worlds-best-and-worst-places-be-mentally-ill.

52. Ibid.

53. Franco Basaglia, "Breaking the Circuit of Control," in *Critical Psychiatry: The Politics of Mental Health*, ed. D. Ingleby (Harmondsworth, UK: Penguin, 1981), 190–191.

54. Portacalone et al., "A Tale of Two Cities."

55. Davidson, Rakfeldt, and Strauss, *Roots of the Recovery Movement*, 175.

56. Ibid., 176.

57. Portacalone et al., "A Tale of Two Cities."

Chapter 6. Beyond Treatment

1. R. E. Drake, Patricia E. Deegan, and C. Rapp, "The Promise of Shared Decision Making in Mental Health," *Psychiatric Rehabilitation Journal* 34, no. 1 (2010), http://dx.doi.org/10.2975/34.1.2010.7.13.

2. Richard Warner and James M. Mandiberg, "Social Networks, Support and Early Psychosis," *Epidemiology and Psychiatric Sciences* 22, no. 2 (2013): 151–154.

3. Richard Warner and James M. Mandiberg, "An Update on Affirmative Businesses or Social Firms for People with Mental Illness," *Psychiatric Services* 57, no. 10 (2006): 1488–1492.

4. Richard Warner, "The Importance of Service-User Communities: Is Mainstreaming Always the Answer?" *European Psychiatry* 30, no. 1 (2015): 167.

5. James M. Mandiberg, "Another Way: Enclave Communities for People with Mental Illness," *American Journal of Orthopsychiatry* 80, no. 2 (2010): 170–171.

6. Warner and Mandiberg. "Social Networks, Support and Early Psychosis," 151.

7. Mandiberg, "Another Way," 176.

8. Ibid., 173.

9. R. Vorspan, "Attitudes and Structure in the Clubhouse Model," *Fountain House Annual* 4, no. 1 (1986): 1–7; J. H. Beard, R. Propst, and T. Malamud, "The Fountain House Model of Psychiatric Rehabilitation," *Psychiatric Rehabilitation Journal* 5 (1982): 47–53; S. B. Anderson, *We Are Not Alone: Fountain House and the Development of Clubhouse Culture* (New York: Fountain House, 1998); Alan Doyle, Julius Lanoil, and Kenneth Dudek, *Fountain House: Creating Community in Mental Health Practice* (New York: Columbia University Press, 2013). I am particularly indebted to Alan Doyle, Julius Lanoil, and Kenneth Dudek in this section for their extraordinary portrait of Fountain House in *Fountain House.*

10. Ian McCabe, *Carl Jung and Alcoholics Anonymous: The Twelve Steps as a Spiritual Journey of Individuation* (New York: Taylor and Francis, 2015).

11. Ibid., 47.

12. Doyle, Lanoil, and Dudek, *Fountain House.*

13. A. Doyle, J. Rivera, and Fang-pei Chen, Fountain House: A Working Community That Brings Hope to Mind, lectures, Columbia University, 2014, https://www.youtube.com/watch?v=pIm2UEThBTA.

14. Susser, quoted in Doyle, Lanoil, and Dudek, *Fountain House,* xxvi.

15. International Center for Clubhouse Development, "How Clubhouses Can Help," http://www.iccd.org/how.html.

16. International Center for Clubhouse Development, "History," http://www.iccd.org/history.html.

17. International Center for Clubhouse Development, "The International Standards," http://clubhouse-intl.org/resources/quality-standards/.

18. International Center for Clubhouse Development, "How Clubhouses Can Help."

19. Southeast Recovery Learning Community, http://www.southeastrlc.org/.

20. George W. Fairweather et al., *Community Life for the Mentally Ill: An Alternative to Institutional Care* (Chicago: Aldine, 1969).

21. Henry David Thoreau, *Walden* (Seattle: Create Space, 2017), 89.

22. Jack Forbes, *Columbus and Other Cannibals: The Wetiko Disease of Exploitation, Imperialism, and Terrorism* (New York: Seven Stories Press, 2008), xi.

23. Mary Field Belenky et al., *The Development of Self, Voice, and Mind* (New York: Basic, 1997).

24. Harold Searles, *The Non-Human Environment in Normal Development and in Schizophrenia* (New York: International Universities Press, 1960), 6.

25. G. Zilboorg, *A History of Medical Psychology* (New York: Norton, 1941).

26. Mindy Fullilove, *Root Shock: How Tearing Up City Neighborhoods Hurts America, and What We Can Do About It* (New York: One World, 2005), 120.

27. Fullilove pieced together the systematic destruction of 2,500 neighborhoods in 993 American cities during the period of urban renewal. Eighty percent of them were neighborhoods of color. Ibid.

28. Ibid., 14.

29. D. W. Winnicott, *Playing and Reality* (New York: Routledge, 2005).

30. Gould Farm, "We Harvest Hope: The Gould Farm Story," www.gould.org.

31. *Care Farms of the Netherlands,* dir. David Heine and Kas Struik, An Aspect Production, 2012.

32. "Warrior Expeditions," https://warriorexpeditions.org/.

33. In "A Tale of Two Cities," Portacolone and colleagues explore the feasibility of embodying the Trieste model in San Francisco. They conclude that there are a set of structural supports that are necessary for the success of the model. Is there affordable housing? Is public support adequate to live above the poverty level? Can medical reimbursement be determined by level of care and quality of relationship, instead of by efforts to eliminate or reduce symptoms? Can continuity of care and the expansion of what constitutes care shift, so that assistance with "housing, meaningful work, meaningful relationships, space for creativity, love, and recreation" becomes possible? Given the poverty suffered by those living on Social Security, the inadequacy of healthcare, the lack of affordable housing, and the prevalence of drugs and dual diagnoses in the San Francisco area, their answer was that the context would not presently support a Trieste model, though it is clear it would be far superior than the homelessness, poverty, and incarceration that people suffering from mental illness now experience.

Chapter 7. Pathways Through Mutual Accompaniment to Solidarity

1. Oliver, *Witnessing*, 219.

2. Freire, *Pedagogy of the Oppressed*, 180.

3. Mark Potter, "Solidarity as Spiritual Exercise: Accompanying Migrants at the US/Mexico Border," *Political Theology* 12, no. 6 (2011): 835.

4. Ibid.

5. Lynd, *From Here to There*.

6. Staughton Lynd and Alice Lynd, "Liberation Theology for Quakers," in Staughton Lynd, *Living Inside Our Hope: A Steadfast Radical's Thoughts on Rebuilding the Movement* (Ithaca, NY: Cornell University Press, 1997), 63.

7. Mary Watkins, "Notes from a Visit to Several Zapatista Communities: Toward Practices of Nomadic Identity and Hybridity," *Psychological Studies* 57, no. 1 (2012): 1–8.

8. The delimited sites of the *caracoles* are akin to what Homi Bhabha calls "interstitial spaces," "third spaces," or "in-between spaces," which he defines as "provid[ing] the terrain for elaborating strategies of selfhood—singular or communal—that initiate new signs of identity, and innovative sites of collaboration, and contestation, in the act of defining the idea of society itself." Bhabha, *The Location of Culture* (New York: Routledge, 1994), 1.

9. Freire, *Pedagogy of the Oppressed*, 24.

10. John Dixon et al., "'What's So Funny 'Bout Peace, Love and Understanding?' Further Reflections on the Limits of Prejudice Reduction as a Model of Social Change," *Journal of Social and Political Psychology* 1, no. 1 (2013): 1.

11. Eve Tuck, "Suspending Damage: A Letter to Communities," *Harvard Educational Review* 79, no. 3 (2009): 412.

12. Wilson, *Research Is Ceremony*.

13. bell hooks, *Outlaw Culture: Resisting Representations* (New York: Routledge, 2006), 193–201.

14. Mary Annette Pember, "This November, Try Something New: Decolonize Your Mind," *Yes! Magazine*, November 13, 2017, http://www.yesmagazine.org/people-power/this-november-try-something-new-decolonize-your-mind-20171113.

15. Teju Cole, "The White-Savior Industrial Complex," *The Atlantic*, March 21, 2012, https://www.theatlantic.com/international/archive/2012/03/the-white-savior-industrial-complex/254843/.

16. Flaherty, *No More Heroes*, 199.

17. Julia Kristeva, *Powers of Horror: An Essay on Abjection* (New York: Columbia University Press, 1982), 135–136.

18. Albert Memmi, *The Colonizer and the Colonized* (Boston: Beacon Press, 1991), 81.

19. Oliver, *Witnessing*, 219.

20. bell hooks, *Outlaw Culture: Resisting Representations* (New York: Routledge, 2006), 248.

21. Quoted in Michelle Alexander, *The New Jim Crow: Mass Incarceration in the Age of Colorblindness* (New York: New Press, 2012), 229.

22. Ibid., 222.

23. Lasch-Quinn, *Black Neighbors*, 112.
24. Robin DiAngelo, "White Fragility," *International Journal of Critical Pedagogy* 3, no. 3 (2011): 54–70.
25. Lauren Mizock and Konjit V. Page, "Evaluating the Ally Role: Contributions, Limitations, and the Activist Position in Counseling and Psychology," *Journal for Social Action in Counseling and Psychology* 8, no. 1 (Summer 2016): 24.
26. Indigenous Action Media, "Accomplices Not Allies: Abolishing the Ally Industrial Complex: An Indigenous Perspective and Provocation," http://www.indigenousaction.org/accomplices-not-allies-abolishing-the-ally-industrial-complex/.
27. Addams, *Twenty Years*, 109, 126, 90.
28. Tomlinson and Lipsitz, "American Studies as Accompaniment."
29. Addams, *Twenty Years*, 125.
30. Kelly Oliver, *Subjectivity Without Subjects: From Abject Fathers to Desiring Mothers* (Lanham, MD: Rowman and Littlefield, 1998), 175.
31. Flaherty, *No More Heroes*, 47; Cole, "The White-Savior Industrial Complex."
32. Etienne Roy Grégoire and Karen Hamilton, "International Accompaniment, Reflexivity and the Intelligibility of Power in Post-Conflict Guatemala," *Journal of Genocide Research* 18, nos. 2–3 (2016): 189–205. doi: 10.1080/14623528.2016.1186896.
33. Nelson Maldonado-Torres, *Against War: Views from the Underside of Modernity* (Durham, NC: Duke University Press, 2008), 151.
34. Gustavo Gutiérrez clarifies that the preferential option for the poor is not to exclude the non-poor but to work toward a universality of love, reversing the usual starting point among the privileged that too often ends up excluding the least powerful. Griffin and Block, eds., *In the Company of the Poor*, 149.
35. Quoted in Jon Sobrino, "On the Way to Healing America: Humanizing a 'Gravely Ill World,'" *America*, October 29, 2014, http://americamagazine.org/issue/way-healing.
36. Hedges and Sacco, *Days of Destruction, Days of Revolt*.
37. Helen Merrell Lynd, *On Shame and the Search for Identity* (New York: Science Editions, 1961), 232.
38. For an in-depth treatment of restorative, reintegrative, and generative shame, see Edward S. Casey and Mary Watkins, *Up Against the Wall: Re-Imagining the U.S.-Mexico Border* (Austin: University of Texas Press, 2014), and John Braithwaite, *Crime, Shame, and Reintegration* (Cambridge: Cambridge University Press, 1989).
39. Christopher LeBron, *The Color of Our Shame: Race and Justice in Our Time* (New York: Oxford University Press, 2013).

40. Potter, "Solidarity as Spiritual Exercise," 836.

41. Ibid.

42. John Braithwaite, *Crime, Shame and Reintegration* (New York: Cambridge University Press, 1989).

43. Dorothy Day, *House of Hospitality* (Huntington, IN: Our Sunday Visitor, 2015), 270.

44. Lynd, *On Shame*, 231, 22, 20.

45. Sobrino, quoted in Griffin and Block, eds., *In the Company of the Poor*, 41.

46. Gloria Anzaldúa, *Borderlands/La Frontera* (San Francisco: Aunt Lute Books, 1999), 107, 243.

47. Mel Mariposa, "A Practical Guide to Calling In," *Consent 101*, May 29, 2016, https://the consentcrew.org/2016/05/29/calling-in/.

48. Potter, "Solidarity as Spiritual Exercise," 836.

49. Staughton Lynd, quoted in Lynd, *From Here to There*, 21, 20.

50. Ibid., 18.

51. Alexander, *The New Jim Crow*.

52. Geoffrey Nelson and Isaac Prilleltensky, *Community Psychology: In Pursuit of Liberation and Well-Being* (New York: Palgrave-Macmillan, 2005); Isaac Prilleltensky and Geoffrey Nelson, *Doing Psychology Critically: Making a Difference in Diverse Settings* (New York: Palgrave Macmillan, 2002).

53. Nelson and Prilleltensky, *Community Psychology*, 145.

54. Ibid.

55. Tuck, "Suspending Damage," 409.

56. Geraldine Moane, "Making Connections: Systems of Resistance," *Irish Journal of Feminist Studies* 6 (2000): 221–226.

57. Mary Pipher, *The Middle of Everywhere: Helping Refugees Enter the American Community* (New York: Houghton Mifflin, 2002).

58. Walter Mignolo, "Geopolitics of Sensing and Knowing: On (De)Coloniality, Border Thinking, and Epistemic Disobedience," European Institute for Progressive Cultural Policies, September 2011, http://eipcp.net/transversal/0112/mignolo/en.

59. Santiago Castro-Gomez, "The Missing Chapter of Empire: Postmodern Re-Organization of Coloniality and Post-Fordist Capitalism," *Cultural Studies* 21, nos. 2–3 (2007): 428–448. doi: 10.1080/09502380601162639.

60. Walter Mignolo, "Epistemic Disobedience, Independent Thought and De-Colonial Freedom," *Theory, Culture and Society* 26, nos. 7–8 (2009), http://waltermignolo.com/wp-content/uploads/2013/03/epistemicdisobedience-2.pdf.

61. Walter Mignolo, "The Communal and the De-Colonial," *Turbulence*, 2010, http://turbulence.org.uk/turbulence-5/decolonial/.

62. Mignolo, "Epistemic Disobedience."

63. According to Mignolo, "The Communal and the De-Colonial," "Evo Morales has been promoting the concept of 'the good living' (*sumaj kamaña* in Quechua, *sumak kawsay* in Quichua, *allin kausaw* in Aymara or *buen vivir* in Spanish). 'The good living'—or 'to live in harmony'—is an alternative to 'development.' While development puts life at the service of growth and accumulation, *buen vivir* places life first, with institutions at the service of life. That is what 'living in harmony' (and not in competition) means."

64. Nancy Scheper-Hughes, "The Primacy of the Ethical: Propositions for a Militant Anthropology," *Current Anthropology* 36, no. 3 (June 1995): 409–430; René Lorau, "Lavoratori del negativo, unitevi!" in *Crimini di pace,* ed. F. Basaglia and F. O. Basaglia (Turin, Italy: Einaudi, 1975), https://archive.org/stream/ AAVVCriminiDiPace.RicercheSugliIntellettualiESuiTecniciComeAddetti Alloppressione./AAVV%20-%20Crimini%20di%20pace.%20Ricerche%20 sugli%20intellettuali%20e%20sui%20tecnici%20come%20addetti%20 all%27oppressione._djvu.txt.

65. Scheper-Hughes, "The Primacy of the Ethical," 420.

66. Merrill Singer and Hans Baer, *Critical Medical Anthropology* (Amityville, NY: Baywood, 1995), 36.

67. Lynd and Grubačić, *Wobblies and Zapatistas*, 123–124.

68. Ibid., 58–59.

69. Mary Watkins and Nuria Ciofalo, "Creating and Sharing Critical Community Psychology Curriculum for the 21st Century," *Global Journal of Community Psychology Practice* 2, no. 2 (2011), http://www.gjcpp.org/pdfs/2011-0002-Final-20111104.pdf. Nuria Ciofalo and I have addressed these issues from our own experience crafting a masters and doctoral level program in critical community psychology, liberation psychology, Indigenous psychologies, and eco-psychology.

70. Jack Zimmerman and Gigi Coyle, *The Way of Council* (Las Vegas: Bramble Books, 1996); David L. Cooperirder and Diana Whitney, *Appreciative Inquiry: A Positive Revolution in Change* (Oakland, CA: Berrett-Kohler, 2005); Patricia Mathes Cane, *Capacitar: Healing Trauma, Empowering Wellness; A Multicultural Popular Education Approach to Transforming Trauma* (Santa Cruz, CA: Capacitar International, 2011). For Public Conversation, see Parker Palmer, *A Hidden Wholeness: The Journey Toward an Undivided Life* (San Francisco: Jossey Bass, 2004), and Alternatives to Violence Project, https:// avpusa.org/.

71. Helene Lorenz and Susan James, "Decoloniality Dialogues in CLE," in *Hearing Voices* (Carpinteria, CA: Pacifica Graduate Institute, 2017), 41–43.

72. Eve Tuck and K. Wayne Yang, "Decolonization Is Not a Metaphor," *Decolonization: Indigeneity, Education and Society* 1, no. 1 (2012): 3.

73. Eduardo Galeano, quoted in David Barsamian, *Louder Than Bombs: Interviews from the Progressive Magazine* (Boston: South End Press, 2004), 146.

74. Fanon, *Wretched of the Earth*, 239.

75. Scheper-Hughes, "The Primacy of the Ethical," 420.

76. Martin Luther King, Jr., "Remaining Awake Through a Great Revolution," National Cathedral, Washington, DC, March 31, 1968.

77. Kei Williams, "The Movement for Black Lives Now," Museum of the City of New York, September 19, 2017; Curtis Ogden, "Moving from Inclusion to Collaborative Solidarity," Interaction Institute for Social Change, October 22, 2015, http://interactioninstitute.org/moving-from-inclusion-to-collaborative-solidarity/.

78. Tuck and Yang, "Decolonization," 26.

79. Chris Moore-Backman, "How Can I Offer Reparations in Direct Proportion to My White Privilege?" *Yes! Magazine*, October 25, 2017, http://www.yesmagazine.org/issues/just-transition/how-i-can-offer-reparations-in-direct-proportion-to-my-white-privilege-20171025?utm_medium=email&utm_campaign=YTW_20171027&utm_content=YTW_20171027+Version+A+CID_3fd59f130afe6e2467 3b0ab1909ec8f3&utm_source=CM&utm_term=How%20I%20Can%20 Offer%20Reparations%20in%20Direct%20Proportion%20to%20My%20 White%20Privilege.

Chapter 8. Nonhuman Animal Accompaniment

1. In appreciation of Animal sentience, existence of their cultures, and sovereignty, Animal species names are capitalized as they are for various human cultures (e.g., Italian, Maori).

2. G. A. Bradshaw, "Elephant Trauma and Recovery: From Human Violence to Trans-Species Psychology" (Ph.D. diss., Pacifica Graduate Institute, 2005); Bradshaw, *Elephants on the Edge*.

3. G. A. Bradshaw and Mary Watkins, "Trans-Species Psychology: Theory and Praxis," *Spring: A Journal of Archetype and Culture* 75 (2006): 69–94.

4. Bradshaw, *Elephants on the Edge*.

5. Melinda A. Novak et al., "Stress, the HPA Axis, and Nonhuman Primate Well-Being: A Review," *Applied Animal Behaviour Science* 143, no. 2 (2013): 135–149.

6. Michael Slusher, *They All Had Eyes: Confessions of a Vivisectionist* (Danvers, MA: Vegan, 2016), Kindle edition, loc. 2567.

7. Survival International, https://www.survivalinternational.org/uncontactedtribes.

8. Bradshaw, "Elephant Trauma and Recovery"; G. A. Bradshaw et al., "Elephant Breakdown," *Nature* 433, no. 7028 (2005): 807.

9. G. A. Bradshaw and Robert M. Sapolsky, "Macroscope: Mirror, Mirror," *American Scientist* 94, no. 6 (2006): 487–489; G. A. Bradshaw, and Barbara L. Finlay, "Natural Symmetry," *Nature* 435, no. 7039 (2005): 149.

10. Martín-Baró, *Writings for a Liberation Psychology*.

11. James Lovelock and James E. Lovelock, *Gaia: A New Look at Life on Earth* (Oxford: Oxford Paperbacks, 2000); Arne Naess, "The Shallow and the Deep, Long-Range Ecology Movement: A Summary," *Inquiry* 16, nos. 1–4 (1973): 95–100; Alf Hornborg, "Vital Signs: An Ecosemiotic Perspective on the Human Ecology of Amazonia," *Sign Systems Studies* 29, no. 1 (2001): 121–151; Vine Deloria, Jr., *The World We Used to Live In: Remembering the Powers of the Medicine Men* (Golden, CO: Fulcrum, 2006); Marisol de la Cadena, *Earth Beings: Ecologies of Practice Across Andean Worlds* (Durham, NC: Duke University Press, 2015); Inge Bolin, "Chillihuani's Culture of Respect and the Circle of Courage," *Reclaiming Children and Youth* 18, no. 4 (2010): 12.

12. Lucy Hastings, Hastings Family Correspondence, 1838, 1855–1874 (Transcriptions), http://digicoll.library.wisc.edu/cgi-bin/WI/WI-idx?type=browse&scope=WI.Hastings.

13. Brian R. Ferguson, "Born to Live: Challenging Killer Myths," in *Origins of Altruism and Cooperation*, ed. Robert W. Sussman and C. Robert Cloninger (New York: Springer, 2011), 249–270; Darcia Narvaez, "The 99 Percent—Development and Socialization Within an Evolutionary Context: Growing Up to Become 'A Good and Useful Human Being,'" in *War, Peace and Human Nature: The Convergence of Evolutionary and Cultural Views*, ed. D. Fry (New York: Oxford University Press, 2013), 341–356.

14. "Memorial for a Brave and Inspirational Makah Elder," Sea Shepherd, http://www.seashepherd.org/news/memorial-for-a-brave-and-inspirational-makah-elder/.

15. Vine Deloria, Jr., personal communication with author, November 2003.

16. Quoted in Peter Nabokov, *Native American Testimony: A Chronicle of Indian-White Relations from Prophecy to the Present, 1492–2000* (New York: Penguin, 1999), 86.

17. Quoted in Bradshaw, *Carnivore Minds*, 54.

18. Robert Jay Lifton, *The Nazi Doctors: Medical Killing and the Psychology of Genocide* (New York: Basic, 1986).

19. Nicholas Kristof, "A Farm Boy Reflects," *New York Times*, July 31, 2008, http://www.nytimes.com/2008/07/31/opinion/31kristof.html?pagewanted=print&_r=0.

20. "Humane Farm Animal Care," Certified Humane, https://certifiedhumane.org/raising-awareness-farm-animals-food-production.

21. "Did You Hear the Cows Cry?" Edgar's Mission, 2014, https://www.edgarsmission.org.au/37923/hear-cattle-cry/.

22. Dave Rogers, "Strange Noises Turn Out to Be Cows Missing Their Calves," *Newbury Port Daily News*, October 23, 2013, http://www.newburyportnews.com/news/local_news/strange-noises-turn-out-to-be-cows-missing-their-calves/article_d872e4da-b318-5e90-870e-51266f8eea7f.html.

23. Personal communication with author, 2017.

24. Personal communication with author, 2016 (quotations); United Poultry Concerns, "Free Range Chicken Slaughter," 2012, https://vimeo.com/34968183.

25. Slusher, *They All Had Eyes*, loc. 2046.

26. Ibid., loc. 2418.

27. Virgil Butler, quoted in "Whistleblower on the Kill Floor: Interview with Virgil Butler and Laura Alexander," *Satya*, February 2006, http://www.satyamag.com/feb06/butler.html.

28. Andrew Sharo, personal communication with author, November 19, 2017.

29. Narvaez, "The 99 Percent."

30. Personal communication with author, May 2012.

31. Karen Davis, "Nicholas Kristof's March 14 Article, 'To Kill a Chicken,'" All-Creatures.org, March 15, 2015, http://www.all-creatures.org/articles/ar-nicholas-kristoff-chicken.html.

32. Wayne Hsiung, quoted in Jasmin Singer and Mariann Sullivan, "An Interview with Wayne Hsiung," Our Hen House, 2014, http://www.ourhenhouse.org/WayneHsiungEpisode245.pdf.

33. Lovelock and Lovelock, *Gaia;* Naess, "The Shallow and the Deep"; Bradshaw, *Carnivore Minds*, 121; John Seed et al., *Thinking Like a Mountain* (Gabrioloa, BC: New Society, 1988).

34. Harold Brown, quoted in Gypsy Carmen Wulff and France Mary Chambers, eds., *Turning Points in Compassion: Personal Journeys of Animal Advocates* (Sydney: SpiritWings Humane Education, 2015), 3.

35. Calvin Luther Martin, foreword, in Bradshaw, *Elephants on the Edge*, ix–xvi.

36. Justo Oxa, quoted in Bradshaw, *Carnivore Minds*, 121.

37. Douglas K. Candland, *Feral Children and Clever Animals: Reflections on Human Nature* (Oxford: Oxford University Press, 1995).

38. G. A. Bradshaw et al., "Developmental Context Effects on Bicultural Post-trauma Self Repair in Chimpanzees," *Developmental Psychology* 45, no. 5 (2009): 1376.

39. Personal communications with author, January 2017.

40. Nikki Evans and Claire Gray, "The Practice and Ethics of Animal-Assisted Therapy with Children and Young People: Is It Enough That We Don't Eat Our Co-Workers?" *British Journal of Social Work* 42, no. 4 (2012): 600–617.

41. Charlie Russell, personal communication with author, 2015 (quotations); Charlie Russell and G. A. Bradshaw, *Learning Nature's Language* (in process).

42. Steven Wise, quoted in Marc Bekoff, "The Nonhuman Rights Project: An Interview with Steve Wise," *Psychology Today*, December 6, 2016; https://www.psychologytoday.com/blog/animal-emotions/201612/the-nonhuman-rights-project-interview-steven-wise.

43. Carol Buckley and G. A. Bradshaw, "The Art of Cultural Brokerage: Recreating Elephant-Human Relationship and Community," in *Minding the Animal Psyche,* ed. G. A. Bradshaw and Nancy Cater (New Orleans: Spring, 2010), 35–59.

44. Mary-Jayne Rust, and Nick Totton, eds., *Vital Signs: Psychological Responses to Ecological Crisis* (London: Karnac Books, 2012), 193–194; Jerome S. Bernstein, *Living in the Borderland: The Evolution of Consciousness and the Challenge of Healing Trauma* (New York: Routledge, 2006).

45. Joe Wood, personal communication with author, March 2017.

46. Lauren Bailey, personal communication with author, December 15, 2017.

47. Lauren Bailey, personal communication with author, February 2017.

48. Clare Mann, *Vystopia: The Anguish of Being Vegan in a Non-Vegan World* (Sydney: Communicate31 Pty, 2018).

49. Quoted in G. A. Bradshaw, "Handling It," *Psychology Today,* June 1, 2014, https://www.psychologytoday.com/blog/bear-in-mind/201406/handling-it.

50. Molly Flanagan, personal communication with author, November 2017.

51. Corey Rowland, personal communication with author, November 2017.

52. The SAVE Movement, http://thesavemovement.org/.

53. Victoria, "Interview with Anita Krajnc," My Non Leather Life, April 10, 2013, http://mynonleatherlife.com/2013/04/10/10-questions-for-anita-krajnc-founder-of-toronto-pig-save/.

54. Toronto Pig SAVE, *Crime of Compassion,* 2015, https://www.youtube.com/watch?v=ekhIzpKkHZo.

55. Quoted in Karen Brulliard, "Three Elephants in Connecticut Just Got a Lawyer," *Washington Post,* November 11, 2014, https://www.washingtonpost.com/

news/animalia/wp/2017/11/14/three-elephants-in-connecticut-just-got-a-lawyer/?utm_term=.6c7d77b0adf2.

56. Ibid.; Daniella Silva, "Connecticut Judge Denies Petition to Grant Elephants Legal 'Personhood,'" Associated Press, December 29, 2017, https://www.nbc-news.com/news/us-news/connecticut-judge-denies-petition-grant-elephants-legal-personhood-n833351.

57. Steven Wise, quoted in Bekoff, "The Nonhuman Rights Project."

58. Victoria, "Interview with Anita Krajnc."

59. Andrew Sharo, personal communication with author, November 19, 2017.

60. Corey Rowland, personal communication with author, November 2017.

61. Lauren Bailey, personal communication with author, December 15, 2017.

62. SafeHaven Small Breed Rescue, http://www.safehavensmallbreedrescue.org/index.html.

63. Teri Walters, personal communication with author, November 2017.

64. Corey Rowland, personal communication with author, November 2017.

65. Corey Rowland, personal communication with author, April 2017.

66. Liberation Pledge, http://www.liberationpledge.com/.

67. Victoria, "Interview with Anita Krajnc."

68. Andrew Sharo, personal communication with author, November 19, 2017.

69. Victoria, "Interview with Anita Krajnc."

70. Ibid.

71. Wayne Hsiung, quoted in Singer and Sullivan, "An Interview with Wayne Hsiung."

72. "Interview with lauren Ornelas," *Even,* 2016, http://www.all-creatures.org/articles/even-lauren-ornelas.html. Ornelas spells her first name with a lowercase "l."

73. Wolf Patrol, https://wolfpatrol.org/.

74. Ibid.

75. Wolf Patrol, "Wolf Patrol Challenged to Fight to the Death," https://www.youtube.com/watch?v=9YfboOBRoSo; Wolf Patrol, "Wolf Patrol Conflict with Hunters near Laona, Wisconsin / Cameras Seized by Police," https://www.youtube.com/watch?v=22XLlDZbwk (part 1); https://www.youtube.com/watch?v=dmSbijdztMQU (part 2); https://www.youtube.com/watch?v=yQuRHlk6ooY (part 3).

76. Kevin Tucker, "The Forest Beyond the Field: The Consequences of Domestication," Black and Green Press, 2015, http://www.blackandgreenpress.org/2015/01/the-forest-beyond-field-consequences-of.html; Darcia Narvaez, *Neurobiology and the Development of Human Morality: Evolution, Culture, and Wisdom* (New York: Norton, 2014).

Chapter 9. Earth Accompaniment

1. Thomas Berry, foreword, in Cormac Cullinan, *Wild Law: A Manifesto for Earth Justice,* 2nd edition (White River Junction, VT: Chelsea Green, 2011), 20.

2. Christopher Stone, "Should Trees Have Standing? Toward Legal Rights for Natural Objects," *Southern California Law Review* 45 (1972): 452.

3. Vandana Shiva, *Earth Democracy: Justice, Sustainability, and Peace* (Cambridge, MA: South End Press, 2005).

4. Ibid., 9–11, 5, 6–7.

5. Ibid., 5.

6. Ibid., 11.

7. Stone, "Should Trees Have Standing?" 456.

8. Ibid., 489.

9. American Society of International Law, https://www.asil.org/eisil/world-charter-nature.

10. "Universal Declaration of the Rights of Mother Earth," April 22, 2010, https://therightsofnature.org/wp-content/uploads/FINAL-UNIVERSAL-DECLARATION-OF-THE-RIGHTS-OF-MOTHER-EARTH-APRIL-22-2010.pdf.

11. Constitution of the Republic of Ecuador, 2008, http://pdba.georgetown.edu/Constitutions/Ecuador/english08.html.

12. Rights for Nature Articles in Ecuador's Constitution, http://therightsofnature.org/wp-content/uploads/pdfs/Rights-for-Nature-Articles-in-Ecuadors-Constitution.pdf.

13. Petition to the Inter-American Commission on Human Rights Seeking Relief from Violations Resulting from Global Warming Caused by Acts and Omissions of the United States, http://www.inuitcircumpolar.com/uploads/3/0/5/4/30542564/finalpetitionsummary.pdf.

14. Eleanor Ainge Roy, "New Zealand River Granted Same Rights as Human," *Guardian*, March 16, 2017, https://www.theguardian.com/world/2017/mar/16/new-zealand-river-granted-same-legal-rights-as-human-being.

15. Te Urewera Act, 2014, http://www.legislation.govt.nz/act/public/2014/0051/latest/DLM6183601.html.

16. Michael Safi, "Ganges, Yamuna Rivers Granted Same Legal Rights as a Human Being," *Guardian,* March 21, 2017, https://www.theguardian.com/world/2017/mar/21/ganges-and-yamuna-rivers-granted-same-legal-rights-as-human-beings.

17. Cullinan, *Wild Law*, 30.

18. Julie Turkewitz, "Corporations Have Rights. Why Not Rivers?" *New York Times*, September 26, 2017, https://www.nytimes.com/2017/09/26/us/does-

the-colorado-river-have-rights-a-lawsuit-seeks-to-declare-it-a-person.html?_r=0.

19. Mari Margill and Ben Price, "Pittsburgh Bans Natural Gas Drilling," *Yes! Magazine*, November 16, 2010, http://www.yesmagazine.org/people-power/pittsburg-bans-natural-gas-drilling.

20. John Vidal and Owen Bowcott, "ICC Widens Remit to Include Environmental Destruction Cases," *Guardian*, September 15, 2016, https://www.theguardian.com/global/2016/sep/15/hague-court-widens-remit-to-include-environmental-destruction-cases.

21. Ken Saro-Wiwa, *A Month and a Day and Letters* (Banbury, UK: Ayebia Clarke, 2005), 3.

22. Bob Herbert, "Unholy Alliance in Nigeria," *New York Times,* January 26, 1996, A27.

23. Nixon, *Slow Violence*, 108.

24. Íde Corley, Helen Fallon, and Laurence Cox, eds., *Silence Would Be Treason: Last Writings of Ken Saro-Wiwa* (Dakar, Indonesia: Council for the Development of Social Science Research, 2013), 47.

25. Ken Saro-Wiwa interviewed on *Without Walls: The Hanged Man—Nigeria's Shame,* channel 4 (UK), November 15, 1995.

26. Nixon, *Slow Violence,* 113.

27. Ibid., 109.

28. Saro-Wiwa, *A Month and a Day,* 123.

29. Kai Erikson, *A New Species of Trouble: The Human Experience of Modern Disasters* (New York: Norton, 1994).

30. Kai Erikson, *Everything in Its Path: Destruction of Community in the Buffalo Creek Flood* (New York: Simon and Schuster, 1976), 154.

31. Erikson, *A New Species,* 240, 242.

32. Ibid., 21.

33. Saro-Wiwa, *A Month and a Day,* 48–49.

34. Rob Nixon, "Environmental Martyrdom and Defenders of the Forest," lecture, Princeton Environmental Institute, 2017.

35. Nixon, *Slow Violence,* 133.

36. Sarah MacDonald, "Irish Archive Recalls Environmental Activist Ken Saro-Wiwa's Life Through Death Row Letters," *National Catholic Reporter,* May 10, 2016, https://www.ncronline.org/blogs/eco-catholic/irish-archive-recalls-environmental-activist-ken-saro-wiwa-s-life-through-death.

37. John Vidal, "Niger Delta Oil Spill Clean-Up Launched—But Could Take a Quarter of a Century," *Guardian,* June 1, 2016, https://www.theguardian.com/global-development/2016/jun/02/niger-delta-oil-spill-clean-up-launched-ogoniland-communities-1bn.

38. Naomi Klein, *This Changes Everything: Capitalism Vs. the Climate* (New York: Simon and Schuster, 2015).

39. Sebastião Salgado, *From My Land to the Planet* (Rome: Contrasto, 2014), Kindle edition, loc. 949.

40. Ibid., loc. 974.

41. Instituto Terra, www.institutoterra.org.

42. Salgado, *From My Land to the Planet,* loc. 1000.

43. Daniela Aparicio, "Cosmovision Lenca," September 4, 2014, https://prezi.com/oiplfv8k2o5k/comovision-lenca/.

44. Ibid.

45. COPINH—Consejo Cívico de Organizaciones Populares e Indígenas de Honduras, https://copinh.org/.

46. Amnesty International, "Defending Human Rights in Honduras Is a Crime," November 22, 2013, https://www.amnesty.org/en/latest/news/2013/11/honduras-human-rights-defenders-under-threat/; "Honduras Police Arrest Executive in Killing of Berta Cáceres, Indigenous Activist," *New York Times*, March 3, 2018, A14, https://www.nytimes.com/2018/03/03/world/americas/honduras-berta-caceres.html.

47. Berta Cáceres, "Acceptance Speech," Goldman Environmental Prize, San Francisco, 2015.

48. Aldo Leopold, *A Sand County Almanac* (New York: Oxford University Press, 1949), 1.

49. Carl Anthony, "Ecopsychology and the De-Construction of Witness," in *Ecopsychology: Restoring the Earth, Healing the Mind,* ed. C. Roszak, M. Gomes, and A. Kanner (San Francisco: Sierra Club Books, 1995), 277.

50. Nixon, *Slow Violence*, 2, 6.

51. Paloma Pavel, ed., *Breakthrough Communities: Sustainability and Justice in the Next American Metropolis* (Cambridge, MA: MIT Press, 2009).

52. Andy Fisher, *Radical Ecopsychology: Psychology in the Service of Life,* 2nd edition (Albany: SUNY Press, 2013), xxix, 239.

53. Joanna Macy and Chris Johnstone, *Active Hope: How to Face the Mess We're In Without Going Crazy* (New York: New World Library, 2012).

54. I refer (in order) to the works of Harry Grammer, Soula Pefkaros, Pesach Chananiah, Chenoa Siegenthaler, Weston Pew, Samantha Gupta, and Gabrielle Zhuang.

55. Robert Greenway, "Robert Greenway: The *Ecopsychology* Interview," *Ecopsychology* 1, no. 1 (March 2009): 47–52. doi: 10.1089/eco.2009.0008.

56. Andy Fisher, personal communication with author, December 12, 2017. See also http://andyfisher.ca/blog/what-ecopsychology.

57. Quoted in Clyde Haberman, "The Lasting Legacy of a Fighter for the Amazon," *New York Times,* November 27, 2016, https://www.nytimes.com/2016/11/27/us/chico-mendes-amazon-retro-report.html.

58. Pope Francis, *Encyclical Letter Laudato Si' of the Holy Father Francis, on Care of Our Common Home* (Huntington, IN: Our Sunday Visitor, 2015), 159, https://laudatosi.com/watch.

59. Philippe Descola, "Societies of Nature and the Nature of Society," in *Conceptualizing Society,* ed. Adam Kuper (New York: Routledge, 1992), 107–126.

60. Philippe Descola, *Beyond Nature and Culture* (Chicago: University of Chicago Press, 2014), 123.

61. Salgado, *From My Land,* loc. 1014.

62. Sebastião Salgado and Lelia Wanick Salgado, *Genesis* (Berlin: Taschecn, 2013).

63. Salgado, *From My Land,* loc. 1084, 1607.

64. Fisher, *Radical Ecopsychology,* 241.

65. Descola, *Beyond Nature and Culture,* 195.

66. Francis, *Encyclical Letter Laudato Si',* 104, 35.

67. Thomas Berry, *The Dream of the Earth* (San Francisco: Sierra Club Books, 1990), 169.

Chapter 10. Mutual Accompaniment and the Commons-to-Come

1. Casey and Watkins, *Up Against the Wall.*

2. Wikipedia, "Separation Barrier," https://en.wikipedia.org/wiki/Separation_barrier.

3. Aimé Césaire, *Discourse on Colonialism* (New York: Monthly Review Press, 2001).

4. This is the pattern for colonialism that was then exported into the southern hemisphere. Now, as neoliberal capitalism suffuses the United States, we witness daily shipwreck in the news, in the internal colonies in the United States that Chris Hedges and Joe Sacco have so poignantly described in *Days of Destruction, Days of Revolt,* including Camden, New Jersey; Flint, Michigan; Ferguson, Missouri; South Central, Los Angeles; Appalachia; and Pine Ridge, South Dakota. The list is long and growing.

5. The Irish watched while food grown in Ireland was exported. Charles Trevelyan, who was the assistant secretary to the English Treasury, saw the Irish as morally evil and greeted the famine as a stroke of providence whose function was to curb Irish population growth. Eamon O'Kelly, "Why Didn't the English Transport Food from England During the Irish Potato Famine? Could the Monarch Have Intervened? *Quora,* https://www.quora.com/

Why-didn%E2%80%99t-the-English-transport-food-from-England-during-
the-Irish-potato-famine-Could-the-monarch-have-intervened.

6. Peter Ackroyd, *Revolution: The History of England from the Battle of the Boyne to the Battle of Waterloo* (New York: St. Martin's Press, 2017); William Gibson, *A Brief History of Britain, 1660–1851,* vol. 3 (Boston: Little, Brown, 2011), 142.

7. Gary Snyder, *The Practice of the Wild* (New York: Farrar, Straus, and Giroux, 1990), 39.

8. Raj Patel and Jason W. Moore, *A History of the World in Seven Cheap Things: A Guide to Capitalism, Nature, and the Future of the Planet* (Berkeley: University of California Press, 2017).

9. Snyder, *The Practice of the Wild,* 34.

10. Ibid., 40.

11. Ibid., 31.

12. Quoted in Thomas Power O'Connor, *The Home Rule Movement: With a Sketch of Irish Parties from 1843 and an Addition Containing a Full Account of the Great Trial Instigated by the London "Times"* (London: Benzinger Brothers, 1891), 173.

13. The open space movement of 1869 halted this practice, preserving the Epping Forest against the wishes of fourteen manor lords. Nevertheless, because of the enclosures, England has the least forest and wildlife of all nations of Europe, according to Snyder, *The Practice of the Wild,* 34.

14. This dynamic continues to unfold in our current world, as commons are erased. For instance, in Mexico, as a result of trade agreements in the North American Free Trade Agreement (NAFTA) that allowed U.S. farmers to dump subsidized corn on the Mexican market, Mexican farmers were unable to compete and had to leave their land to survive. Many tried to gain employment in the vast *maquiladores,* the industrial plants created in the new "free" trade zones, which require cheap labor; others risked the perilous passage to the United States.

15. Peter Linebaugh, *Stop Thief! The Commons, Enclosures, and Resistance* (Oakland, CA: PM Press, 2014), 2.

16. Ibid.

17. In the United States, we are witnessing the development of the largest prison population per capita in the world. Private prison corporations have been pleased to expand their services into the development of a gulag archipelago of 250 private detention centers for people awaiting asylum adjudication and for those confronting the life-wreck possibilities of deportation, separating parents and children, wives and husbands.

18. Allan Greer, "Commons and Enclosures in the Colony of North America," *American Historical Review* 117, no. 2 (2012): 379.

19. Ibid., 369.
20. Ibid., 372, 369.
21. Cronon, *Changes in the Land*, 67.
22. Greer, "Commons and Enclosures," 376, 371.
23. Brooks, *The Common Pot*, xli, 251, 5; Greer, "Commons and Enclosures," 376.
24. Brooks, *The Common Pot*, 45.
25. Ibid., 70.
26. Lisa T. Brooks and Cassandra M. Brooks, "The Reciprocity Principle and Traditional Ecological Knowledge: Understanding the Significance of Indigenous Protest on the Presumpscot River," *International Journal of Critical Indigenous Studies* 3, no. 2 (2010): 12.
27. Ibid., 14.
28. William Apess, *On Our Own Ground: The Complete Writings of William Apess, A Pequot,* ed. Barry O'Connell (Amherst: University of Massachusetts Press, 1992).
29. Brooks, *The Common Pot*, 200.
30. Ibid., 218.
31. Cornelia H. Dayton and Sharon V. Salinger, *Robert Love's Warnings: Searching for Strangers in Colonial Boston* (Philadelphia: University of Pennsylvania Press, 2014).
32. Césaire, *Discourse*, 43.
33. Forbes, *Columbus and Other Cannibals*.
34. Ibid., 24.
35. Alnoor Ladha and Martin Kirk, "Seeing Wetiko: On Capitalism, Mind Viruses and Antidotes for a World in Transition," *Cosmos Journal,* Spring/Summer 2016, https://www.kosmosjournal.org/article/seeing-wetiko-on-capitalism-mind-viruses-and-antidotes-for-a-world-in-transition/.
36. Jason W. Moore and Kamil Ahsan, "Capitalism in the Web of Life: An Interview with Jason Moore," *Viewpoint Magazine,* September 28, 2015, https://www.viewpointmag.com/2015/09/28/capitalism-in-the-web-of-life-an-interview-with-jason-moore/.
37. Patel and Moore, *A History of the World*.
38. Nelson Maldonado-Torres, "Outline of 10 Theses on Coloniality and Decoloniality," Frantz Fanon Foundation, 12–13, http://frantzfanonfoundation-fondationfrantzfanon.com/IMG/pdf/maldonado-torres_outline_of_ten_theses-10.23.16_.pdf.
39. Jacques Derrida, "9/11 and Global Terrorism: A Dialogue with Jacques Derrida," in *Philosophy in a Time of Terror: Dialogues with Jurgen Habermas and Jacques Derrida,* ed. Giovanna Borradori (Chicago; University of Chicago

Press, 2003), http://www.press.uchicago.edu/books/derrida/derrida911.html; Jacques Derrida, *Rogues: Two Essays on Reason* (Palo Alto, CA: Stanford University Press, 2005).

40. Nelson R. Mandela, "Experience Ubuntu Interview," interview by Tim Modise, May 24, 2006, http://en.wikipedia.org/wiki/File:Experience_ubuntu. ogg.

41. Desmond Tutu, *No Future Without Forgiveness* (New York: Doubleday, 2000), 32.

42. Gloria Anzaldúa, "(Un)natural Bridges, (Un)safe Spaces," in *This Bridge We Call Home: Radical Visions for Transformation,* ed. Gloria Anzaldúa and Analouise Keating (New York: Routledge, 2002), 3–4.

43. Freire, *Pedagogy of the Oppressed,* 61.

44. Gustavo Esteva, "Commoning in the New Society," *Community Development Journal* 49, no. 1 (2014): 154.

45. Snyder, *The Practice of the Wild,* 38.

46. Thich Nhat Hanh and Daniel Berrigan, *The Raft Is Not the Shore: Conversations Toward a Buddhist Christian Awareness* (Maryknoll, NY: Orbis, 2001), 129.

47. Here I follow Hussein Bulhan's grasp of "understanding" as comprehending from below, from "how colonized peoples in these distant peripheries live." Bulhan, "Stages of Colonialism in Africa," 240.

48. Shiva, *Earth Democracy,* 142, 109.

49. Freire, *Pedagogy of the Oppressed,* 49.

50. Snyder, *The Practice of the Wild,* 27.

51. Staughton Lynd applauds the small-scale successes of accompaniment, having seen how they can lead to wide-scale change. He gives the example of his and Alice Staughton's work at the Ohio State Penitentiary, which has led to positive changes in super maximum security prison conditions across the United States. Staughton Lynd and Alice Lynd, *Moral Injury and Nonviolent Resistance: Breaking the Cycle of Violence in the Military and Behind Bars* (Oakland, CA: PM Press, 2017).

52. Magón was a critical anarcho-syndicalist thinker who aided the Mexican revolution.

53. When the United States replaced the separation wall with a larger and more militarized wall in 2011, the mural was removed.

54. Casey and Watkins, *Up Against the Wall,* 207–226.

Acknowledgments

By now it will not surprise you that of all the gifts I have had the grace to receive, I value accompaniment most. During the decade I have been at work on these ideas, I have been blessed by the daily accompaniment of Ed Casey, my philosopher husband. His interest, love, and encouragement have lifted the burden of excess solitude that prolonged writing entails. His wise and sensitive intelligence has made sharing these ideas a generative life dialogue that I treasure beyond words.

In my experience, every book project has its own dark tunnel, where another's capacity to hold the potential significance of the project shines a light so one can continue despite one's own shadow of doubt. While in the tunnel of this book, I turned to Gay Bradshaw for help and encouragement, and thank her for her ever-generous response. I am also deeply grateful she agreed to contribute a chapter about trans-species accompaniment, a form of accompaniment that is essential but well beyond my own experience and knowledge.

Ignacio Dobles Oropeza, Glenn Adams, and the rest of the editorial board of the *Journal of Social and Political Psychology*, where my first essay on psychosocial accompaniment appeared, were enormously helpful and generous in their incisive critique. Their assistance helped inform the transformation of that early piece into this book. As I was finishing this book, I reached out to a number of treasured colleagues for their feedback on particular chapters where their knowledge is invaluable. I am grateful for their helpful and incisive comments, which greatly assisted me in strengthening the text: Alexandra Adame, John Becknell, Deanne Bell, Gay Bradshaw, Ed Casey, Nuria Ciofalo, Andy Fisher, Michael Kearney, Lynne Layton, Jancis Long, Jim Mandiberg, Dennis Rivers, David Schwartz, Mimi Simon, Elizabeth Stone, Janet Surrey, David Walker, and Fred Wertz.

I appreciate those who reviewed this book for Yale Press and am thankful for the time they took to offer their extremely helpful comments and encouragement, including Chakira Haddock-Lazala, Darcia Narvaez, Tod Sloan, and Peter Westoby.

I thank Jean Thomson Black, senior executive editor at Yale University Press, for taking a leap of faith and tucking this book under her wing.

I have been blessed to be able to explore the practice of mutual accompaniment with hundreds of graduate students at Pacifica Graduate Institute for the last twenty-four years—first in the original Depth Psychology Program and, for the last nine years, in its Community, Liberation, Indigenous, and Eco-Psychologies specialization. I am grateful for what these students and their visionary scholar-activist work have taught me. Through their creative energies and life commitments, I have had the gift of seeing the commons-to-come become a loving and lively reality in so many varied corners of our shared world.

Index